THE MINOR GESTURE

THOUGHT IN THE ACT   *A series edited by Erin Manning and Brian Massumi*

THE MINOR GESTURE

ERIN MANNING

DUKE UNIVERSITY PRESS DURHAM AND LONDON 2016

Designed by Amy Ruth Buchanan
Typeset in Arno and Avenir by Graphic Composition, Inc.,
Bogart, Georgia

Library of Congress Cataloging-in-Publication Data
Names: Manning, Erin, author.
Title: The minor gesture / Erin Manning.
Other titles: Thought in the act.
Description: Durham : Duke University Press, 2016.
Series: Thought in the act | Includes bibliographical references and
index.
Identifiers: LCCN 2015046671 (print) | LCCN 2015048953 (ebook)
ISBN 9780822361039 (hardcover : alk. paper)
ISBN 9780822361213 (pbk. : alk. paper)
ISBN 9780822374411 (e-book)
Subjects: LCSH: Perception (Philosophy) | Self (Philosophy)
| Cognitive neuroscience—Philosophy. | Autism. | Political
psychology.
Classification: LCC B828.45 .M366 2016 (print) |
LCC B828.45 (ebook) | DDC 128—dc23
LC record available at http://lccn.loc.gov/2015046671

Cover art: Nathaniel Stern and Erin Manning,
Weather Patterns: The Smell of Red. Installation,
Glasshouse, New York, 2014. Photo by Leslie Plumb.
Courtesy of the artists and Leslie Plumb.

CONTENTS

There's something about writing books that is out of time. As though the writing only really knows what it's after once it has begun to make its way into the world. For me, thinking too has always had this quality: thinking thickens in its encounter with the futurity that orients it. This futurity in thinking's presentness is part of what keeps thinking lithe: thinking is always out of sync with itself.

The best kind of encounter with thinking's outside is the kind that deeply listens to what writing is trying to do, almost thinking beyond what the author is capable of thinking, then returning that thinking, almost beyond what the reader can think, to the author. In this gesture of encounter, no one is trying to convince anyone: thought is thinking collectively at its limit.

Going through the review process for *The Minor Gesture*, I had the luck of encountering thinking at the limit. In an affirmative gesture—what I call "affirmation without credit" in the postscript—the reviewers took time to think-with the text in a gesture of writing-with, returning *The Minor Gesture* to me with the richness of an engagement that was capable of opening my thinking beyond where I thought it could go. In this return, I received not a simple account of how writing performs knowledge, but something much more important: an engagement with how thinking does its work, in the writing.

What struck me, in reading these reviews (can these still be called reviews?), was how fragile this gesture of writing-with made me feel. The fragility, I think, has to do with writing pushed to a limit where it is truly in contact with the tremulousness of thinking in the act. Bringing thought into contact with its limit this way is a minor gesture. It is a minor gesture in that it activates a tendency already in germ and emboldens it toward an altering of what that tendency can do. A thought less concerned with the certainty of what it knows is more open to the minor in thinking, more open to the force of the as-yet-unformed coursing through it. This minor tendency values the *force* of form, not just the form knowledge takes.

The Minor Gesture engages directly with this tension between knowledge and value. What else could be at stake in the encounter if it weren't organized around the certainty of knowing? What might become thinkable if knowledge weren't so tied to an account of subject-driven agency? And, what else might value look like if it weren't framed by judgment?

A minor gesture that activates the collectivity at the heart of thought effects change. It affects not only what the text can become: it alters to the core what thinking can do. It gives value to the processual uncertainty of thought as yet unformed, and gives that thought the space to develop collectively.

For their elegant engagement with collective thinking in the act, I thank these reviewers by name: Greg Seigworth and Fred Moten. Thank you for inviting me to think beyond the limit of what seemed thinkable, and for thinking there with me.

I also thank the SenseLab, with whom the thinking never stops, whether we are making or moving or talking or writing. My life is changed, continuously, by the thinking that moves us.

And, as always: thank you to Brian Massumi. Even when we're not writing together I hear the speculative force of our collective thinking in my words. You have taught me that we never write alone.

INTRODUCTION

In a Minor Key

This book begins in a minor key and works to create a field of resonance for the minor. It does so through the concept of the minor gesture. The minor gesture, allied to Gilles Deleuze and Félix Guattari's concept of the minor, is the gestural force that opens experience to its potential variation. It does this from within experience itself, activating a shift in tone, a difference in quality.

A minor key is always interlaced with major keys — the minor works the major from within. What must be remembered is this: neither the minor nor the major is fixed in advance. The major is a structural tendency that organizes itself according to predetermined definitions of value. The minor is a force that courses through it, unmooring its structural integrity, problematizing its normative standards. The unwavering belief in the major as the site where events occur, where events make a difference, is based on accepted accounts of what registers as change as well as existing parameters for gauging the value of that change.[1] Yet while the grand gestures of a macropolitics most easily sum up the changes that occurred to alter the field, it is the minoritarian tendencies that initiate the subtle shifts that created the conditions for this, and any change. The grand is given the status it has not because it is where the transformative power lies, but because it is easier to identify major shifts than to catalogue the nuanced rhythms of the minor. As a result, these rhythms are narrated as secondary, or even negligible.

The minor is a continual variation on experience. It has a mobility not given to the major: its rhythms are not controlled by a preexisting structure, but open to flux. In variation is in change, indeterminate. But indeterminacy, because of its wildness, is often seen as unrigorous, flimsy, its lack of solidity mistaken for a lack of consistency. The minor thus gets cast aside, overlooked, or forgotten in the interplay of major chords. This is the downside of the minor, but also its strength: that it does not have the full force of a preexisting status, of a given structure, of a predetermined metric, to keep it alive. It is out of time, untimely, rhythmically inventing its own pulse.

The minor isn't known in advance. It never reproduces itself in its own image. Each minor gesture is singularly connected to the event at hand, immanent to the in-act. This makes it pragmatic. But the minor gesture also exceeds the bounds of the event, touching on the ineffable quality of its more-than. This makes it speculative. The minor gesture works in the mode of speculative pragmatism. From a speculatively pragmatic stance, it invents its own value, a value as ephemeral as it is mobile. This permeability tends to make it ungraspable, and often unrecognizable: it is no doubt difficult to value that which has little perceptible form, that which has not yet quite been invented, let alone defined. And so the minor gesture often goes by unperceived, its improvisational threads of variability overlooked, despite their being in our midst. There is no question that the minor is precarious.

And yet the minor gesture is everywhere, all the time. Despite its precarity, it resurfaces punctually, claiming not space as such, but space-of-variation. The minor invents new forms of existence, and with them, in them, we come to be. These temporary forms of life travel across the everyday, making untimely existing political structures, activating new modes of perception, inventing languages that speak in the interstices of major tongues. The minor gesture's indeterminacy, and even its failure to thrive, is what interests me here. For there is no question, it seems to me, that we put too much credence in that which persists, in the edifices rebuilt daily by technocrats. There must be other ways of living?

In its movement, the minor gesture creates sites of dissonance, staging disturbances that open experience to new modes of expression. In making felt the event's limit, the operational interval where the event exceeds the sum of its parts, the minor gesture punctually reorients experience. The event here is defined according to a Whiteheadian concept of the actual occasion. Actual occasions are the coming-into-being of indeterminacy where potentiality passes into realization (Whitehead 1978: 29). When speaking of the event's potentiality, I am lingering on the side of the as-yet-undetermined share of the actual occasion. I am focusing on the phase of realization of the event, of experience, where it has not yet fully become this or that. The minor gesture is active in this indeterminate phase of the event. This is not to underestimate the necessity of an event's coming to form. As Alfred North Whitehead emphasizes, it is the event's atomicity, its capacity to be fully what it is, that ultimately opens the way for the potential of what is to come: without atomicity, in an arena of pure becoming, there would be no "elbow room in the universe," no opening for the disjunctions through which difference is produced (1967: 195). The emphasis here is not on the continuity of becoming, an infinitely open account of process, but on the becoming of continuity: process punctuated. The event and the minor gesture are always in co-composition, the minor gesture punctuating process, moving the welling event in new and divergent directions that alter the orientation of where the event might otherwise have settled.

By making everything an event, by emphasizing that there is nothing outside of or beyond the event, the aim is to create an account of experience that requires no omnipresence. The event is where experience actualizes. Experience here is in the tense of life-living, not human life per se, but the more-than human: life at the interstices of experience in the ecology of practices.[2] From this vantage point of an ecology of practices, it is urgent to turn away from the notion that it is the human agent, the intentional, volitional subject, who determines what comes to be.[3] It is urgent to turn away from the central tenet of neurotypicality, the wide-ranging belief that there is an independence of thought and being attributable above all to the human, a better-than-ness accorded to our neurology (a neurology, it must be said, that reeks of whiteness, and classism). Neurotypicality, as a central but generally unspoken identity politics, frames our idea of which lives are worth fighting for, which lives are worth educating, which lives are worth living, and which lives are worth saving.[4]

Despite its role as a founding gesture of humanism, of individualism, neurotypicality remains for the most part in the background of our everyday lives. Certainly, activists who fight for neurodiversity are very aware of how neurotypicality frames experience. But for the rest of us, neurotypicality as such tends to be backgrounded, and so we underestimate both its force and its pervasiveness. Issues that most readily define neurotypicality as foundational are often seen as given. We pay them little attention: we don't tend, for instance, to question the abortion of vast numbers of Down syndrome fetuses.[5] Or we don't think of mental illness as on a spectrum with our own neurology. Or we ignore how pervasive it is not to create robust accommodations for difference and rarely organize events with accommodation in mind.[6] We don't concern ourselves with the fact that, too often, people with disabilities, intellectual or physical, are offered palliative care instead of life-sustaining treatment for diseases.[7] We too often see all of these scenarios—if we do see them at all—simply as aspects of existence at this current juncture: they are what they are, and surely they have come to be for a reason.[8] Neurotypicality tells us what is in our best interest, and we tend to accept it wholesale. It is for this reason that neuro-typicality as foundational identity politics is rarely named as such. When do we question what we mean by independence, by intelligence, by knowl-edge? When do we honor significantly different bodies and ask what they can do, instead of jumping to the conclusion that they are simply deficient?[9] When is the fat body, the immobilized body, the blind body, the deaf body, the old body, the spastic body celebrated? Yours, mine, the life of the autis-tic, still taught in segregated classrooms, yours, mine, the life of the schizo-phrenic, of the psychotic, the depressed, institutionalized and out of sight, yours, mine, the First Nations, disenfranchised by a settler colonialism that refuses to recognize political practices neurodiverse at their core, yours, mine, the drug addict, the drunk, the black man, treated last in the emer-gency ward (if treated at all), yours, mine, the transgender, the transsexual, the gay or lesbian, our rights too rarely recognized as they should be, yours, mine, lives deemed less worthy, less worthy not just because of our visible difference, but because we have already been classed as less-than, as less educable, as less desirable, as less knowledgeable, as less valuable. We have already been situated, aligned in opposition to the dominant ideal of life, to the majoritarian discourse of neurotypicality, and we fall short.

I define this framing of existence as neurotypical not to underestimate other forms of oppression, including racism, classism, sexism. My hope is to underscore the mutual indebtedness of the narrative of neurotypicality and the framing of certain bodies and certain forms of life as less worthy. Take blackness. Neurotypicality, Fred Moten suggests, is another name for antiblackness.[10] The neurotypical stages the encounter with life in such a way as to exclude what cannot fit within its order, and blackness, or what Moten describes as "black sociality," always ultimately exceeds capture.

In a videotaped conversation entitled "Do Black Lives Matter" between himself and Robin D. G. Kelley, Moten speaks of the concept of black so-ciality in the context of the 2014 murders of Michael Brown and Eric Gar-ner.[11] He explains:

> We need to understand what the state is defending itself from and I think that in this respect, the particular instances of Michael Brown's murder and Eric Garner's murder are worth paying some attention to.

Because what the drone, Darren Wilson [the police officer], shot into that day was insurgent Black life walking down the street. I don't think he meant to violate the individual personhood of Michael Brown, he was shooting at mobile Black sociality walking down the street in a way that he understood implicitly constituted a threat to the order he represents and that he is sworn to protect. Eric Garner on the everyday basis initiated a new alternative kind of marketplace, another mode of social life. That's what they killed, OK? So when we say that Black lives matter I think what we do sometimes is obscure the fact that it's in fact Black life that matters. That insurgent Black social life still constitutes a profound threat to the already existing order of things.

Insurgent Black life is neurodiverse through and through. This is its threat, that it cannot be properly regulated, that it exceeds the bounds of the known, that it *moves* too much—"I don't need to disavow the notion that black people have rhythm."[12] Blackness, life-living, is life at the limit.[13] Moten continues: "Antiblackness is antilife. Somewhere along the line black flesh held the responsibility of protecting generativity. . . . Life is Black life. . . . When you say Black life matters, you are saying life matters, and when you say life matters, you are saying Black life matters." That neurotypicality as founding identity politics discounts black life implies, at the limit, that it discounts all life, all generative force, all unbounded, unpredictable, rhythmic, insurgent life.

Neurodiversity is the path I choose here to explore insurgent life. Encouraged by neurodiversity activism, I take neurodiversity as a platform for political change that fundamentally alters how life is defined, and valued. I do this with the neurodiversity movement's call in mind: to honor complex forms of interdependence and to create modes of encounter for that difference.[14] One of the compelling tenets of the movement for neurodiversity is that it explicitly calls for social and medical services. Many classical autistics, for instance, cannot live without facilitation. They need assistance. And so they not only want to be seen as valuable in their difference, they also want their need for facilitation to be seen as a necessary and honored aspect of social life. The neurodiversity movement celebrates the relational force of facilitation broadly defined. This emphasis on relation is central to my discussion of facilitation in chapter 7.

The neurotypical, as real contributor to society and to humanity in general, is strongly paired with a notion of independence understood according to normative definitions of ability and able-bodiedness framed by what I call the volition-intentionality-agency triad. Despite several decades of the Disability Act, what Guattari would call "normopathy" continues to rule, not only defining value in terms of normative criteria of functioning, but also reducing the importance of relation by placing facilitation on the side of lack: those who need facilitation demonstrate a lack of intelligence, a lack of will, a lack of agency.[15] The neurotypical is the very backbone of a concept of individuality that is absolutely divorced from the idea that relation is actually what our worlds are made of. The neurotypical does not need assistance, does not need accommodation, and certainly does not need facilitation. The neurotypical is independent through and through.

The approach I am taking here, in my calling into question the centrality of neurotypicality as grounding structure for existence as we practice it, might be called schizoanalytic, not because there is an encounter with schizophrenia per se, but because the account involves an engagement with the cleaving of experience. A working definition of schizoanalysis for the purposes of this project might be: the active operation that creates schisms, in an ecology of practices, opening up the event to its potential for a collectivity alive with difference. A concept that composes well with the activity of this cleaving is *agencement*. *Agencement*, as Guattari writes, is a junction that "secretes [its own] coordinates, [that] can certainly impose connections, but [does] not impose a fixed constraint" (2013: 24). Mobilizing the cleave of the event, its internal schism, *agencement* foregrounds not the agency of an individual acting on the event, but those very operations that "secrete their own coordinates" *in the event*, affecting how it comes to expression. A schizoanalytic approach, as I will elaborate in chapter 8, affirms these complex ecologies that could not come into existence without the schisms that radically alter the operational quality of the event.

As the postscript will emphasize, a schizoanalytic approach has a belief in the world. In this sense it is Nietzschean: "Was that life? Well then, once more!" (1954: 157). The world it believes in is a world where to act is an inherently affirmative gesture that cannot be distinguished from the in-act of the event. What acts at the heart of the event is the minor gesture. This is not to say that the minor gesture is inherently positive, or good. The minor gesture, like schizoanalysis, is operational. It shifts the field, altering the valence of what comes to be. It is affirmative in its force, emphatic in its belief. Yet it would be to radically misunderstand the cut of difference to ignore the pull of the tragic, as Nietzsche makes clear in drawing a connection between affirmation and tragedy. This is further developed in the postscript.

Deleuze's words should also be heeded: "It is not the marginal who create the lines; they install themselves on these lines and make them their property, and this is fine when they have that strange modesty of people of the line, the prudence of the experimenter, but it is a disaster when they slip into a black hole from which they no longer utter anything but the micro-fascist speech of their dependency and their giddiness: 'We are the avant-garde,' 'We are the marginal'" (2007: 139, translation modified). The minor gesture is not the *figure* of the marginal, though the marginal may carry a special affinity for the minor and wish to compose with it. The minor gesture is the force that makes the lines tremble that compose the everyday, the lines, both structural and fragmentary, that articulate how else experience can come to expression. To compose with the minor gesture requires, as Deleuze cautions, the prudence of the experimenter, a prudence awake to the speculative pragmatism at the heart of the welling event. Study and research-creation, both developed in the first chapter, are techniques for experimental prudence, a prudence patient enough to engage with that which experimentation unsettles, a prudence attuned to the force of the in-act. But beware: this is not the prudence of a passive outlier! This is a tentativeness in the act that jumps at the chance to discover what else the event can do. It is a prudence that composes at the edges of the as-yet-unthought in the rhythm of the minor gesture.

The minor gesture is the activator, the carrier, it is the *agencement* that draws the event into itself. It moves the nonconscious toward the conscious, makes felt the unsayable in the said, brings into resonance field effects otherwise backgrounded in experience. It is the forward-force capable of carrying the affective tonality of nonconscious resonance and moving it toward the articulation, edging into consciousness, of new modes of existence.

This capacity to actualize, at the edge of the virtual where the actual is not-yet, is what makes the minor a *gesture*: the minor is a gesture insofar as it punctuates the in-act, leading the event elsewhere than toward the governant fixity of the major, be it the major in the name of normative political structures, of institutional life, of able-bodiedness, of gender conformity, of racial segregation. This book celebrates the fragility and the persistence of the minor gesture, perceiving in it more potential than in the self-directed "I" that stands outside experience and speaks the major languages of the brands of individualism and humanism that frame neurotypicality as the center of being.

The register of the minor gesture is always political: in its punctual reorienting of the event, the minor gesture invents new modes of life-living. It moves through the event, creating a pulse, opening the way for new tendencies to emerge, and in the resonances that are awakened, potential for difference looms. This is how I am defining the political: the movement activated, in the event, by a difference in register that awakens new modes of encounter and creates new forms of life-living. Life-living in its usage throughout refuses to privilege *this* life, this human life, at the expense of different forms and forces of life, even as it recognizes the importance of the punctuality of *this* singular event we call our life. Life-living is a way of thinking life with and beyond the human, thinking life as more-than-human. Deleuze's concept of *a life* resonates strongly here, *a life* defined in his last ode to living as the flux of liveliness coursing through existence unlimited.[16] The conjunction between the minor gesture and life-living is a political ecology that operates on the level of the in-act, asking at every juncture what else life could be. How *this* singular life-orientation carries existence, and where its minor gestures may lead, is always, for me, a political question.

The political opening that lurks here is built of a procedural architecture called the undercommons, a concept coined by Fred Moten and Stefano Harney.[17] The undercommons is not a given site, not a place predefined, not even a recognizable enclave we could return to having found it once. The undercommons is an emergent collectivity that is sited in the encounter. Allied to the minor gesture, it is an activator of a tendency more than it is an offering of a commonality. What makes it a commons is not the existing gathering but its speculative presence as an ecology of practices. The undercommons is a tentative holding in place of fragile comings-into-relation, physical and virtual, that create the potential to reorient fields of life-living—a belief in the ineffable and its powers of resistance keep it alive.

In Moten and Harney's reading of the undercommons, the university looms large as a site in need. The academic institution also has a major role to play with respect to the policing of neurotypicality. For this reason, like Moten and Harney, I will first dwell on the example of what an undercommons might look like in the context of academia before then opening the undercommons beyond the strictures of the academic institution to what else study looks like in the everyday.

Neurotypicality involves a hierarchization of knowledge, based as it is on a belief that favors normative forms of instruction and segregates knowledge according to accepted ideas of what serves society best. Most accepted approaches to learning assume neurotypicality with regard to processing information, thereby segregating not only neurodiverse learners, but also predefining what counts as knowledge.[18]

In *The Undercommons*, Moten and Harney foreground the university as an institutional system that, in the neoliberal economy, thrives on a belief that knowledge can be encapsulated and marketed. There is no question that this tendency has become more marked in the last decades, with funding for the humanities, social sciences, the theoretical sciences, and studio arts (to name only the most obvious examples) continuously under threat due to their so-called uselessness in the economic marketplace. With the increased pressure of bringing funds to the university through grant-writing comes the generalization of knowledge and the emphasis on disciplinary framing. The shift looks something like this: in order to get grants, scholars and artists within the university are asked to frame their own work according to perceived use-value (read: grant-value). This tends to hierarchize certain forms of knowledge over others, though these hierarchies can turn around quite quickly, given the mobility of capital. Paired with the increased financial instability of the university, which leads to fewer positions being created and thus fewer differences within the ranks, this can have the effect of narrowing knowledge to what are perceived to be the needs of the discipline (now redefined according to granting categories), often acting against the very openings learning can facilitate.

Critique tends to lead the way. Learning is a fragile enterprise that can too easily be sidetracked by the encroachment of what is set up, in advance, as relevant or irrelevant. In the name of critique, this fragility is often framed and deadened through the crafting of questions that already have answers, or whose answers are close at hand, contained within preexisting academic discourse. "The critical academic questions the university, questions the state, questions art, politics, culture. But in the undercommons it is 'no questions asked'" (Moten and Harney 2013: 38). The mode of critique that operates as an academic trope stifles the very opening through which fragile new modes of existence can come to expression. What if knowledge were not assumed to have a form already? What if we didn't yet know what needed to be taught, let alone questioned?

The undercommons opens the way for the crafting of problems greater than their solutions. Here I am following Henri Bergson, who suggests that the best problem is the one that opens up an intuitive process, not the one that already carries within itself its fix. A solvable problem was never really a problem, Bergson reminds us. Only when a question is in line with the *creation of a problem* is it truly operational. Most academic questions are of the solvable, unproblematic sort. What the undercommons seeks are real problems, problems intuited and crafted *in the inquiry*. Bergson writes:

> It is the clarity of the radically new and absolutely simple idea, which catches as it were, an intuition. As we cannot reconstruct it with pre-existing elements, since it has no elements, and as on the other hand, to understand without effort consists in recomposing the new from what is old, our first impulse is to say it is incomprehensible. . . . One must . . . distinguish between the ideas which keep their light for themselves, making it penetrate immediately into their slightest recesses, and those whose radiation is exterior, illuminating a whole region of thought. (2007: 23)

The challenge, as Bergson underscores, involves crafting the conditions not to *solve* problems, or to resolve questions, but to illuminate regions of thought through which problems-without-solutions can be intuited. Problems "must be given time. The philosopher has not always the patience. How much simpler it is to confine oneself to notions stored up in language!" (2007: 24). The call made by the undercommons is that we refrain from taking on problems that are already recognizable, available, but work instead, collectively, to invent open problems that bring us together in the mode of active inquiry. We must be careful, though, in doing so, not to create false problems. "False problems are of two sorts, 'nonexistent problems,' defined as problems whose very terms contain a confusion of the 'more' and the 'less'; and 'badly stated' questions, so defined because their terms represent badly analyzed composites" (Deleuze 1988: 17). False problems, like the questions the undercommons does not ask, bring us up against "an illusion that carries us along, or in which we are immersed, inseparable from our condition" (Deleuze 1988: 20). False problems and badly stated questions maintain the status quo. Academic critique and debate are too often played out at the level of false problems and badly stated questions.

To explore regions of thought that open onto new kinds of problematic processes, I begin the book with an account of research-creation. Research-creation is the term given, in Canada, to academic work that is evaluated both for a creative, usually artistic contribution, and a written, more theoretical or philosophical one.[19] On the surface, research-creation is a term without much traction, more a funding category than a conceptual approach. Since 2003, however, when the term came into general usage in Canada, the SenseLab has taken it on as a problem, asking how the hyphen between research and creation opens up the differential between making and thinking.[20] This differential, we argue, needs to be kept alive in its difference—philosophy does not require artistic practice any more than art requires philosophy. Different practices must retain their singularity. At the same time, when they do come together, as with research-creation, it is important to inquire into what the hyphenation does to their singularity. We find research-creation to be a fertile field for thinking this coming-into-relation of difference. Problems that arise include: How does a practice that involves making open the way for a different idea of what can be termed knowledge? How is the creation of concepts, in the context of the philosophical, itself a creative process? How can we bring the different registers of art and philosophy, of making-thinking, together in ways that are capable of honoring their difference? In what ways does the hyphen make operational interstitial modes of existence? Here, as we have done at the SenseLab for the past decade, I take research-creation as one of the most lively current modalities, in the academic institution, of problem-making, and I explore how it creates fields of inquiry for reframing how knowledge is practiced beyond typical forms of academic use-value, including the value we place on linguistic expression and language-based evaluation. Research-creation, I argue in chapter 1, has no method to follow, and no ready-made modes of evaluation.

The term Moten and Harney propose for the crafting of problems is *study*, emphasizing that study is not a place where everyone "dissolves into a student" but where there is the acknowledgment that there is no way "of being intellectual that isn't social." In a conversation between himself, Stevphen Shukaitis, and Stefano Harney, Moten explains:

> When I think about the way we use the term "study," I think we are committed to the idea that study is what you do with other people. It's talking and walking around with other people, working, dancing, suffering, some irreducible convergence of all three, held under the name

of speculative practice. The notion of a rehearsal—being in a kind of workshop, playing in a band, in a jam session, or old men sitting on a porch, or people working together in a factory—there are these various modes of activity. The point of calling it "study" is to mark that the incessant and irreversible intellectuality of these activities is already present. These activities aren't ennobled by the fact that we now say, "oh, if you did these things in a certain way, you could be said to be have been studying." To do these things is to be involved in a kind of common intellectual practice. What's important is to recognize that that has been the case—because that recognition allows you to access a whole, varied, alternative history of thought. (Moten and Harney 2013: 109–110)

Whether we call it study or we call it research-creation and engage directly with knowledge as it is being reframed in pockets of academic discourse, what matters is that there is an explicit disavowal of method as generator of knowledge. For method, aligned as it is to the major, is what seeks to capture the minor gesture, what seeks to capture study, and silence it.

With the undercommons as beacon for emergent collectivity, and study, or research-creation, as its mode of engagement, this book attempts to get away from asking questions that already contain their answers. "What I would want to do is not so much keep producing questions but to step to the side of the question a bit and think through the importance of study—that it might be possible to imagine a form of movement or political mobilization that would be driven by or centered on the activity of study in a way that does not require the figuration of the student, or potentially some sort of reification of the figure of the student" (Bousquet, Harney, and Moten 2009: 160). Study, like research-creation, refutes the "subject" of study, and in so doing it also refuses the "object of study." It does so by always beginning with the creation of a problem that is truly productive of inquiry. In so doing, it opens the field of experience to the more-than of objects or subjects preformed. Study is an act that delights in the activation of the as-yet-unthought. It is an activity of *immanent* critique, as I argue in chapter 1, an act that only knows the conditions of its existence from within its own process, an act that refuses to judge from without. Study, research-creation—these are pragmatically speculative practices that, while absolutely entrenched in their own process of making-time, *here, now,* remain untimely. For as practices, they activate event-time, the time unparsed of the intuitive, a concept I explore further in chapter 2, inventing problems that have no home, no reference yet. Such problems need a collective to answer them; they need the undercommons. They require study. And, it bears repeating: what emerges from study will never be an answer. What emerges will be patient experimentation. What emerges will be another mode of encounter, another problem, another opening onto the political as site as yet undefined.

WHAT ART CAN DO

To begin with research-creation is to immediately situate the force of the minor gesture in the activity of the differential. The differential, the active hyphen that brings making to thinking and thinking to making, ensures that research-creation remain an ecology of practices. This ecology of practices needs a punctual proto-event such as the minor gesture to bring its potential into focus. The minor gesture activates the differential such that the ecology's incipient heterogeneity becomes operational. When this happens, something has begun to take form that exceeds the registers of making on one end and thinking on the other. A movement of thought, as Bergson might say, becomes active, and in this activity a new register begins to take shape. This new register is neither art per se nor philosophy: it is study, it is practice, it is speculation.

In most cases research-creation as an academic category is directly concerned with *artistic* practice. Combined with study, however, the emphasis moves toward the exploration of how modes of making and thinking become consolidated in emergent, collective forms of practice that are artful, if not necessarily artistic in the strong sense. The artful, or what Raymond Ruyer (1958) calls "the aesthetic yield," is defined throughout as the in-act of the more-than where the force of form remains emergent. Artful practices honor complex forms of knowing and are collective not because they are operated upon by several people, but because they make apparent, in the way they come to a problem, that knowledge at its core is collective. Practices that think multiply are many: they can be activist practices, environmental practices, social practices. They can involve child-rearing, social work, teaching, playing. They can take place on a park bench, in the city, in the classroom, in the kitchen. To think multiply is to think in the register of the hyphen, of the differential, in the complex field of study opened up by the undercommons.

In chapter 2, where the concept of the artful takes form, I propose we work not with the current and most typical definition of art, which tends still to foreground an object, but with an aspect of its medieval definition:

art as *the way*. By focusing on process instead of form, it becomes possible not only to raise the issue of the object—to ask how a focus on the object is similar in many ways to situating the subject as initiator of experience—but to explore how time is engaged in the artistic process. Following Bergson, I turn to intuition, and its manner of making time. I argue that intuition is as key to a process as any other building-block and that through intuition, as allied to the creation of a problem, the artful comes to expression.

What art can do when it tweaks toward the artful, what research-creation can do when the differential is activated by a minor gesture, is to make felt the intervals, the openings and captures within a process that is on its way to becoming a practice. This is explored in more detail in chapter 5.

The artful, in my reading of it, is aligned to what I have elsewhere called "autistic perception."[21] Autistic perception is the opening, in perception, to the uncategorized, to the unclassified. This opening, which is how many autistics describe their experience of the world, makes it initially difficult to parse the field of experience. Rather than seeing the parts abstracted from the whole, autistic perception is alive with tendings that create ecologies before they coalesce into form. There is here as yet no hierarchical differentiation, for instance, between color, sound, light, between human and nonhuman, between what connects to the body and what connects to the world. When we engage in practice, when we are subsumed by process, we often seek this kind of perception, and it is available to us all: autistic perception does not belong exclusively to autistics. The difference is that, except in extreme circumstances, most of us parse experience before having a direct experience of the field in its complexity. The autistic, on the other hand, directly perceives the complexity before (and between) the parsings.

In the chapters that follow, the artful is always colored by the edgings into perceptibility of autistic perception. I focus on autistic perception not only to honor neurodiversity, to take into account modes of existence I consider key to making our worlds richer, but to make a political case for the necessity of creating techniques and minor gestures that open existence to its perceptual more-than. This is not to deny that autistic perception, for all its perceptual wonders, also makes typical aspects of everyday life difficult to manage. For instance: crossing a street, it is always safer to have been capable of parsing cars from sidewalks from humans. After all, we live in a world that privileges forms of perception where the part can quickly and easily be singled out from the whole. By foregrounding the inheritance of autistic perception in the artful, we are reminded that the qualitative openings in experience activated by autistic perception have a value in their own right. The problem is not with autistic perception but with how we constitute and value the frameworks of everyday living.

Frameworks of everyday living are also of the event. And so, like all events, they can be modulated by minor gestures. They can be opened up to their potential in ways that intervene into capitalist time. They can become forms of resistance. They can do so, for instance, by altering rhythms, reducing our alignment to the homogeneity of capitalist speed. Altering the speed at which the everyday tends to function creates openings for neurodiverse forms of perception. It also makes time for modes of encounter otherwise elided. This call for the coursing of minor gestures within frames of everyday life involves crafting techniques that create the conditions not for slowness exactly, but for the opening of the everyday to degrees and shades of experience that resist formation long enough to allow us to see the potential of worlds in the making. This involves becoming more attuned to event-time, the nonlinear lived duration of experience in the making. For it is in event-time that the minor gesture tunes the event to what it can do.

A politics allied to study, engaged in the crafting of problems that open up the time of the event, is an affirmative politics, not in the sense that it is optimistic, but in the sense that it begins with the in-act and embraces the force of the *what else* at the heart of all speculative pragmatisms. Such a politics emphasizes the techniques and conditions that lead to the creation of new problems, rather than promising an already-constituted field replete with form and content. Form and content are short-lived, and this makes them false starters. In a politics attuned to emergent difference, we must begin instead in the midst, where force has not yet tuned to form. In this middle, where the event is still welling, there is potential for new diagrams of life-living to be drawn.

IN THE ACT

Alternative diagrams for life-living must resist returning to a model of inside-outside where the human subject is situated as the motivator of experience. This is our habit: to make the work about us. When we do so, we set up conditions that are only generative as regards what we perceive as our own well-being. Framing our approach to the political this way, we place the subject, the human, in the position of agency, promoting the act in terms of the volitional thrust of our own intentionality. Even when we give voice to those silenced, even when we speak in the name of the multitude, even when we talk about the "agency" of an artistic process, even when we try to give agency to an oppressed people, we assume a mediation between an act and its unfolding, most often attributing the push to action to ourselves as a species, while still retaining a strong sense that the world is ultimately led and enhanced by the neurotypical few. This is the problem with agency: it makes the subject the subject of the action. What if the act did not fully belong to us?

Around the turn of the twentieth century, both Bergson and William James become invested in this problem of the act. What is it, they ask, that makes us so certain that the act is volitionally directed by a human subject? What is it that gives us the strong sense that the act's effort belongs to us? And why is it so threatening, I might add, to think that within the act there is a considerable involuntary share of activity?

In chapter 6, I explore James's account of the feeling of effort in detail. Here I will turn to Bergson's analysis of the same question. The feeling of effort, Bergson suggests, seems to be allied to a muscular sensation: the magnitude associated with an effort is quantified according to the degree of muscular sensation a given activity demands. This suggests that the feeling of effort is allied to consciousness: what we name effort has something to do with a conscious estimation of intensity. Even when the effort is in vain—as in, for instance, picking up what we thought was a heavy box of books but was actually an empty box—the *feeling* of effort remains. Effort would therefore seem to be aptly connected to a willful movement undertaken, its intensive magnitude linked to the expectation of the amount of muscular contraction needed to follow through with the act.

And yet, as both Bergson and James point out, there is an issue with the above analysis. First, intensity cannot be quantified. It is but a shading, a coloring, of the event, in the event. If intensity is felt to have magnitude, the magnitude can only be qualitative. A quantification cannot therefore be assigned to intensity per se, but must instead be connected to a sense of what the intensity represented, after the fact. What this means is that there is an alliance between the feeling of effort and how the event has come to be known in retrospect. This knowing-in-retrospect is the work consciousness does in the parsing of an event.[22] Bergson writes: "But just as consciousness . . . concentrates on a given point of the organism the increasing number of muscular contractions which take place on the surface of the body, thus converting them into one single feeling of effort, of growing intensity, so it will hypostatize under the form of a growing desire the gradual alterations which take place in the confused heap of coexisting psychic states" (2007: 9). What is felt as quantitative effort is felt consciously, backgrounding not only the qualitative complexity in the event, but intensity's own qualitative multiplicity. In the parsing that occurs with consciousness, a certain poverty of complexity has been chosen over the confused heap. This leads to the intervals of sensation — its degrees and multiplicities — being flattened into one single overarching feeling. The transition from the complexity of a purely qualitative experience to the feeling of effort occasioned in the conscious accounting of the act makes the intervals of sensation appear "as different intensities of one and the same feeling, which is thus supposed to change in magnitude" (Bergson 2007: 11). Whereas in the nonconscious welling event, every shift caused a change in nature, in turn causing a qualitative transformation in the field of experience, with the onset of consciousness the tendency is to backgrid effect onto cause, creating a solid accounting of change that organizes the event within a temporal grid. This solid accounting is quantifiable only because it can be said to be the same or different — in time, in space, in effect — from the last solid accounting of experience. "Consciousness, accustomed to think in terms of space and to translate its thoughts into roots, will denote the feeling by a single word and will localize the effort at the exact point where it yields a useful result: it will then become aware of an effort which is always of the same nature and increases at the spot assigned to it, and a feeling which, retaining the same name, grows without changing its nature" (Bergson 2007: 26). With consciousness, the feeling tends to move from the event into the subject, where the effort's magnitude is directly aligned to experiences parsed, past and present.

If the feeling of effort is tied to consciousness, it follows that it must be tied to volition. The argument would look like this: when a movement is made consciously, we know the effort contained because movement is volitional, and as such, it belongs to us. A volitional movement, because it is intentional, and because it comes from us, must therefore already include within its parameters the knowledge of how much effort is necessary to carry it out. This effort is learned and comes through repetition. Once the movement becomes a habit it is practiced volitionally, that is, intentionally. We thus have agency over it.

We tend to divide movement into two general categories: reflexes or automatic movements, on the one hand, and directed or volitional movements, on the other. We are taught that reflex, which is considered in-stinctual and therefore less refined than volitional movement, is a direct, nonconscious response *in the event* to a cause. A parent running into the street to grab their child before it gets hit by a car is engaged in automatic movement, suddenly capable of amazing acts of strength and stamina, all of which take place nonconsciously. Directed, or volitional movement, on the other hand, is defined as strategized movement. Because it is consid-ered to be beyond instinct, directed movement is said to be more free than automatic movement. After all, it is conscious, and consciousness is said to be a prerequisite for freedom. One sign of this freedom is that volitional movement is said to be able to resist the strict overlay of cause onto effect. For instance, during a game, a soccer player might be taught a strategy that includes moving in a certain way on the field, but she is equally expected to be able to consciously, that is, volitionally, alter course if necessary. Indeed, the soccer player's talent is often measured by this "free act" of movement she is expected to be able to undertake in the split second of a change in play. This differentiation between conscious and nonconscious movement, between so-called "free" movement, on the one hand, and automatic or reflex movement, on the other, is problematic for several reasons. First, it hierarchizes forms of movement according to conscious behavior, ignoring the complex tendings within consciousness that open it to nonconscious inflections. Second, it classifies as primitive forms of movement that are alive *in the event*, thus situating autistic perception, for instance, on the side of reflex and neurotypical perception on the side of volition, thereby fur-ther cementing the hierarchy. It also confuses two levels of cause and effect in its account of freedom.

In the moving, in the act, we are in an immanent cause-effect relation. The soccer player's active response to a change in play is an account of cause-effect, but one where cause-effect is still in transformation, affected by emergent improvisational movement operations. How the shift in play will affect the game is not strategized consciously by the moving soccer player; the cause-effect scenario is not measured in the doing. Something altogether different is at stake: the soccer player is in the field, is moved by the field; her movement not a *response* to the play so much as the acti-vation of a new field of relation. The talent ascribed to the soccer player is ultimately due not to her volitional ability to move, but to her capacity to effect cause *in the event*, opening the field to its potential through intuitive realignings activated by mobile cues, leading to a (re)directing of the game. All movement works this way, as I argue in chapter 5. When we believe we have consciously affected the direction of an event, when we feel that an event has been moved by our volition alone, it is because a backgridding onto the event has taken place that has made sense of the play-by-play. This is usually how we explain our actions, but it is not how we act. How we act is based on a continuous interplay of conscious and nonconscious movement with nonconscious movement playing a vital part, especially as regards movement's creative potential.

In our everyday movements, especially in relation to movements that have become habitual, a movement might nonetheless *feel* completely volitional. When this is the case, what has happened is that we've experienced a sense of déjà-felt, in the event. This déjà-felt occurs in the interstices of the conscious and the nonconscious, directing the event to its familiarity-in-feeling. What is important to realize, and what I explore further in chapter 7, is that the feeling of volition is not volition itself. The feeling of volition is more aptly defined as a certain recognition, in the moving, of our having already moved "just this way." But movement-moved is never twice the same: it is always altered by the ecologies that create *this* singular field of relation, and that influence how it will unfold *this* time. Volitional movement understood as movement belonging to the subject and fully directed by the subject is, therefore, impossible. Such an account of volition, as suggested above, can only be narrated after the fact. This post facto narration of our movements as volitional is of course more straightforward if the act maintains a certain similarity across variations. Major movements— movements that have a form that can easily be recognized, such as getting on the bus—are therefore more easily post-identified as "volitional" than are minor gestures.

Throughout, I consider movement as *decisional* rather than volitional, decision defined here not as external to the event but as the cut, in the event, through which new ecologies, new fields of relation are crafted. The soccer player's reorienting of the field was decisional in *just this way*. Nonconscious movement is decisional in the sense that it is capable of altering the course of the event *in the event*. Elsewhere, I've called the attunement, in the event, toward decisional movement, choreographic thinking, emphasizing the ability of movement to cue and align in spacetimes of composition in ways that open experience to new registers.[23] Reflective consciousness actually gets in the way of this process, as dancers and athletes will attest to. Movement-moving is at its most creative, its most operational, when not curtailed by the imposition of narratives of volition and intentionality.

Affect is one of the most habitual ways we experience the nonvoluntary in the act. Bergson writes: "The intensity of affective sensations might . . . be nothing more than our consciousness of the involuntary movements which are being begun and outlined" (2007: 35). The force of the affective moves us. When this movement tunes toward an experience that can be defined as such, the conscious share of the nonconscious has briefly made itself felt. Degrees of parsing are possible here. There can, for instance, be a feeling, irreducible to definition but nonetheless semi-consciously ascertained, affectively felt but unarticulated, of an uneasiness or a tremulousness. Or, in cases where affect tunes to emotion, there can be a clearer parsing into the language of a singular feeling. In the second instance, where affect tunes to emotion, there is a shadowing over of the intensity of affect, though an affective trace still remains.

In the case of affect, the involuntary tends to be recognized and even accepted, but only insofar as it is considered to have no *real* effect on our modalities of existence. For we know well that affect is considered lower on the scale than reason or rationality. All is well with affect as long as ultimately we can hold it back and use our volition to steer our feelings, imposing decision from without. The problem should be clear by now. In transposing reason onto affect we are trying to have it both ways: we want to feel the ineffable, yet deceive ourselves into thinking we can sideline the ineffable and leave the bubbling ground of the welling event when it suits us. We want to believe we can decide where the event will take us. This is a mirage that underestimates the force of the nonvoluntary in our daily lives.

Because we have little by way of evaluative strategies for the nonvoluntary, because the nonvoluntary resists method, and, in many cases, language, there remains a firm belief that it is of lesser value than conscious, so-called volitional experience. Yet nonconscious experience is full of knowledge: it is, after all, the site of decision. No decision, as mentioned above, is made outside the event's welling.[24] Both Carl Schmitt and Whitehead, in their different ways, emphasize that decision is the cut that opens the event to a new field of relation, not the act that precedes or follows the event. Decision is not what happens after the affective opening of the event to its potential, but what cleaves the event, in the event. The minor gesture is a decisional cut.

The decisional cut is everywhere active. Take the example of picking up milk at the corner store. You might assume that this simple act is completely volitional. But much is left open to the event's own process of decision, even in what seems to be such a simple, habitual act. You may not have realized, for instance, the way your movement was immanently directed and shaped not by your will alone, but by the pull of the corner store, or what James calls the "terminus," a pull that doesn't necessarily include a direct follow-through. For while the store did get you up, while its immanent directionality did incite directional mobility, it is possible that in this corner store instance you're still in your living-room because on the way to the door a song began to play on the radio that brought the couch into focus and you found yourself lying down to listen to it instead of getting milk. Likely, when asked, you will say that you decided to lie on the couch, that you didn't *really* need the milk, but in fact the event decided and you followed, open to the nature of the event-based improvisation that is part of all our daily choreographies.

I emphasize the nonvolitional in the act because so much is taken for granted in the name of neurotypicality, in the name of volition, of intentionality, of agency. For those who pass as neurotypical, for whom movement usually reads as volitional, it seems absolutely acceptable to have listened to the song on the couch instead of walking to the corner to get milk. But for the autistic or anyone else for whom activation and impulse control may be an issue, the daily experience of *not* ending up where our movement seemed initially to be directed is not only deeply frustrating, but can also be taken as a sign of our lesser value as human beings: anything that makes us less independent in the eyes of a world that takes intentionality and volition as a normative standard tends to decrease our perceived value as contributors to society.[25]

One reason we identify nonvoluntary movement as other to neurotypical movement is because we have a tendency to see movement as continuous, a view perpetuated by the habit of backgridding the event in consciousness, thereby introducing homogeneity into the activity after the fact. Movement is of course anything but continuous, its activity constantly inflected by the improvisatory quality of a response, in the event, to cues and alignments. Just think of the last time you moved on a crowded sidewalk. It's amazing how few people we bump into in the welter of crowds moving!

Bergson uses music as an example. For some of us, it is very difficult to select out sensory input. To listen to music might be to hear it as a many-times-unfolding, untimely complexity. It might mean you hear not the tune as such, or the measure, but the music's differential, its composite and rhythmic force of form. For those of us less attuned to autistic perception, however, this is likely not how we hear it. What we hear instead is a more homogenized version: we consciously reduce the sensation of sound's intensity to a quantitative magnitude that is averaged out. "Thus when we speak of the intensity of a sound of medium force as a magnitude, we allude principally to the greater or less effort which we should have ourselves to expend in order to summon, by our own effort, the same auditory sensation" (Bergson 2007: 44). This averaging out through consciousness distances us from sound as pure quality: "The sound would remain a pure quality if we did not bring in the muscular effort which produces it or the vibrations which explain it" (2007: 46). In the parsing of sound, the music's qualitative nuance is diminished.

To hear the differential of music's immanent rhythms, to participate directly in the quality of its sounding, it is necessary to hold back the conscious ordering of sensation. It is necessary to increase the duration of the experience of direct perception, thereby honing autistic perception. For Bergson, this means doing away with the idea that sensation can be measured, which also means: articulated, identified, parsed. Parsing, so allied with the neurotypical, not only reduces our capacity to feel the complexity of the event in the event, it perpetuates the hierarchy of conscious experience over nonconscious experience, reason over affect. "What strengthens the illusion on this point is that we have become accustomed to believe in the immediate perception of a homogeneous movement in a homogeneous space" (2007: 49). By situating the event outside of its activity, we become accustomed to neutralizing the force not only of what the event can do, but what the event *is doing*. In Bergson's account, this involves a post facto spatialization of duration, of event-time.

Continuing with his example of music, Bergson writes: "As I interpret this new series . . . as a continuous movement, and as this movement has the same direction, the same duration and the same velocity as the preceding, my consciousness feels itself bound to localize the difference between the second series of sensations and the first elsewhere than in the movement itself" (2007: 49–50). What if instead of parsing movement, we dwelt in movement-moving? This would allow us to be more attuned to the differential at the heart of the event, to its immanent contrast. If we did so, we would no longer be able to believe in pure continuity and would perhaps refrain from our tendency to homogenize experience. And we would begin to more easily perceive minor gestures at work.

Minor gestures recast the field, open it to contrast, make felt its differential. They do so by activating, in the event, a change in direction, a change in quality. The activation of a change in quality is what Bergson defines as freedom. Freedom is here not linked to human volition, nor is it allied to intentionality or agency. Freedom is instead allied to the in-act, to the decisional force of movement-moving, to the *agencement* that opens the event to the fullness of its potential. Freedom is how the event expresses its complexity, in the event.

Bergson's concept of freedom does not separate out activity from the in-act. In doing so, it radically repositions volition as an aspect of experience, active in the act, no longer the external director of experience mediated. Without a hierarchy of conscious versus nonconscious experience, a more complex compositional field of experience emerges. Here there is still room for mutation, for difference, for an opening toward the as-yet-unseen, the as-yet-unthought, the as-yet-unfelt. In these interstices of the as-yet, minor gestures proliferate and can be harnessed toward the reorienting of experience. This is freedom, for Bergson, defined against the usual definition of the free act, which would separate freedom from the in-act, placing freedom side by side with a voluntarist notion of decision. This more typical definition of freedom has us standing outside the event. We are free because we are rational, because we orient the act, because we have agency, because we resist the affective forces of those passions and desires that would steer us in the wrong direction. In this usual definition of freedom, as Bergson says, "we give a mechanical explanation of a fact, and then substitute the explanation for the fact itself" (2007: 181). This is not the way Bergson conceptualizes freedom. As he writes, "Time is not a line along which one can pass again" and therefore "freedom must be sought in a certain shade or quality of the action itself and not in the relation of this act to what it is not or to what it might have been" (2007: 181–183).

Freedom, for Bergson, is dynamic, ecological. Freedom is a quality of the act, an ethos in the act's opening onto experience. Not all events are free, but in every event we find the germs of freedom. These germs must be tended, must be sown in ways that allow the act to create problems that will in turn generate modes of action, of activity, of activism that create new modes of existence. The minor gesture tends the germs of experience in-forming, opening the act to its potential. In this sense, the minor gesture is a force for freedom. For the gesture is only a minor gesture insofar as it opens the way, insofar as it creates the conditions for a different ecology of time, space, of politics. The minor gesture, we must remember, is defined by its capacity to vary, not to hold, not to contain. It acts on, moves through, its gesturing always toward a futurity present in the act, but as yet unexpressed. This is its force, this is its call for freedom.

In the chapters that follow, this is the operative question: what kinds of practices can be crafted that are generative of minor gestures? What might a politics of the minor gesture act like, *here, now*, in the event? And how can we articulate the delicate contrast carried by the minor gesture without flattening out difference, homogenizing experience?

This poses a significant challenge: how to articulate modes of existence, to articulate fields of experience, that operate as much in the nonconscious as in the conscious realms, how to do so in a language that operates chiefly within the realm of the conscious. Perhaps the first step is not to be too certain of the frame that would separate the nonconscious from consciousness. States of consciousness, Bergson writes, "are processes and not things; . . . if we denote them each by a single word, it is for the convenience of language; that they are alive and therefore constantly changing; that, in consequence, it is impossible to cut off a moment from them without making them poorer by the loss of some impression, and thus altering their quality" (2007: 196). Minor gestures operate at this cusp where the nonconscious and the conscious co-compose, where language operates "beneath the words," as autistic Amelia (formerly Amanda) Baggs might say (2010). From this position of indeterminacy, of the ineffable, how to make intelligible the singularity of what cannot be measured or categorized but is felt and, in some sense, known? Here, where there is no perceptible difference, as Bergson says, "between foreseeing, seeing and acting," the minor gesture is key. For the minor gesture can open the way for a different kind of knowing, a knowing in the event, in nonlinear event-time, a knowing that, while impossible to parse, delights in the force of conceptual invention (2007: 198). The minor gesture is an ally of language in the making.

"Freedom" may not be a word to hold onto. For now, I use it as a placeholder to remind us that volition and freedom need not be thought of as complementary. I use it also because the neurodiverse are rarely considered free in a world where freedom is usually associated with independence. A serious taking into account of the nonvoluntary aspect of freedom Bergson foregrounds might ultimately make the neurodiverse free, free to be different, free to need and receive facilitation, free to perceive the complexity of experience on their own terms, and free, also, to move, to live, to love in unpredictable ways. For freedom is not to be found in the ordering of experience, in its measure, but in the dynamic intensity of the event's unfolding. This unfolding affects us, moves us, directs us, but it does not belong to us. Freedom is transversal to the human: it cuts across human experience but is not defined by it. As Bergson writes: "The process of our free activity goes on, as it were, unknown to ourselves, in the obscure depths of our consciousness at every moment of duration" (2007: 237). The heterogeneity of the noncontinuous nature of experience is certainly not easy to articulate, but it is rich, infinitely so. To hear it, it is necessary to refrain from setting experience apart from the in-act.

AGAINST METHOD

Some of the major disasters of mankind have been produced
by the narrowness of men with a good methodology.
—Alfred North Whitehead, *The Function of Reason*

The question of inter- and transdisciplinarity has recently opened up in academic circles to what we in Canada call "research-creation." Research-creation, also called "art-based research," was adopted into academic language through the very question of methodology. Starting out as a funding category that would enable artists teaching in universities who didn't have PhDs to apply for large academic grants, the apparition of research-creation as a category was more instrumental than inventive.[1] For weren't artists already involved in research? Wasn't art practice always engaged in forms of inquiry? Wasn't it a mode of knowledge in its own right? The issue was not, it seems to me, one of simply acknowledging that artists were also researchers, but an institutional tweaking of that already-existent research category into modes of knowledge more easily recognized by the academic institution. To be an artist-researcher would now mean to be able to organize the delineations between art practice and research methodology for the purposes of a grant that would then, inasmuch as grants ordinarily function this way, orient the research toward "academic" aims.

The issue here is complex. It touches not only on the question of how art itself activates and constitutes new forms of knowledge *in its own right* but, perhaps most importantly, incites us to inquire into the very question of how practices produce knowledge, and whether those forms of knowledge can engagingly be captured within the strictures of methodological ordering. While I believe that this is a question that could be posed to all forms of knowledge (following philosophers like Henri Bergson, William James, and Alfred North Whitehead, who all, in their own ways, inquire into the methodological frameworks of science, psychology, and philosophy), here I will focus strictly on the question of research-creation and its relationship to what Moten and Harney call "study," emphasizing research-creation's inherent transversality.

Unlike the definition used by Canadian funding agencies and propagated in many of our institutions, which sees the research component as extra to the artistic practice, thereby emphasizing what has come to be known as the theory-practice split, I would like to take seriously that research-creation in its hyphenation of research with creation proposes singular forms of knowledge which may not be intelligible within current understandings of what knowledge might look like.[2] Taking as my inspiration the myriad colleagues and students whose work has moved me to rethink how knowledge is crafted, and taking also my own practice as a starting point, I would like to suggest that research-creation does much more than what the funding agencies had in store for it: it generates new forms of experience; it tremulously stages an encounter for disparate practices, giving them a conduit for collective expression; it hesitantly acknowledges that normative modes of inquiry and containment often are incapable of assessing its value; it generates forms of knowledge that are extralinguistic; it creates operative strategies for a mobile positioning that take these new forms of knowledge into account; it proposes concrete assemblages for rethinking the very question of what is at stake in pedagogy, in practice, and in collective experimentation. And, in so doing, it creates an opening for what Moten and Harney conceptualize as the undercommons: it creates the conditions for new ways of encountering study—forms and forces of intellectuality that cut across normative accounts of what it means to know.

New forms of knowledge require new forms of evaluation, and even more so, new ways of valuing the work we do. In the case of research-creation, which inevitably involves a transversal engagement with different disciplines, this incites a rethinking of how artistic practice reopens the question of what these disciplines—anthropology, philosophy, art history, cinema, communications, biology, physics, engineering—can do. Here, my focus will be on philosophy, which has a history of launching its speculative apparatus in relation to artistic practice. How, I will ask, can the rethinking of how knowledge is created in the context of artistic practice become an opening to thinking philosophy itself as a practice of research-creation? How, following Gilles Deleuze, might a resituating of research-creation as *a practice that thinks* provide us with the vocabulary to take seriously that "philosophical theory is itself a practice, just as much as its object? It is no more abstract than its object. It is a practice of concepts, and we must judge it in light of the other practices with which it interferes" (1989: 280, translation modified)?[3]

To make this move requires orienting the concept of art toward the transversality of study, thereby tuning making toward a practice of incipient thought. This involves a rethinking of the concept of thought itself. To follow through with this proposition, it will be necessary, as I do in chapter 2, to turn to the medieval definition of art—defined as "the way," "the manner"—locating art not at the level of the finished object, but in its trajectory. As regards thought, it will be necessary to reorient it to the relational field of the occasion, refraining from delimiting it to predominant notions of intellectuality which tend to place thought squarely within the linguistic limits of intelligibility. Staging a critique of neurotypicality as begun in the introduction, it will also be necessary to undo thought of its dependence on the human subject. This will mean opening thought toward the movement of thought, engaging it at the immanent limit, where it is still fully in the act.

Four propositions to begin:

1. If "art" is understood as a "way" it is not yet about an object, about a form, or content.
2. Making is a thinking in its own right, and conceptualization a practice in its own right.
3. Research-creation is not about objects. It is a mode of activity that is at its most interesting when it is constitutive of new processes. This can only happen if its potential is tapped in advance of its alignments with existing disciplinary methods and institutional structures (this includes creative capital).
4. New processes will likely create new forms of knowledge that may have no means of evaluation within current disciplinary models.

IMMANENT CRITIQUE 1—ON MATTER

In *Modes of Thought*, Whitehead protests what he calls "the bifurcation of nature" (1938: 30). The tendency to separate out the concept of matter from its perception or to make a constitutive difference between "nature apprehended in awareness and the nature which is the cause of awareness" leads to a splintering of experience (1938: 30). What emerges is an account of experience that separates out the human subject from the ecologies of encounter: "The problem is to discuss the relations inter se of things known, abstracted from the bare fact that they are known" (1938: 30). To posit two systems—one "within the mind" and one "without the mind"—is a methodological posture still very much alive in the critical apparatus of the disciplinary model. What we know is what can be abstracted from experience into a system of understanding that is decipherable precisely because its operations are muted by their having been taken out of their operational context. Whitehead explains: "The reason why the bifurcation of nature is always creeping back into scientific philosophy is the extreme difficulty of exhibiting the perceived redness and warmth of the fire in one system of relations with the agitated molecules of carbon and oxygen, with the radiant energy from them, and with the various functionings of the material body. Unless we produce the all-embracing relations, we are faced with a bifurcated nature; namely, warmth and redness on one side, and molecules, electrons and ether on the other side" (1938: 32). The unquantifiable within experience can only be taken into account if we begin with a mode of inquiry that refutes initial categorization. Positing the terms of the account before the exploration of what the account can do only results in stultifying its potential and relegating it to that which already fits within preexisting schemata of knowledge. Instead of holding knowledge to what can already be ascertained (and measured), we must, as William James suggests, find ways to account not only for the terms of the analysis, but for all that transversally weaves between them. James calls this "radical empiricism."

Radical empiricism begins in the midst, in the mess of relations not yet organized into terms such as "subject" and "object." In this mess, everything that happens is real, be it the redness of the fire or its molecular makeup. James calls this field of relations "pure experience," pure understood not in the sense of "purity" but in the sense of *immanent to actual relations.* Pure experience is on the cusp of the virtual and the actual: in the experiential register of the not-quite-yet. It is *of* experience in the sense that it affectively contributes to how experience settles into what comes to be. As with Deleuze's actual-virtual distinction, pure experience is the in-folding of potential that keeps actual experience open to its more-than. The virtual is never the opposite of the actual—it is how the actual resonates beyond the limits of its actualization. In this relational field of emergent experience, there is no preestablished hierarchy, nor is there a preconstituted subject-position external to the event. There are only emergent relations. James writes: "Nothing shall be admitted as fact . . . except what can be experienced at some definite time by some experient; and for every feature of fact ever so experienced, a definite place must be found somewhere in the final system of reality. In other words: Everything real must be experience-able somewhere, and every kind of thing experienced must somewhere be real" (1996: 160).

To reorient toward the radically empirical is to profoundly challenge the knower-known relation as it is customarily defined. Neither the knower nor the known can be situated in advance of the occasion's coming to be—both are immanent to the field's composition. Nor can the knower-known relation be classified independently of the ecologies that compose it, including those whose register is unquantifiable, such as the quality or affective tonality of experience. Like Deleuze's insistence that the virtual, while not actual, is real, radical empiricism emphasizes that experience is made up of more than what actually takes form. Experience is alive with the more-than, the more-than as real as anything else directly experienced.

James calls the in-act of experience "something doing" (1996: 161).[4] When something *does*, new relational fields are forming, and with them, new modes of existence. A new mode of existence brings with it modalities of knowledge. These modalities of knowledge are not yet circumscribed— they are transversal to the modes of operation active in the relational field. They are still in-act. This is the force of radical empiricism: it gives us a technique to work with the in-act at the heart of experience, providing subtle ways of composing with the shifting relations between knower and known. It is important to reiterate: the knower is not the human subject, but the way relations open themselves toward systems of subjectification.[5]

Similar to Whitehead's notion of the "superject"—which emphasizes that the occasion of experience is itself what proposes its knower-known relations, resulting in a subject that is the subject *of the experience* rather than a subject external to the experience—radical empiricism refutes the notion that experience is constituted before all else of human relations. In Whitehead's terms: "An actual entity is at once the subject experiencing and the superject of its experiences" (1978: 43). An occasion of experience produces the means by which it will eventually define itself as this or that. It is an occasion of experience, not the human subject external to that ex-perience, that creates the conditions for subjectivity, a subjectivity that can never be disentangled from how the event came to fruition. A radically empirical approach takes this as its starting point, giving us the means to consider how relations themselves field experience.

To engage the field of relation as an ecology where knowledge occurs, to place knowledge outside the register of existing knower-known relations, allows us to consider the importance of what escapes that register. The ineffable felt experience of the more-than is also a kind of thinking, a kind of knowledge in the making, and it changes experience. That it cannot be systematized or hierarchized does not make it less important to the realization of the event. This is the force of radical empiricism: it propels us into the midst, opening the way for an account of study that embraces the value of what must remain ineffable.

IMMANENT CRITIQUE 2—ON REASON

The question of knowledge—of its role in experience, of its value, and of its accountability—is, in our philosophical age, still a question of reason. Despite decades of engagement in transdisciplinary thought, disciplines still tend to order knowledge according to specific understandings of what constitute proper methods, policing these methods through long-standing systems of peer and institutional review. Disciplines also tend, in too many cases, to suggest that interdisciplinary research and especially transversal modes of thought are by nature weak because of their inability to secure robust methodologies that prove that knowledge was indeed formally attained. Method, here, is aligned to a making-reasonable of experience. At its worst, it is a static organization of preformed categories. At its best, it is an inquiry into the formation of categories that will, in the future, stand in as organizational strategies for academic thought.

Method's alignment to reason is about setting into place hierarchies of relevance whose work it is to include that which is seen to advance knowledge. The problem is that in this activity of assuming in advance that we know what constitutes knowledge, there is a danger of not hearing the voices that, as Amelia Baggs might say, lurk beneath the words. These excluded voices include that which makes language tremble, the voice of knowledges not yet parsed for the academic establishment. I think here of the call of indigenous philosophy (as story, as performance, as practice) as proposed by thinkers such as Leanne Simpson, Audra Simpson, Peter Kulchyski and others, the call of autistics and other disability activists who invite us to hear what has been silenced by neurotypicality, such as Baggs, Tito Mukhopadhyay, DJ Savarese, Melanie Yergeau and others, especially those whose nonspeaking voices are rarely included in what we understand as knowledge-formation, the call of artists whose work moves us toward aesthetico-political issues within drawing firm territorial lines, despite the political urgency their work addresses, such as Cecilia Vicuña, Elisapee

Ishulutaq, Mona Hatoum, and others, and the call of scholars who seek to listen and write across the uneasy resonances of knowledges in the making. It's not that these voices are never heard. It's that what they make palpable, what they make heard, unmoors the very edifice on which method is built. They unsettle thought and, in so doing, question the place reason still plays within the methods that direct our belief in what constitutes knowledge.

In working as an apparatus of capture, method gives reason its place in the sun: it diagnoses, it situates, it organizes, and ultimately it surveys and judges. Methods, we hear, are ever-changing, and this is surely the case. But any ordering agenda that organizes from without is still active in the exclusion of processes too unintelligible within current understandings of knowledge to be recognized, let alone studied or valued. Despite its best intentions, method works as the safeguard against the ineffable: if something cannot be categorized, it cannot be made to account for itself and is cast aside as irrelevant. The consequences are many: knowledge tends to be relegated to the sphere of "conscious knowledge," backgrounding the wealth of the relational field of experience in-forming; the force of change that animates a process is deadened; the uneasiness that destabilizes thinking is backgrounded or effaced completely.

A standardized methodological approach begins to unravel if we ask not how knowledge can be organized, but what knowledge *does*. This radically empirical question is at the heart of Whitehead's 1929 book *A Function of Reason*. What at first reads as a very strange account of reason, where reason is defined in relation to appetition and the more-than, *The Function of Reason* is an extraordinary feat of recontextualizing method beyond what Whitehead suggests is its superficial ordering of knowledge (1929: 10). Critical at its core of Kant's notion of reason and indebted both to Plato and Ulysses—"the one shares Reason with the Gods, the other shares it with the foxes" (1929: 10)—*The Function of Reason* is a book I return to every time I want to rethink the way study can orient and invent movements of thought.

Whitehead begins by defining the function of reason in opposition to "the godlike faculty which surveys, judges and understands," as "the art of life" (1929: 4). The Kantian definition of reason, which has left its imprint on contemporary understandings of reason, is here cast aside for a strange and compelling account of reason as the appetite for the cut of difference.

Two kinds of reason are at stake in Whitehead's account: pragmatic and speculative. On the one hand, reason is the decision-like function that cuts into a process to facilitate its actualization. On the other hand, reason is what activates the more-than of a process, opening it to its potential. Drawing out the bold lines of his analysis, what emerges in Whitehead's *The Function of Reason*, I believe, is a call for a speculative pragmatism, speculative in the sense that the process remains open to the more-than, and pragmatic in the sense that it is completely invested in its "something doing."

In the crafting of his account of the function of reason, Whitehead begins with a definition of life. The art of life, he writes, is "first to be alive, secondly to be alive in a satisfactory way, and thirdly to acquire an increase in satisfaction" (1929: 8). The main point Whitehead seeks to make here is that the lively push to acquiring an increase in satisfaction cannot be limited to a doctrine of the "survival of the fittest."[6] "In fact life itself is comparatively deficient in survival value. The art of persistence is to be dead. Only inorganic things persist for great lengths of time. A rock survives for eight hundred million years; whereas the limit for a tree is about a thousand years, for a man or an elephant about fifty or one hundred years, for a dog about twelve years, for an insect about one year" (1929: 5–6). "Why," he asks, "has the trend of evolution been upwards? The fact that organic species have been produced from inorganic distributions of matter, and the fact that in the lapse of time organic species of higher and higher types have evolved, are not in the least explained by any doctrine of adaptation to the environment, or of struggle" (1929: 7). Reason, he suggests, may be one way to account for the upward evolution, and, in particular, to the increase of satisfaction occasioned by the art of living. His conclusion: the function of reason is to direct the otherwise anarchic field of relation toward its actualization (1929: 1). Reason is that which "realizes the possibility of some complex form of definiteness, and concurrently understands the world as, in one of its factors, exemplifying that form of definiteness" (1929: 9).

The question of the anarchic share of existence is key here. What is it that creates the conditions for "the adventure of living better?" Whitehead asks (1929: 19). The adventure of living better is achieved through the tightrope of a constant realignment of the anarchic and the cut of actualization. Reason is not simply the pull toward the categorization that comes with forms of definiteness. It is the active differential at play in the between of anarchy and organization. Reason, as Whitehead defines it, is a decisional force that remains operative precisely because it carries the more-than of the anarchic. Method, on the other hand, allied as it is with the more Kantian definition of reason, is a cut that stills. Method stops potential on its way, cutting into the process before it has had a chance to fully engage with the complex relational fields the process itself calls forth. As Whitehead so forcefully writes: "The birth of a methodology" is "in its essence the discovery of a dodge to live" (1929: 18).[7] He continues:

> Each methodology has its own life history. It starts as a dodge facilitating the accomplishment of some nascent urge of life. In its prime, it represents some wide coordination of thought and action whereby this urge expresses itself as a major satisfaction of existence. Finally it enters upon the lassitude of old age, its second childhood. The larger contrasts attainable within the scope of the method have been explored and familiarized. The satisfaction from repetition has faded away. Life then faces the last alternatives in which its fate depends. . . . When any methodology of life has exhausted the novelties within its scope and played upon them up to the incoming of fatigue, one final decision determines the fate of a species. It can stabilize itself, and relapse so as to live; or it can shake itself free, and enter upon the adventure of living better. (1929: 18–19)

A process must determine its own reason. Any attempt to chart in advance the interplay between the anarchic fullness of experience welling and the cut of actualization into determinateness of an event's coming-to-be, stems the potential for difference. This renders experience stillborn: an event accounted for outside its own evolution is an event that has already been taken out of its liveness and organized within the bounds of preexisting forms of knowledge. Life cannot be lived better in retrospect, as Nietzsche warns.

Whitehead's account of reason does not deny definiteness or organization. Neither does it suggest that experience does not create categories of existence. The issue is how this happens. Hence Whitehead's emphasis on function. Experience in Whitehead's account, as in James's, is not delimited from outside its own process: conditions must be invented, in the event, to make it operational. New modes of experience are created from the perspective of the event itself. This making-operational, from within the event, is what produces not only new modes of life, but livelier living. Reason is not the ability to judge from without, but the event's own ability to parse "the welter of the process" (1929: 9). If we do not proceed against method, acknowledging the event's own potential for activating the differential between the actual and the more-than, Whitehead warns that "varied freshness [will be] lost, and the species [will live] upon the blind appetitions of old usages" (1929: 19).

On the continuum of reason as defined by Whitehead we find another key concept of his process philosophy: mentality. Mentality is the force that propels the physical beyond its mere life toward quality of existence. Each occasion of experience, for Whitehead, is both physical and mental. What is crucial is to understand that the mental and the physical are not mind/body (or body and consciousness) but differential aspects of one complex relational process directed by the occasion's coming to be. The physical is that which persists in conformity with past forms. The mental is what troubles the conformity, opening the event to its more-than. "Mental experience," Whitehead writes, "is the experience of forms of definiteness in respect to their disconnection from any particular physical experience, but with abstract evaluation of what they can contribute to such experience" (1929: 32).

In relation to the function of reason, Whitehead defines mentality as the "urge towards some vacuous definiteness," a taking-into-account of what otherwise will likely remain unaccounted for (1929: 32). This is where appetition comes in: "This urge is appetition. It is emotional purpose: it is agency" (1929: 32). Appetition is the drive that propels the cut, the *agencement* that activates the ineffable within a process where, as James would say, everything is real, including the force of the more-than. With appetition comes, as the function of reason, an appetite for new forms of knowledge, new ways of coming-to-be. The appetite for more life, as Nietzsche might say.

Whitehead's process philosophy never privileges the human realm. Experience is experience; different kinds of experience have different effects. When exploring what an occasion of experience can do, appetition is a productive place to begin, for it reminds us that the urge is part of the process: the urge has an effect on where the event can take us. Whitehead sees reason both as the appetition that creates the initial opening onto the process, and as the decision that cuts into it to align it in a certain direction toward specific ends. Where mentality can open a process to anarchy, revealing the open-endedness of its proposition, appetition of a second order can lend the process a sense of organization. This is not the same kind of organization as method. It doesn't seek to deny the anarchic share of the process—it mutually includes it (1929: 33). This mutual inclusion is felt as the carrying-over into experience of the beneath of words, the pulling-in of the ineffable more-than. This tunes the occasion to its differential, foregrounding contrast, the force of form that always resonates on the edges of the gesture toward the ordering we call categories. The function of reason is not to judge the categories, but to effect a canalization that can momentarily contain the anarchy. Reason as appetition allows the occasion to become self-regulatory, inducing "a higher appetition which discriminates among its own anarchic productions" (1929: 34). The mutual inclusion of the anarchic share tunes the event away from mere life toward life's more-than.

IMMANENT CRITIQUE 3—ON THOUGHT

In the final pages of his account of the function of reason, Whitehead writes: "The quality of an act of experience is largely determined by the factor of the thinking which it contains" (1929: 80). Challenging the habit of situating facts above thinking—"the basis of all authority is the supremacy of fact over thought"—Whitehead inquires into the tendency to place thought outside experience, suggesting that this is precisely what is wrong with any concept of method (1929: 80). How might the fact of this occasion—what it does, how it feels, where it moves—be separated out by its thinking when thought itself "is a factor in the fact of experience" (1929: 80)?

Whitehead's process philosophy is a critique of pure feeling that reinvents the function of reason. By definition, this will imply sidling thought and feeling, and locating thinking-feeling at the heart of all process. Indeed, every occasion of experience prehends the world through a process "of feeling the many data, so as to absorb them into the unity of one individual 'satisfaction'" (1978: 65). Feeling here suggests an operation that moves incipient experience from the objectivity of data to the subjectivity of the actual occasion, data understood here not as packets of information but as the traces of past events which can be taken up or prehended to form a new occasion of experience. "Feelings," Whitehead writes, "are variously specialized operations, effecting a transition into subjectivity" (1978: 65). The subjectivity feeling-thoughts effect is not that of a preexisting human subject, but the subjectivity *of the occasion as such*—its superject. Like Bergson's intuition, which is the art in which the very conditions of experience are felt, feeling opens the event to the as-yet-unthought within thought itself.[8]

Thought taken beyond reflective consciousness reminds us that conscious thought is but the pinnacle of an experience that, in order to become conscious, has divested itself of much of its potential. As Nietzsche writes: "The logic of our conscious thinking is only a crude and facilitated form of the thinking needed by our organism, indeed by the particular organs of our organism. For example, a thinking-at-the-same-time is needed of which we have hardly an inkling" (2003: 8). A thought that has little inkling of itself is a thought in the act, a thinking in the making of an occasion of experience. It is an incipient activity that summons intensities toward a coming-to-expression, a thinking directly imbued with rhythm, with feeling. Marking a difference between recognizing and knowing—*erkennen* and *kennen*—Nietzsche plays with the strange untimeliness of thought in-forming, reminding us that with nonconscious thinking-feeling there is often a sense of recognition despite a lack of knowing in the strong sense (2003: 14). Knowing is incipient to the experience at hand, actively felt but often indecipherable in linguistic terms, alive only in its rhythms, in its hesitations, in its stuttering.

And all of this, to return to my mantra, not in the preexisting subject. "I don't concede," Nietzsche writes, "that the I is what thinks. I take the *I itself to be a construction of thinking*, of the same rank as 'matter,' 'thing,' 'substance,' 'individual,' 'purpose,' 'number': in other words to be only a regulative fiction with the help of which a kind of constancy and thus 'knowability' is inserted into, *invented into*, a world of becoming" (2003: 20–21). "I" is the movement of thought destabilized by the act, the coming-into-itself of a capacity to regulate experience, but only until it is destabilized again by the minor gestures coursing through the event.

This does not of course mean that there is no "I." It just means that the "I" cannot be located in advance of the event, that the "I" is always in the midst, active in the relational field as one of the vectors of the in-act of experience. "I am" is always, to a large degree, "was that me?"

IMMANENT CRITIQUE 4—ON TECHNIQUE

I began with research-creation—with study—and with the question of what art can do. While I think method everywhere needs to be rethought in relation to its capacity to produce knowledge (rather than simply reproduce it), this rethinking is perhaps most productive in areas that are still by their very nature under redefinition. Research-creation is one of those areas, coming as it does out of a long and rich experiment in transdisciplinarity.

It's probably fair to say that method has never managed to gain a stronghold in transdisciplinary research, though there have been many attempts to couple the inter- or trans- with method. These attempts, usually organized around introducing students to their "field" through the academic proseminar, have largely focused on bringing together texts from different disciplines to explore a variety of accounts of how a disciplinary problem has historically been addressed, hoping to provide categories that will assist the student in locating their research within existing realms of knowledge. The supposition behind such courses is that they enliven cultural debate by situating the thinker in a community of thought, thereby opening up discussion to a plurality of modes of doing and thinking. In the best cases, this would then lead to an understanding of how a field or two have dealt with interdisciplinarity, giving the student a sense of the limits of inquiry. When this works, the student has not felt pressure to adopt one approach over others or to cradle the analysis with an already-existing framework.

Still, the question begs: do these approaches to learning accomplish much beyond teaching us to think in terms of disciplinary or scholarly limits? What is made unthinkable by an approach to learning that begins by delimiting, by sequestering modes of knowing from modes of making, including the making of concepts?

A speculative pragmatism takes as its starting point a rigor of experimentation. It is interested in the anarchy at the heart of all process, and is engaged with the techniques that tune the anarchical toward new modes of knowledge and new modes of experience. It is also committed to what escapes the order, and interested in what this excess can do. It implicitly recognizes that knowledge is invented in the escape, in the excess.

What mobilizes the rigor of a speculative pragmatism therefore cannot be a method imposed on the process from without. The rigor must emerge from within the occasion of experience, from the event's own stakes in its coming-to-be. Technique is necessary. In philosophy, one technique is close reading. This proposition of Bertrand Russell's is key: "In studying a philosopher, the right attitude is neither reverence nor contempt, but first a kind of hypothetical sympathy, until it is possible to know what it feels like to believe in his theories, and only then a revival of the critical attitude, which should resemble, as far as possible, the state of mind of a person abandoning opinions which he has hitherto held" (1996: 47).

A process of close reading involves a technique that opens philosophy to "a hypothetical sympathy." This sympathy, aligned as it is with Bergson's notion of intuition (which understands sympathy to be the vector through which intuition becomes operative), involves exploring, from within the process of study, what the work does, asking the work to open itself to its own field of relations. How are these relations posited? What do they do?

How does the rhythm, the cadence, the intensity of the text compose with its words? Where does thought-feeling escape or resist existing forms of knowledge? All of this before even beginning to explore the question of "where I stand," which arguably, is the least interesting question of all. For "where I stand," similar to the ubiquitous "object of study," is too often the question that stops the process, that takes the writing out of the act, that aligns it to disciplinary method and, by extension, to institutional power. We all do this, of course, to a certain degree, but it seems to me that what study can do exceeds the kind of self-situating that too often becomes the death-knell of creative acts of reading (and, of course, of making). Another kind of stand must be taken, one that erupts from the midst, one that engages sympathetically with the unknowable at the heart of difference, one that heeds the uneasiness of an experience that cannot yet be categorized. Otherwise we find ourselves right back where we started: outside looking in at what is already recognizable, at what is already knowable.

Taking a stand in the midst is a messy proposition—the image that comes to mind is of being barefoot in a pile of grapes, assisting them in their process of fermentation. In the grapes, the process is directly felt, if not quite understood in its minutiae, and, to push the image further, it will no doubt leave stains. Reading or making are as messy, as uneasy-making, as exciting as pounding the grapes, provided that we take this situatedness seriously. For it is in the midst of the field of relations, in the undercommons, that practices are at their most inventive, at their most intense. This is also, of course, the place of risk. All that work, and the wine may still turn. Or just never be any good. The same goes for the sympathetic reading that creates a concept, or the artistic process that activates an object. These may go nowhere. But what they will do, no matter what, is create a process and, even better, a practice, and it is this that will have made a difference. For it will have made felt the urge of appetition, and with it the work's affirmation of the not-yet.

Speculative pragmatism means taking the work's affirmation, its urge of appetition, at face value, asking what thought-feeling does *in this instance*, and how it does it. It means inquiring into the modes of existence generated by the act of "hypothetical sympathy," honoring the minor gestures produced at this interstice, and seeing what these open up, in a transversal maneuvering. It is about balancing several books, or several passages, or several ideas, or several textures, at the edge of the desk, on the floor of the studio, and wondering how else they might come together, and what else, together, they might do. It is about asking, as Russell does, "what it would *feel* like to believe in his or her theories," a task speculative at best, and taking this speculation to its pragmatic limit: what can it do to thought, to a thinking in action? This is immanent critique.

IMMANENT CRITIQUE 5—ON RESEARCH-CREATION

Technique touches on how a process reveals itself as such. Dance technique involves the honing of repetitive movements, but it also encourages the experimentation of what else those movements can do. Painting involves techniques for mixing color, for composition and form, but it also generates techniques of exhibition invested in mobile reorientations of what painting can do. This is not method: it is more dynamic than method, open to the shift caused by repetition, engaged by the ways in which bodies change, environments are modulated and modulating, and ecologies are composed. The painter-paint-canvas ecology is an ever-changing one, from sitting to standing to looking to feeling to touching to seeing. The writer-keyboard-book ecology also inventively alters its technique from the necessity to get another cup of tea to the rereading of the passage that gets things going to the habit of starting with a citation, to the terror and excitement of the writing itself.

Technique is necessary to the art of thought—to thought in the act— but it is not art in itself. Elsewhere, I have proposed that technicity may be one way to talk about what art can do in its outdoing of technique.[9] Technicity would be the experience of how the work opens itself to its potential, to its more-than. This quality of the more-than that is technicity is ineffable—it can be felt, but it is difficult to articulate in language.

Since it works, as radical empiricism does, in the complex field of conjunctions opened up by the transitions in experience, research-creation can make technicity palpable across registers. It can make felt the force of transition and dissonance active in the conjunction. James writes: "Against [the] rationalistic tendency to treat experience as chopped up into discontinuous static objects, radical empiricism protests. It insists on taking conjunctions at their 'face-value,' just as they come. Consider, for example, such conjunctions as 'and,' 'with,' 'near,' 'plus,' 'towards.' While we live in such conjunctions our state is one of *transition* in the most literal sense" (1996: 236).

Transition doesn't mean pure unconstrained becoming. It means flow and cut, discontinuity and difference. Transition is the swerve of experience through which continuity expresses itself. Continuity becomes; it is not becoming that continues. Emphasizing the cut of process, James reminds us that process grows from discontinuity: "One more will continue, another more will arrest or deflect the direction, in which our experience is moving even now. We cannot, it is true, *name* our different living 'ands' or 'withs' except by naming the different terms towards which they are moving us, but we *live* their specifications and differences before those terms explicitly arrive" (1996: 238).

What the conjunction between research and creation does is make apparent how modes of knowledge are always at cross-currents with one another, actively reorienting themselves in transversal operations of difference, emphasizing the deflection at the heart of each conjunction. The conjunction is never neutral: it works the work, actively adjusting the immanent coupling of research and creation, asking how the thinking in the act can be articulated, and what kind of analogous experience it can be coupled with, asking how a making is a thinking in its own right, asking what else that thinking can do.

The analogous experience that perhaps most strongly connects to the way in which making and thinking compose in research-creation is philosophy's crafting of concepts. Philosophy is here understood not as a discipline but as a force of appetition, as a "hypothetical sympathy" in the intuitive making. Philosophy understood as a practice at crosscurrents with other practices. Philosophy as study.

As study, what philosophy can do is attend to the appetitions of other practices, composing with their thinking in the act. No method will ever assist philosophy in this enterprise, nor will any method be able to bring the complexity of divergent appetitions together as though they were one. Thought must not be mapped onto practice: it is an emergent, incipient tendency to be discovered in the field of activation of practices co-composing. To map thought in advance of its speculative propositions would diminish the force of study and reduce the operation to the status of the creation of false problems and badly stated questions. In study, what is prized is not the homogenization of thinking-doing, the superimposition of one practice onto the other as though they were the same, but the creation of conditions for encountering the operative transversality of difference at the heart of all practice.

What is at stake is the very redefinition of knowledge. For what research-creation does is ask us to engage directly with a process which, in many cases, will not or cannot be articulated in language. Philosophically, this involves an opening toward a speculative pragmatism that defies existing understandings of where knowledge is situated and what it can do. Innate knowledge—intuition, speculation—is frowned upon within methodological approaches, unless they can somehow be quantified. We need look no further than our own PhD programs in research-creation to see that our emphasis on the written document is about situating incipiency, locating intuition, managing speculation.

Research-creation does not need new methods. What it needs is a re-accounting of what writing can do in the process of thinking-doing. At its best, writing is an act, alive with the rhythms of uncertainty and the openings of a speculative pragmatism that engages with the force of the milieu where transversality is at its most acute. These, however, are not, generally speaking, the documents we require from students of research-creation. What we require, in the name of the academic institution, are documents that facilitate the task of our evaluation of their projects, writing that describes, orients, defends. This is the paradox: we are excited by the openings research-creation provides and yet remain largely unwilling to take them on their own terms and experiment with them as new modes of existence and new forms of knowledge. We remain held by existing methods because we remain incapable (or unwilling) to evaluate knowledge on its own incipient terms, or, better, to engage productively with new concepts of value.

The challenge that research-creation poses is one that touches at the very core of what the university has come to recognize as knowledge. By inadvertently acknowledging that nonlinguistic practices are forms of knowledge in their own right, we face the hurdle that's been with us all along: how do we evaluate process?

IMMANENT CRITIQUE 6—ON METAMODELING

Several decades ago, Félix Guattari faced similar questions. Having gone through a lengthy analysis with Jacques Lacan and having himself entered the field of psychiatry, he began to ask himself whether the models at hand would be capable of supporting (let alone creating) new modes of existence. "From the start, psychoanalysis tried to make sure that its categories were in agreement with the normative models of the period," he writes (1984: 85). Everywhere around him, the emphasis was on language. What of the modes of articulation, he wondered, that precede or exceed language? What about modes of subjectivity that cannot be made sense of through the split between subject and object, analyst and analysand? And, in thinking against method, how might we get beyond transference, the keystone of psychoanalysis, itself such a powerful model? "Regardless of the particular psychoanalytic curriculum, a reference to a pre-determined model of normality remains implicit within its framework. The analyst, of course, does not in principle expect that this normalization is the product of a pure and simple identification of the analysand with the analyst, but it works no less, and even despite him . . . as a process of identification of the analysand with a human profile that is compatible with the existing social order" (in Genosko 1996: 65–66).

Schizoanalysis was Guattari's antimodel proposition. He called it a "metamodel." A metamodel, for Guattari, is a nonmodel that upsets existing formations of power and knowledge, challenging the tendency of models to "operate largely by exclusion and reduction, tightly circumscribing their applications and contact with heterogeneity" (Genosko and Murphie 2008). Metamodeling makes felt lines of formation. It does not start from one model in particular, but actively takes into account the plurality of models vying for fulfillment. Metamodeling is against method, active in its refutation of preexisting modes of existence, meta in the sense of mapping abstract formative conjunctions in continuing variation. As Gary Genosko and Andrew Murphie write: "Metamodeling de-links modeling with both its representational foundation and its mimetic reproduction. It softens signification by admitting a-signifying forces into a model's territory; that is, the centrality and stability of meaningfulness is displaced for the sake of singularity's unpredictability and indistinctness. What was hitherto inaccessible is given room to manifest and project itself into new and creative ways and combinations. Metamodeling is in these respects much more precarious than modeling, less and less attached to homogeneity, standard constraints, and the blinkers of apprehension" (2008). Whether we call it metamodeling, or whether we think of it as study or call it research-creation or radical empiricism, it is the question of how knowledge is crafted in each singular instance of a practice's elaboration that is key. An engaged encounter with the very constitutive nature of knowledge—be it at the level of new forms of subjectivity, or in the reorientation of how thinking and doing coexist—is necessarily a disruptive operation that risks dismantling the strong frames drawn by disciplines and methodological modes of inquiry. Of course, we've been saying this, in one way or another, for decades. But disciplinarity tends to win out, again and again.[10] This is why we need the undercommons, an emergent site that does more than question the academic institution and its role in society. In the undercommons, where emergent collectivity is the order of the day, appetition trumps nostalgia, inventing metamodels that experiment with how knowledge can and does escape instrumentality, bringing back an aesthetics of experience where it is needed most: in the field of learning.

Such an approach to knowledge in the making can be said to be schizo-analytic. Guattari explains:

> With respect to schizoanalysis . . . it is clear that it cannot pose itself as a general method which would embrace the ensemble of problems and new social practices. . . . Without pretending to promote a didactic program, it is a matter of constituting networks and rhizomes in order to escape the systems of modelization in which we are entangled and which are in the process of completely polluting us, heart and mind. . . . At base, schizoanalysis only poses one question: "how does one model oneself?" . . . Schizoanalysis . . . is not an alternative modelization. It is a metamodelization. It tries to understand how it is that you got where you are. "What is your model to you?" It does not work?—Then, I don't know, one tries to work together. . . . There is no question of posing a standard model. And the criterion of truth in this comes precisely when the metamodeling transforms itself into self-modeling [*automodalisa-tion*], or self-management [*auto-gestion*], if you prefer. (in Genosko 1996: 133; translation modified)

Against method is not simply an academic stance. Much more is at stake here. How you get where you are is an operative question. What models model you? What else can be created, sympathetically, in the encounter? What kind of metamodeling is possible, in the event? What can a minor gesture open up? These questions cannot be abstracted from the question of value as it is defined by current capitalist practices, practices that take knowledge as an instrumental aspect of added-value or, in the artistic realm, prestige-value. How do we operate transversally to such capitalist capture? What new processes of valuation can be explored, and what will be the effect, for knowledge, of such experimentations?

New modes of valuation make apparent the cleft in the very question of what constitutes knowledge, making felt the share of unknowability within knowing. To attend to this cleft in creative and generative ways, we must engage not only the register of conscious knowing, but also that of the in-act of intuition at the edge of the nonconscious that makes felt the ineffability of the event's middling into experience. A leap must be made, and it is a leap that is undoubtedly disorienting. "He who throws himself into the water, having known only the resistance of the solid earth, will immediately be drowned if he does not struggle against the fluidity of the new environment: he must perforce still cling to that solidity, so to speak, which even water presents. Only on this condition can he get used to the fluid's fluidity. So of our thought, when it has decided to make the leap" (Bergson 1998: 193). Research-creation embraces the leap, and radical empiricism proposes a technique to compose with it across transversal fields of inquiry. What emerges across this cleft cannot be mapped in advance. "Thousands and thousands of variations on the theme of walking will never yield a rule for swimming: come, enter the water, and when you know how to swim, you will understand how the mechanism of swimming is connected with that of walking" (Bergson 1998: 193). Making and thinking, art and philosophy, will never resolve their differences, telling us in advance how to compose across their incipient deviations. Each step will be a renewal of how this event, this time, this problem, proposes this mode of inquiry, in this voice, in these materials, this way. At times, in retrospect, the process developed might seem like a method. But repeating it will never bring the process back. For techniques must be reinvented at every turn and thought must always leap.

ARTFULNESS

Emergent Collectivities and Processes of Individuation

> Thanks to art, instead of seeing a single world, our own, we see it multiply.
> —Gilles Deleuze, *Proust and Signs*

PART 1. THE ART OF TIME

The word "art" (*die Art*) in German means "manner" or "mode." While it's true to say that *Kunst* is the term in German currently used for art, might there be a recuperable trace of this early meaning in contemporary notions of artistic practice? Might there be a way to reclaim the processual that has increasingly become backgrounded in the definition of art as tied to an object?

In Romantic languages, where "art" as a word has been retained, mode or manner is eclipsed by a definition of art that emphasizes "the expression or application of human creative skill and imagination." Art is not only reduced entirely to human expression; it is also synonymous, as the *Oxford English Dictionary* (OED) would have it, with "visual form . . . appreciated primarily for [its] beauty and emotional power."[1]

This current definition of art signals the way the object continues to play a key role in artistic practice, holding art to a passive-active organization that segregates maker from beholder. For those whose practice opens the way toward processual concerns, the OED definition will feel outdated. And yet there is no question that the object's hold remains strong. I would therefore like to propose a new definition of art-as-practice that begins not with the object, but with *what else* art can do. I want to propose we engage first and foremost with the manner of practice and not the end-result. What else can artistic practice become when the object is not the goal, but the activator, the conduit toward new modes of existence?

Art, as *a way* of learning, acts as a bridge toward new processes, new pathways. To speak of a "way" is to dwell on the process itself, on its manner of becoming. It is to emphasize that art is before all else a quality, a difference in kind, an operative process that maps the way toward a certain attunement of world and expression.

Art as *way* is not yet about an object, about a form, or a content. It is still on its way. As such, it is deeply allied to Bergson's definition of intuition as the art—the manner—in which the very conditions of experience are felt. Intuition both gets a process on its way and acts as the decisive turn within experience that activates a productive opening within time's durational folds. Intuition crafts the operative problem.

In its feeling-forth of future potential, intuition touches the sensitive nerve of time. Yet intuition is not time or duration per se. "Intuition is rather the movement by which we emerge from our own duration, by which we make use of our own duration to affirm and immediately to recognize the existence of other durations" (Deleuze 1991: 33). Intuition is the relational movement through which the present begins to coexist with its futurity, with the quality or manner of the not-yet that lurks at the edges of experience.[2] This, I want to propose, is art: the intuitive potential to activate the future in the specious present, to make the middling of experience felt where futurity and presentness coincide, to invoke the memory not of what was, but of what will be. Art, the memory of the future.

Duration is lived only at its edges, in its commingling with actual experience. In the time of the event, what is known is not outside the event: it is the mobility of experience itself, experience in the making. To actually measure the time of the event, a backgridding activity is necessary. Such a reconstruction "after the fact" tends to deplete the event-time of its middling, deactivating the relational movement that was precisely event-time's force. Backgridded, experience is reconceived in its poorest state: out of movement.

Out of movement is out of act. For Whitehead, all experience is in-act, variously commingling with the limits of the not-yet and the will-have-been. Experience is (in) movement. Anything that stands still—an object, a form, a being—is an abstraction (in the most commonsense notion of the term) from experience. Such abstractions are not the image of the past (the past cannot be differentiated from the in-act of the future-presenting), but ahistorical cutouts from a durational field already on its way. Time cannot be held, and with its movement, everything changes in kind. "Object and objective denote not only what is divided, but what, in dividing, does not change in kind" (Deleuze 1991: 41).

This is the paradox: for there to be a theory of the "object," the "object" has to be conceived as out of time, relegated beyond experience, unchanging. Yet, in experience, what we call an object is always to some degree not-yet, in process, in movement. In the midst, in the event, we know the object not in its fullness, in its ultimate form, but as an edging into experience. What resolves in experience is not, as Whitehead would argue, first and foremost a chair, but the activity of sitability. It is only after the fact, after the initial entrainment the chair activates, after the movement into the relational field of "sitability," that the chair as such is ascertained, felt in all its "object-like" intensity. But even here, Whitehead would argue, its three-dimensional form cannot be disconnected from the quality of its form-taking. Form is less the endpoint than the conduit.

That form is held, to a certain degree, in abeyance. That the chair does not ultimately settle, once and for all in experience, does not mean that the form we know as "chair" is contained in an unreachable elsewhere. The object *is* the abeyance—the feeling-form (a form felt more than actualized) that cannot be separated out from the milieu, from the field that it co-activates: in this case something like the ecology of comfort, sitability, and desire to sit. Whether the desire to sit errs on the edge of sitability or leans toward plushness of comfort, the experience of chair is never a finite one, it is never contained by the dimensions of the object (or the subject) itself. The object, like the subject, is never it-self.

Art can make this more-than of the object felt. This happens through art's capacity to bring event-time to expression. This crafting of the art of time involves the activation of time's differential. This activation of the dynamic difference, in the event, between what was and what will be, creates a memory of the future.[3] This memory of the future, activated by the minor gesture, is a feltness, in the event, of a tendency. When art is at its most operational, this tendency does not settle in the object. It moves across it, pushing the now of experience in the making to its limit. Here, in the uneasy opening between now and now, art's manner is felt.

All actualization is in fact differentiation. The in-act is the dephasing of the process toward the coming into itself of an occasion of experience. In this dephasing, the differences in kind between the not-yet and the will-have-been are felt, but only at the edges of experience. They are felt in the moving, in their activation of experience's more-than.

To feel in the moving, to activate the more-than that coincides both with object likeness and relational fielding, is to experience the nonlinearity of time where nothing *is* yet, but everything acts.[4] Here, there is no succession in the metric sense. To act is to activate as much as to actualize, to make felt the schism between the virtual folds of duration and the actual openings of the now as quality of passage. On its way.

The emphasis on the ontogenesis of time is important: the quality of the way depends on there not being a notion of time or space that preexists the event of expression art creates. This is not to deny the past, but to say instead that what exists in experience is not a linear timeline but "various levels of contraction" (Deleuze 1991: 74). The manner of existence is how experience contracts, dilates, expands.

The manner of experience is felt qualitatively in its event-time. This qualitative expression of experience in the making is not "objective." There is no perfect standpoint from which to explore it, and its effects are immeasurable. Event-time is in movement, lived, felt. How it connects to what will come to be is how it becomes what it is. In this sense, it is intuitive. The manner created in the practice of artmaking is intuitive chiefly in its way of taking and making time. The art of time is elasticity—not object, not genre, not form, not content. This is not to say that these aspects of artistic practice cannot coincide with part of its process. It is to say that the eventness that is the art of time is before all else an elastic opening onto the qualitative difference intuition activates. The manner of art's making creates robust effects that nonetheless are capable of generating infinite intuitive openings for art's more-than.

The art of time is not about definitions so much as about sensations, about the affective force of the making of time where "we are no longer beings but vibrations, effects of resonance, 'tonalities' of different amplitudes" (Lapoujade 2010: 9; my translations throughout). Nor is the art of time about economy, about marking the worthiness of a given experience, the usefulness of time spent. "We must become capable of thinking . . . change without anything changing" (Lapoujade 2010: 12). Duration is time felt in the beyond of apparent change, independently of any notion of linear succession.

Intuition never stems from what is already conceived. Wary of false problems, it introduces into experience a rift in knowing, a schism in perception. It forces experience to the limits not only of what it can imagine, but what it has technically achieved. For intuition is never separate from technique. It is a rigorous process that consists in pushing technique to its limit, revealing its technicity. Technicity: the outdoing of technique that makes the more-than of experience felt.[5]

A memory of the future is the direct experience of time's differential. "It is a question here of something which has been present, that has been felt, but that has not been acted" (Lapoujade 2010: 21–22). A memory not only of and for the human: a memory active in duration itself, a memory inseparable from duration's relational movement. Not only of and for the human because duration is not strictly speaking of the human—"duration does not attach itself to being—or to beings, it coincides with pure becoming" (Lapoujade 2010: 24).

A memory of the future makes felt the smallest vibrational intervals—human and nonhuman—that lurk at the interstices of experience. Paired with the minor gesture, which assists in making these intervals take expression, a memory of the future intuits them, activating their force of becoming by opening them to the untimeliness of their current rhythms. This is intuition: the captivation, in the event, of the welling forces that activate the dephasing of experience into its more-than. A memory of the future because this more-than cannot quite be captured, cannot be held in the presentness of experience. The memory of the future is an attunement, in the event, to futurity not as succession but as rhythm: the future pulses in experience in-forming. The memory of the future is the recursive experience, in the event, of what is on its way. Déjà-felt.

Bergson calls the mechanism by which this future-feeling arises sympathy—sympathy not "of" the human but *with* experience in the making. "We call intuition that sympathy by which we are transported to the interior of an object to coincide with what it has that is unique and, consequently, inexpressible" (Lapoujade 2010: 53). Sympathy as the motor of excavation allows the movement to be felt, opens experience to the complexities of its own unfolding.

What is intuited is not matter per se: "There is therefore no intuition of matter, of life, of society *in and of themselves*, that is, as nouns" (Lapoujade 2010: 56). There is intuition of forces, of qualities that escape the superficial interrogation of that which has already taken its place. Intuition is always and only compelled by what is on its way.

Deleuze sometimes speaks of the art of time as essence. Essence here has nothing to do with a stable quality. In his early work on Proust, Deleuze speaks of essence as the force of the as-yet-unfelt in experience. Essence is here everything it usually isn't: it is not truth, or origin. Essence is the ultimate difference in kind. Linked to art, essence for Deleuze speaks of the unquantifiable in experience, of that which exceeds the equivalence between sign and sense. "At the deepest level, the essential is in the signs of art" (1972: 13).

The signs of art do not convey meaning, they make felt its ineffability. The essential, the creative sign that does not represent, is a species of time, a durational fold in experience. Its quality of time cannot be abstracted from its coming-into-formation. The field it creates is analogous to its time, a time not of succession but a time-schism. Time, as Deleuze says, "*le temps*," is plural.

A plurality of time in time multiplies experience in the now. This, Deleuze suggests, is what art can do. Art not as the form an object takes, but as the manner in which time is composed. Time, as the force of the differential, has effects. It creates a compositional matrix that transversal-izes the act and the in-act. In time, in the art of time, what is activated is not a subject or an object, but a field of expression through which a different quality of experience is crafted. What art can do is to bypass the object as such and make felt instead the dissonance, the dephasing, the complementarity of the between, of what Deleuze calls the "revelatory" or refracting milieu (1972: 47). It does so when it is capable of making operative its minor gesture. The refraction produces not a third object but a quality of experience that reaches the edgings into form of the material's intuition. When this occurs, matter intuits its relational movement, activating from within its qualitative resonance an event that makes time for that which cannot quite be seen but is felt in all its uncanny difference. Intuition, in its amplification of the technicity of a process, in its capacity to think the more-than as memory of the future, forecasts what Deleuze calls "an original time" which "surmounts its series and its dimensions," a "complicated time" "deployed and developed," a time devoid of preconceptions, a time that makes its own way (1972: 61).

Tuning into the art of time involves crafting techniques that open art to its minor gestures. It requires an attentiveness to the field in its formation. This attention is ecological, collective, in the event. It is relational, relation here understood as the force that makes felt the how of time as it co-composes with experience in the making. It is out of relation that the solitary is crafted, not the other way around: relation is what an object, a subject is made of.

This is what David Lapoujade means when he writes that "at the heart of the human there is nothing human" (2010: 62). The world is made of relation activated by intuition, felt sympathetically on the edges of experience. Here, at the edges, the more-than, the more-than-human tendencies for experience in the making, are lively. "We must move beyond the limits of human experience, sometimes inferior, sometimes superior, to attain the pure material plane, the vital, social, personal, spiritual planes across which the human is composed" (2010: 62). What is at stake in the intuiting of the more-than that art requires in order to activate a minor gesture is not the requalification of subject and object, artist and work, but the shedding of all that preexists the occasion in which the event takes place. Only this, Lapoujade suggests, makes the unrealizable realizable.

The memory of the future, the art of time — these are not quantifiable measures. These are speculative propositions, forces within the conceptual web of experience in the crafting that lurk on the edges of the thinkable. The art of time is the proposition art can make to a world in continual composition. It is also the proposition that opens art to its outside, to art as in-act, to practice as the crafting of emergent collectivities. Instead of immediately turning to form for its resolution, the art of time can ask how techniques of relation become a conduit for a relational movement that exceeds the very form-taking art so often strives toward. Instead of stalling at the object, art as manner can explore how the forces of the not-yet co-compose with the milieu of which they are an incipient mode. It can inquire into the collective force that emerges from this co-composition. It can develop techniques for intuiting how art becomes the basis for creating new manners, new modes of collaboration, human and nonhuman, material and immaterial. It can touch on the technicity of the more-than of art's object-based propositions. It can ask how the collective iteration of a process in the making itself thinks, how it activates the limits of research-creation. It can ask what compels it to think, to become. It can inquire into the forces that do violence to the act of making time, and it can create with the unsettling milieu of a time out of joint, intuiting its limits, limits that often have little to do with form. In so doing, it can create a time for thought "that would lead life to the limit of what it can do," complicating the very concept of life by pushing life "beyond the limits that knowledge fixes for it" (Deleuze 1983: 101). Art as technique, as way.

This way is relational. It is of the field, in the milieu. Art: the intuitive process for activating the relational composition that is life-living, for creating a memory of the future that evades, that complicates form. The art of time: making felt the rhythm of the differential, the quality of relation. It is not a question, once again, of slow time, or quick time, of lingering or speeding. It is a question of moving experience beyond the way it has a habit of taking, of discovering how the edges of life-living commingle with the force of that which cannot yet be perceived, but is nonetheless felt. The art of time involves taking a risk, no doubt, but risk played out differently, at the level not of identity or being: risk of losing our footing, risk of the world losing its footing, on a ground that moves and keeps moving. Here, in the crafting of an undercommons where movement predates form, where expression remains lively at the interstices of the ineffable, the field of relation itself becomes "inventor of new possibilities of life," possibilities of life we can only intuit in the art of time (Nietzsche 1996: 3).

PART 2. THE ART OF PARTICIPATION

If the art of time, or art as manner, invents new possibilities for life-living, it does so because of its continual investment in the question of practice. Practice, as that which moves technique toward technicity, cannot be reduced to an individual. Practice is transversal to the field of experience.

Gilbert Simondon speaks of the individual as the point of inflection of a process of individuation. For Simondon, the individual is emergent, not preconstituted. In Simondon's vocabulary, there is an intrinsic relationship between individuation (the process), the preindividual (the force of form), and the individual (the turning point that opens the process toward new individuations). The individual (the singularity of a process) is never the starting point—it is what emerges from the middling of individuation. The individual is how the event expresses itself, never what sets it in motion.

The individual, emergent from the process, cannot be fully abstracted from the force of the preindividual, the virtual excess or more-than that accompanies all processes of force taking form. If the more-than of a process's individuality accompanies all comings-to-form, this means that there is no phase of a process that isn't actively in excess of the form it takes. A process is thus by its very nature collective. It is an ecology of practices. Whereas in many readings of collectivity, the multiple refers to the sum of individual parts (thereby subsuming the collective to the individuals within it), for Simondon individuation is always transindividual. Individuals do emerge from it, but the process can never be returned to the sum of its parts. Even the individual, when abstracted, cannot simply be reduced to a sum, for it continues to carry its preindividual charge, a charge that "contains potentials and virtuality," which means it is susceptible to continuous changes in kind (Simondon 2005: 248; my translation).

Simondon uses the concept of the transindividual to describe the collectivity at the heart of all individuations, before and beyond any speciating into individuals. He mobilizes the transindividual to make apparent that any shift in the event is a shift in the ecology of which it is composed. The transindividual is the concept that most underscores the fact that all events are collaborative, participatory.

Participation is key to the art of time. In the OED's normative account of art as object, art has two times: the time of making, and the time of the spectator's appreciation of that making. Maker and spectator are the two limits of the process. While this account is complicated in participatory art and in collective artistic processes of all kinds, the question remains: to what degree does art retain this original dichotomy between maker and spectator/public/participant even in the cases where the participatory aspect of the work is absolutely central to what makes the work work? To what degree does the maker continue to see themselves as the central pivot (or to what degree does the curator still see the maker as the central pivot)? To what degree do we continue to hold onto the idea of the artist as solitary genius?

When a process is delimited by the belief that there is a preexisting individual creating at its center, the collective becomes an afterthought. The participatory is left to the end, and with this, a decisive stage of the event is muted. In segregating participation from the work, in making participation the afterthought of a practice already under way, what we do is set apart integral aspects of a process. The real work is seen as that which emerges before the event opens to the public. Practice thus separates itself from techniques for activation. When this happens, the participatory is set up in an uneasy dichotomy between what becomes the inside and the outside of a process. An expectation emerges that places the public in a position of uneasy judgment. On the one hand, the public becomes the judge of the work, and on the other hand, the artist becomes judge of the public's judgment. Even in the best of situations, a certain prescribed hierarchy cannot but emerge. Not only does this deaden the force of what a practice can do, it limits participation to a predefined definition of a public, which inevitably orients participation to human intervention, curtailing the more complex ecology of participation. As activator after the event, this human presence now has the task of bringing into being this new phase of the practice. While this can be successful in the sense that it can produce new modes of encounter that begin to make felt how the work is open to a reorientation, too often in this context the conditions have not been created that would allow the work to really extend beyond it-self. The concept of the transindividual makes felt the limitations of this view. From the perspective of transindividuation, participation is always already there, active as the more-than at the heart of the event in its formation. Participation is not the way the outside adds itself to a process already under way, but the operational multiplicity of a practice in its unfolding. Participation is not what the artist wishes the public would do (I have certainly succumbed to this in my own practice), but the activity of the work's potential as opened up by the process itself.[6] Though this more-than, this participatory activity, is highlighted in participatory art, it is important to recall that all events are transindividual at their core, and by extension, all artistic processes are capable of mobilizing this transindividual share.

Participation understood as immanent to the event raises a completely different set of expectations. Now, practice is considered immanent to the ecologies of an ever-shifting process. This radically alters the conditions of the work. Now, the problem is not how the participant can reanimate a process, but how the process itself as emergent practice can make felt its own participatory or transindividual nature. The practice shifts from seeing the object as endpoint to exploring how to prolong the art of time in the event such that new forms of collaboration can be engendered. Whether we are talking about the making of an artwork or the setting into place, through a process artfully in-act, of activist practices of emergent collectivity, what matters is less how the work defines itself than how it is capable of creating new conduits for expression and experimentation. Participation thus conceived is a putting into relation of an *agencement*, a mobilizing-toward, in the event, that doesn't begin and end with the human individual.

Simondon writes: "Couldn't we conceive of individuation as being . . . a process intrinsic to the formation of individuals, never achieved, never fixed, never stable, but always realizing, in their evolution, an individuation that structures them without eliminating the associated charge of the preindividual, constituting the horizon of transindividual Being from which they detach themselves?" (2005: 13). The transindividual, it bears repeating, "is neither raw sociality nor the interindividual; it presupposes a veritable operation of individuation from a preindividual reality" (2005: 13). Preindividual reality, the charge of the more-than that accompanies all processes of individuation, creates not an individual formed once and for all, but a metastability that expresses "a quantum condition, correlative of a plurality of orders of magnitude" (2005: 13). It is from the perspective of this metastability that the crafting, in an artistic process, of the art of participation can begin, a crafting that takes the event as participatory at its core, a process always in co-composition across the scales and times of its making.

Limits of Existence
To explore the art of participation, it is necessary to return to a few key issues raised earlier around the notion of the art of time:

1. What is activated by an artwork is not its objecthood (an object in itself is not art). Art is the way, the manner of becoming that is intensified by the coming-out-of-itself of an object. It is the object's outdoing as form or content.
2. Intuition is the work that sets the process of outdoing on its way.
3. The manner of becoming makes time felt in the complexity of its nonlinear duration. This is an activation of the future—the force of making-felt what remains unthinkable (on the edge of feeling).
4. The activation of the manner of becoming is another way of talking about the work's technicity, or its more-than. This more-than is a dephasing of the work from its initial proposition (its material, its conditions of existence).
5. The relational field activated by the work's outdoing of itself is a more-than-human ecology of practices. Relationally, ecologically, the work participates in a worlding that potentially redefines the limits of existence.

Limits of existence are always under revision. The art of participation takes the notion of modes of existence as its starting point, asking how the conditions that orient it toward its more-than modify or modulate how art can make a difference, opening up the existing fields of relation toward new forms of perception, accountability, experience, and collectivity. This aspect of the art of participation cannot be thought separately from the political, even though the work's political force is not necessarily in its content. This is not about making the form of art political. It is about asking how the field of relation activated by art can affect the complex ecologies of which it is part.

Sympathy
Sympathy, for Bergson, is neither the benevolent act that follows the event nor the result of or a response to an already-determined action. Sympathy is the vector of intuition without which intuition would never be experienced as such. An event sympathetic to the force of its intuition becomes

capable of generating minor gestures that open the process to its technicity. Sympathy is what allows the event to express its more-than. It is what opens the event to what intuition has called forth: "We call intuition that sympathy by which we are transported to the interior of an object to coincide with what it has that is unique, and, consequently, inexpressible" (Lapoujade 2008: 11).

It is impossible to think intuition and sympathy as wholly separate from one another, but neither should we consider them the same. Intuition touches on the differential of a process, and sympathy holds the contrasts in the differential together, such that, coupled with the minor gesture, the ineffable becomes expressive. Sympathy, allied with the minor gesture, is the conduit for the expression of a certain encounter already held in germ. Where intuition is the force of expression or prearticulation of an event's welling into itself, sympathy, calling forth the minor gesture, is the way of its articulation.

Sympathy is a strange term for this process, so connected is it in our everyday language with the sense of applying a value-judgment to a pre-existing process. It may therefore not hold the power as a concept to make felt the force of what it does, or can do. I use it here as an ally to concepts such as concern and self-enjoyment in Whitehead, concepts that remind us that the event has a concern for its own evolution, and that this concern is key to the event outdoing itself. To make sympathy the driver of expression *in the event* is to bring care into the framework of an event's concrescence, to foreground how intuition is a relational act that plays itself out in an ecology that cannot be abstracted from it. Intuition leads to sympathy— *sympathy for the event in its unfolding*. Without sympathy for the unfolding, the event cannot make felt the complexity of durations of which it is composed. Sympathy tends to the complexity of an intuition that lurks at the very edge of thought where the rhythms that populate the event have not yet moved into their constellatory potential.

The Way of Art

If the art of time is inextricably linked to practice as way, then practice and intuition must always be seen as co-operative: intuition is the fold in experience that allows for the staging of a problem that starts a process on its way, or curbs a process into its difference, creating the germ for a practice.

This raises the question of where intuition is situated is relation to practice's inherent double: participation. Is participation also intuitive? I would say that where art as event is mobilized through an intuitive process that crafts and vectorizes the problem that will continue to activate it throughout its life, participation is the sympathy for this process. Participation is the yield in what Ruyer calls the "aesthetic yield." It is the yield both in the sense that it gives direction to a process already under way and that it opens that process to the more-than of its form or content.

Aesthetic yield expands beyond any object occasioned by the process to include the vista of expression generated by practice as event. This is artfulness. Artfulness, the aesthetic yield, is about how a set of conditions coalesce to favor the opening of a process to its inherent collectivity, to the more-than of its potential. The art of participation is the capacity, in the event, to activate its artfulness, to tap into its yield. Artfulness is the force of a becoming that is singularly attendant to an ecology in the making, an ecology that can never be subsumed to the artist or to the individual participant. Artfulness: the momentary capture of an aesthetic yield in an evolving ecology.

The complex ecology of a process outdoing itself that is made operational by the minor gesture is felt, in its intensity, in the artful: the artful is palpably transindividual. In the context of art as manner, artfulness is therefore closer to the differential than to any object, a differential that has been activated through the punctuality of a minor gesture's movement through the process. This is not to suggest that the crafting of operational problems through intuition, the activation of minor gestures through sympathy for the event, the coming-into-expression of artfulness are quickly or easily done: when writing about intuition's role in the crafting of a problem, Bergson speaks of the necessity of a long camaraderie engendered by a relationship of trust that leads toward an engagement with that which goes beyond premature observations and preconceived neutralizing facts (in Lapoujade 2008: 12). Intuition is a rigorous process that agitates at the very limits of an encounter with the as-yet-unthought. Artfulness is the sympathetic expression of this encounter.

Tapping into the differential, artfulness opens the world to the kind of novelty Whitehead foregrounds—a novelty not concerned with the capitalist sense of the newest new, but novelty as the creation of mixtures that produce new openings, new vistas, new complexions for experience in the making. This novelty can never be reduced to art as object: only the artful is truly capable of activating new mixtures.

Artfulness does not belong to the artist, nor to art as a discipline. If it need be attached to something, it could be said to be what the most operational process of research-creation seeks to actualize. Artfulness is the operative expression of worlds in the making, the aesthetic yield that opens experience to the participatory quality of the more-than.

Artfulness emerges most actively in the interstices where the world has not yet settled into objects and subjects. One lively environment for artfulness is the field of direct perception I defined in the introduction as *autistic perception*. When there is artfulness, it is because conditions have been created that enable not only the art of time, but also the art of participation. Autistic perception, the direct participation, in the event, of its welling ecologies, is perhaps the most open register for the experience of the artful. For it is only when there is sympathy for the complexity of the welling event that the more-than of an emergent ecology can truly be perceived. When this happens, a shift is felt toward a sense of immanent movement—and the way at the heart of art is felt. It is not the object that stands out here, not the tree or the sunset or a painting. It is the force of immanent movement the event calls forth that is experienced, a mobility in the making that displaces any discrete notion of subjectivity or objecthood. This does not mean that what is opened up is without a time, a place, a history. Quite the contrary: what emerges at the heart of the artful in the rhythmic time of autistic perception is always singular—*this* process, *this* ecology, *this* feeling. It is how the constellation of emergent factors co-compose, how they are felt in their emergence, that make this singular event artful, an artfulness that will then, in retrospect, carry a history, a commitment to a cause, mobilizing a politics in the making.

Artfulness is an immanent directionality, felt when a work runs itself, or when a process activates its most sensitive fold, where it is still rife with intuition. This modality is beyond the human. Certainly, it cuts through, merges with, captures, and dances with the human, but it is also and always more-than human, active in an ecology of resonances that are most readily perceived by the neurodiverse. The process now has its own momentum, its own art of time, and this art of time, excised as it is from the limits of subject-centered volition, collaborates to create its own way. The force of art as way is precisely that it is more-than-human.[7]

Rhythm is key to this process that flows through different variations of human-centeredness toward ecologies as yet unnamable. Everywhere in the vectorizations of intuition and sympathy are durations as yet unfolded, expressions of time as yet unlived, rhythms still unexpressed. This is what makes an event artful—that it remains on the edge, at the outskirts of a process that does not yet recognize itself, inventing as it does its own way, a way of moving, of flowing, of stilling, of lighting, of coloring, of participating. This is how artfulness is lived—as a field of flows, of differential speeds and slownesses, in discomfort and awe, distraction and attention. Artfulness is not something to be beheld. It is something to move through, to dance with on the edges of perception where to feel, to see, and to become are indistinguishable.

What moves here is not the human per se, but the force of the direction the intuition gave the event in its preliminary unfolding paired with the force of a minor gesture. Techniques are at work, modulating themselves to outdo their boundedness toward a technicity in germ. Thought, intent, organization, consideration, habit, experience—all of these are at work. With them comes the germ of intuition born of a long and patient process now being activated by a sympathy for difference, a sympathy for the event in its uneasy becoming. To touch on the artful is to touch on the incommensurable more-than that is everywhere active in the ecologies that make us and exceed us.

Tweaked toward the artful in the process of making, art becomes a way toward a collective ethos. From the most apparently stable structure to the most mobile or ephemeral process, art that is artful activates the art of participation, making felt the transindividual force of an event-time that catapults the human into our difference. This difference, the more-than at our core, the nonhuman share that animates our every cell, becomes attentive to the relational field that opens the work to its intensive outside. This relational field must not be spatially understood. It is an intensive mattering, an absolute mobility that inhabits the work durationally. It is the art of time making itself felt.

A fielding of difference has been activated, and this must be tended. The art of participation involves creating the conditions for this tending to take place. This tending is first and foremost a tending of the fragile environment of duration generated by the working of the work and activated by the minor gesture. A tending of the work's incipient rhythms. I say fragile because there is so much to be felt in the process of a work's coming to resonance with a world itself in formation.

Sympathy makes felt how the tendency, the way, the direction or incipient mobility, is itself the subject of the work. Sympathy makes tending the subject, undermining the notion that either the work or the human come to experience fully formed. Sympathy: that which brings the force of the more-than to the surface. That which makes felt how the force of experience always exceeds the object. That which generates the opening for the minor gesture to take the work on its way.

Vectors

The art of participation, as mentioned above, does not find its conduit solely in the human. The artful also does its work without human intervention, activating fields of relation that are environmental or ecological in scales of intermixings that may include the human but don't depend on it. How to categorize as human or nonhuman the exuberance of an effect of light, the way the air moves through a space, or the way one artwork catches another in its movement of thought?

Whitehead's notion of vectors is useful in conveying a stronger sense of the more-than-human quality of experience artfulness holds. The vector, in Whitehead's work, is defined as a force of movement that travels from one occasion of experience to another or within a single occasion. What is particular to Whitehead's definition is the way he connects the vector to feeling. "Feelings are 'vectors'; for they feel what is there and transform it into what is here" (1978: 87). It bears repeating that for Whitehead, feelings are not associated with a preexisting subject. They are the force of the event as it expresses itself. Understood as vectors, feelings have the force of a momentum, an intuition for direction.

Whitehead's theory of feeling catapults the notion of human-limited participation on its head. *What the feeling has felt* is how the event has come to expression. The subject, the individual, is its aftermath, how it will have come to know itself. The subject is not limited to the human—it is the marker of a dephasing, in Simondon's terms, in the event. An occasion of experience always holds such a marker—once it has come to concrescence, it will always be what it was. This is what Whitehead calls the superject, or the subject of experience. Making the subject the outcome of the event rather than its initiator reminds us that the subject of an event includes its vector quality—in Massumi's terms, its thinking-feeling. The subject can never be abstracted or separated out from the vector quality, the "feeling-tone" which co-composed it.

The artful is the event's capacity to foreground the feeling-tone of the occasion such that it generates an affective tonality that permeates more than this singular occasion. For this to happen, there has to be, within the evolution of an occasion, the capacity for the occasion to become a nexus that continues to have an appetite for its process. This does not mean to imply that the occasion will not perish. It simply emphasizes that in the perishing, there can be a qualitative shading that persists in occasions to come.

As feeling-tone, vectors attune to the field of relation and tune it to its more-than. In so doing, they activate the collectivity of a given nexus of occasions. What emerges, in the act, is what Whitehead would call a society, a becoming of a wider field of relation that outdoes the atomicity of the occasion's initial coming into being. As Whitehead underscores, this is a rhythmic (and not a linear) process. It swings from the in-itselfness of a given actual occasion, where what is fashioned is simply what it is, to a wider field where the openness to fashioning remains rife with potential not only in the occasion at hand but across the wider expanse of the occasion's nexus. The artful lives at this intersection.

Whitehead talks about this in terms of the creation of worlds—"feeling from a beyond which is determinate and pointing to a beyond which is to be determined" (1978: 163). To be determined here is resolutely to be in potentia—for how a feeling-tone vectorizes cannot be mapped in advance, and whether it lands in a way that activates a worlding cannot be predicted. But it can be modulated through the collaborative, participatory work of the minor gesture, and in the mix the artful can emerge.

Contemplation

A feeling-vector contemplates its passage, attending to the dance of an occasion coming into itself. The occasion cannot be abstracted from its feeling-tone. The contemplation of its becoming cannot be separated out from how it comes into itself.

Artfulness has no use-value—it does nothing that can be mapped onto a process already under way. It has no end point, no preordained limits, no moral codes. But it is conditioning. To say that a process is conditioning is to say that the enabling constraints of its emergence continue to facilitate a propitious engagement with the problem at hand, enabling the passage toward a field that yields. A practice does its work when this yield—already present in germ in the initial problem that activated its process, in the intuition that tapped into how technique might become technicity—is made operational by a minor gesture. Without propitious conditions, the aesthetic does not yield, and the work or event cannot become in excess of the techniques that brought it into being.

Propitious conditions facilitate contemplation. Contemplation, understood as the act of lingering-with, of tending to a process, is a minor form of doing. It attends to the conditions of the work's work. Contemplation is passive only in the sense that this attending provokes a waiting, a stilling, a listening, a sympathy-with. This sympathy is enveloped in the process, sympathetic to the ineffable share of experience emboldened by the minor gesture, attuned to the fragile art of time. Contemplation, operative at the edges of perception where the conscious and the nonconscious overlap, activates times of its own making, sometimes even opening the neurotypical to autistic perception. For contemplation, like intuition and its counterpart, sympathy, activates the differential of an event and, in so doing, becomes responsive to the subtle nuances of experience crafting itself.

Contemplation makes the artful felt. It does so in the event, in the uneasy balance between seeding a practice and becoming-with a practice. Here, in the midst of life-living, artfulness reminds us that the "I" is not where life begins, and the "you" is not what makes it art. Made up as it is of a thousand contemplations, the art of time reminds us that "we [must] speak of the self only in virtue of these thousands of little witnesses which contemplate within us: it is always a third party who says 'me'" (Deleuze 1978: 75). This is why artfulness is rarer than art. For artfulness depends on so many tendings, so many implicit collaborations between intuition and sympathy. And more than all else, it depends on the human getting out of the way.

Artfulness: the way the art of time makes itself felt, how it lands, and how it always exceeds its landing.

WEATHER PATTERNS,

or How Minor Gestures Entertain the Environment

WEATHER PATTERN

The movements of the sun on a terrace in the late afternoon.
The smell of red in the fall.
The weight of closed skies in a dark, february winter.
The moodiness of shadows on fresh snow.
The light after the rain.

MINOR GESTURE

A weather pattern is an artful expression of experience's lively differential.
Perhaps the mention of the smell of red moves you to a September afternoon in the northern autumn. Perhaps this connection is spurred by the
memory of leaves turning red along the street where you lived, or by the
memory of jumping in piles of those crisp leaves and feeling them carry
your weight, or by recalling the feeling of a cool afternoon spent bagging
leaves that left their scent on your hands. The smell of red is all of these
things but none of them alone. The smell of red: a direct feeling of redness
that folds into itself a living memory of a certain quality of air, of a certain
angle of light, of a certain sense of place. The smell of red is less a recollection of something specific than a sense of accompaniment, a living-again
of the activity of a series coming together just this way. The smell of red is
how the weather pattern of autumn makes itself felt.

Every weather pattern includes a minor gesture. The minor gesture is the
pulse of a differential that makes experience in its ecology felt. It is the generative force that opens the field of experience to the ways it both comes
together and subtly differentiates from itself. In the tuning of the season to
fall—which in Canada is also accompanied by a shift in the smell of earth

as the grass begins to dry out and the leaves fall on it and are stepped on, with a shift in light from the fullness of an immersive brightness to the becoming-angled light of winter, with a different sense of warmth on skin as the layers of cotton and wool and silk and leather compose with the winter body, with a shift in the feeling of ground as bare feet in sandals give in to the enclosure of boots—sensations, perceptions, feelings are active at the threshold of a shifting experience that cannot be reduced to one aspect of weather alone (the leaves, the sun, the earth). A weather pattern, when it emerges, is the activating of a certain minor tendency that resonates across time. This tendency is a gesture felt in the event both as absolutely singular and infinitely multiplicitous. The one and the many, the minor gesture has a quality of a resonant multiplicity singularly itself.

The minor gesture emerges from within the field itself: it is a gesture that leads the field of experience to make felt the fissures and openings otherwise too imperceptible or backgrounded to ascertain. A minor gesture is a gesture that tweaks the experiential to make its qualitative operations felt, a gesture that opens experience to its limit.

A minor gesture cannot be known as such. It is what the minor does within the field of experience that makes its gesture felt. In the field of art, the artwork, the object, or even the effect created by an ephemeral composition is not, in itself, a minor gesture. The minor gesture is what *activates* the work under precise conditions, what makes the attunements of an emerging ecology felt, what makes the work work. It is what tunes the work to its processual force, to what Deleuze and Guattari call "material-forces" as opposed to "matter-form," referring to how material is already imbued with force (1987: 95). Introducing into the work's process a kind of continuous variability, a minor gesture makes times felt, but not time as measure: time as duration. This variability, in the event of a work's becoming artful (a work's *faire oeuvre*), makes felt how the work co-composes across the measured time of the object and the a-measure of event-time. The minor gesture foregrounds the art of time. The time of red in fall is felt not simply in calendar-time. It is not simply a feeling of "Oh, here we are again—it's October." The weather pattern comes all of a sudden, just this way, iteratively and yet always as though for the first time. A weather pattern, as activated by a minor gesture, creates a direct feeling of variability, a direct experience, in this case, of the rhythm of time tuning to its difference, made active and palpable by how this red (leaf), this (fall) smell, this (October) slant of sun moves the feeling of summer into the feeling of fall. The minor gesture: not the leaf, not the color or the month or even the season, but the internal variability, active in the differential, that tunes this particular ecology to the felt experience of time shifting.

ARTFULNESS

The minor and the major are not opposed. They are variabilities in differential co-composition. Speaking of minor literatures, Deleuze and Guattari write: "Minor languages are characterized not by overload and poverty in relation to a standard or major language, but by a sobriety and variation that are like a minor treatment of the standard language, a becoming-minor of the major language. . . . Minor languages do not exist in themselves: they exist only in relation to a major language and are also investments of that language for the purpose of making it minor" (1987: 104–105).

In the context of research-creation, the question is how a practice is capable of opening up the field such that minor gestures can emerge, this despite the value placed on the more recognizable and predictable grand gestures. Grand gestures carry with them a degree of the spectacular. They connect into concerns "of the day" in ways that further cement already existent stakes. They give us categories to separate out "good" work from "bad" work, the valuable from the overlookable. They connect to what is considered "current." Both grand and minor gestures are active in and activated by the major languages that seek to frame them, such as the university and the contemporary art institution, and are often interwoven. Despite the ways the grand gesture overshadows the minor, minor gestures nonetheless course through all events. It is therefore less a question of placing one gesture *against* the other than it is of exploring what kinds of conditions foster the capture of the minor by the major. The focus here is not on how to "make" a minor gesture, or how to resist a grand gesture, but on how to develop techniques that allow the singularity of a gesture that opens the work to its workings to come to the fore, how to invent techniques that resist immediate capture by the major.

The minor gesture acts as intercessor to the major, for the major is never fully itself: it is continuously cut through by flows that expose it to its minoritarian tendencies. In the context of the art exhibition, I would like to explore this question through the use of the multiple. I have come to wonder how the gestures both minor and grand are active within the specter of the multiple, an artistic tendency in the past century that has had a strange persistence in our contemporary artistic landscape. What does the foregrounding, in an artistic context, of the multiple do? Is it that the seriality of the multiple shifts the role of the object-as-such? Is it that the multiple activates space in a way that reorients the artistic experience? Does the making of the multiple, in cases where it involves a repetitive and almost ritualized crafting, create a particular sense of duration? I think here of the many hours in my own art practice spent making objects that resemble one another—the two thousand pieces of fabric, for instance, from my work *Folds to Infinity*, which took me seven years to sew—and I wonder to what extent it is less the object that matters than the ritualized gestures that compose it, hour after hour, year after year?[1] Does this ritualizing activity facilitate the shift from the multiple to multiplicity, from the countable to the more-than?

This question takes me to the active passage between ritual and rituality, rituality here connected to everyday repetitive practices that activate a minor transduction in the event, and ritual understood as the more formalized techniques carried through generations that mark rites of passage in a given culture, reorienting not only the individual but the collective as a whole. Rituality is the return, through repetition, to a task that, despite its habitual nature, is nonetheless capable of shifting the field of experience. The morning coffee that opens the way for the day to begin. The cleaning of the desk that creates the conditions for a day of writing. The breathing techniques, for the performer, that facilitate the shift from the street to the theater. Rituality, like ritual, performs a shift in register that opens the way for new modes of becoming. Is rituality also capable of generating a shift in kind that opens the everyday object to its more-than?

In formalized ritual, the ritual object usually has a role to play both within and beyond the ritual. The ritual object is like a time machine: in its ritual activation it energizes experience such that time is felt differently; in its more passive state, when it crosses the threshold back from the formal ritual into the everyday, it carries the traces of this activation in germ, continuing to affect event-time. From the site of the collective ritual gathering to the site where the object is cared for, usually by an elder in the community, there is here a double sense of the collective's commitment not simply to the object as such, but to what the object can do. This capacity to cross the threshold in two directions emphasizes how collectivity is never only active in its present iteration. Collectivity becomes an expression of how time folds.

Through this crossing of the threshold, the ritual object is the force that holds a community together, both past and future. The ritual object, both actively and passively, performs a passage that activates that collectivity, making felt time's spiral: despite their adherence to the inheritance of the past, rituals are ever-changing, altered by the conditions of futurities in the making. It is these futurities in the making, as mobilized by the force of form of the object, that continue to be felt in the object's passage back to the everyday. This is the case even when that passage is virtual, where objects are destroyed in the ritual. This potential, this force of form, is what is cared for by the community between rituals. This explains why the object is considered sacred even when in retreat. This is not usually the case with objects activated in the gallery, particularly those objects that are seen as discardable in advance—elastic bands, plastic cups, candies. The object in this context is only asked to cross the threshold in one direction. If the use of the multiple is in some sense invested in rituality, might there be something to be said for asking how the object can perform its return to the everyday? Can the object carry its more-than beyond the gallery setting? Could the object return to the pantry, to the cupboard, to the closet, to be used again, differently, instead of either going into storage or being discarded?

A ritual object is always singular-multiple in the sense that even if it is used alone, it carries the force of the differential of all past rituals and all future rituals. The object is in this sense less object than stand-in for the unfathomable force of the not-yet. This not-yet is dynamic: it activates time, folding futurity into a pastness that pulls the present into itself. The ritual object is therefore not a thing in itself: its presence is not meaning-oriented in a semiotic sense. It is a carrying-over that acts as transducer for the object's immanent force. The object can therefore never be simply reduced to its form. Nor can it be counted as such (as "this" one). The object is always many, always more than one. The ritual object is less a form than a material-force: it acts as the intercessor into the ritual that opens experience to its differential.

The ritual object's role is to synergize the event, opening the field of experience to the emergent force of *this* singular collective setting in *this* singular spacetime of composition. The object is a dynamic form in the activation of what it will come to be through the rite. What the object will become, what it will be able to do, will depend on how the conditions for the event have been crafted. Techniques for crossing the threshold from the everyday into rituality and back are vital: if the conditions aren't right, the transduction cannot occur. The crossing of the threshold must every time be invented anew. The ritual must be capable of activating not the object-as-such, the activity-in-itself, but the shift in register embodied in the crossing of the threshold. The material quality of the object is important only insofar as it is able to carry experience elsewhere.

If art is one way that the crossing of the threshold occurs, how does the passage from the multiple to multiplicity occur? How does rituality as the force of form that opens the everyday to its more-than exact from ritual a bringing to expression of a minor gesture that is operative in the artistic realm? Can artistic objects carry the double-articulation of ritual objects? For without at least an echo of this double-articulation, it seems to me, the object risks operating only denotatively. The object risks remaining countable, perceived only as the sum of its parts. What is of interest to me is what techniques are necessary to activate the more-than of objectness within the artistic context, what techniques are necessary to give the object the opportunity to take on the aura, as Walter Benjamin (2008) might say, of another kind of newly invented value, a value activated in the setting that transduces the everyday object into an artful one.[2]

Consider the work of Beijing-based artist Song Dong entitled *Waste Not* (2005–). This work is described in the following way:

> *Waste Not* [is] comprised of over 10,000 items ranging from pots and basins to blankets, bottle caps, toothpaste tubes, and stuffed animals collected by the artist's mother over the course of more than five decades. . . . *Waste Not* follows the Chinese concept of *wu jin qi yong* or "waste not," as a prerequisite for survival. The project evolved out of a family necessity and the artist's mother's grief after the death of her husband. . . . The centerpiece of the installation is the architectural armature of the building where the artist was born. A core theme of *Waste Not* is the idea that people, everyday objects and personal stories are not only spiritually rich in thematic material but recognizable evidence of the impact of politics and history on family life.[3]

Having exhibited in proximity to Song Dong's work twice, both at the Sydney and the Moscow Biennales (2012, 2013, respectively), and having had my work next to Song Dong's in the second of these biennales, I have had ample opportunity to explore, in his work, how the multiple might participate in a kind of ritual shift as it enters into the contemporary art exhibition.

Often, the object-as-multiple exhibited in the gallery is used to forecast something that happens elsewhere: as participants in the gallery we are invited to look at the wall label to understand the meaning of the objects in

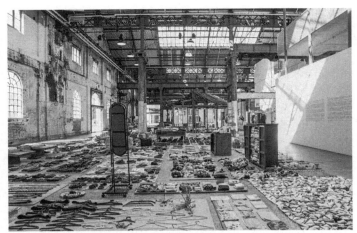

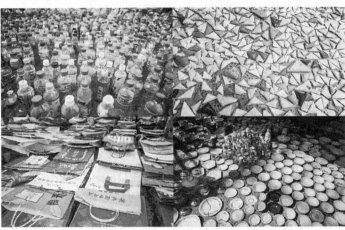

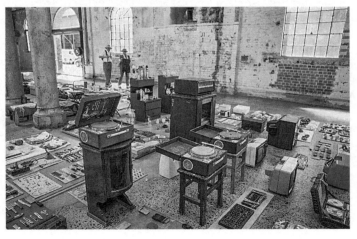

front of us, and it is this added-value of the artist statement that gives us a sense of what the work is meant to denote. Outside of the problem of explanation, which to my mind too often reduces the force of art, denotation is not activation. What rituality does is activate. It does so outside of systems of value imposed on it from elsewhere: rituality is considered a practice precisely because it is capable of inventing forms of value emergent from the ritual itself. In the case of artistic exhibitions, too often capitalist prestige-value frames the work. Just as it was important not to underestimate the crippling agenda of "the object of study" as foregrounded by Moten and Harney in relation to the undercommons, it is important not to deny the disabling force of the statement that promises to encapsulate and direct the art object. For if art needed to be explained in words, it wouldn't need to be art. This is not to say, of course, that words cannot be art. But in this case, when language becomes artful, words operate differently. They are used not to denote but to make felt the beneathness of language in the crafting.

For an object to become artful in the context of the gallery, it must be capable of inventing its own value. Even more so, it must be capable of activating it. It cannot therefore simply be a comment on the art market, or a comment on culture.[4] While it can comment, and art often does in important and unique ways, it has to create a site of encounter that makes the cultural field tremulous, opening it to its minor gestures. The object becomes artful when its value is truly invented in its crossing of the threshold, in the passing from one site to another, and when this value continues to metamorphose in the field of variation the old-new object creates. To become artful, the object must be capable of carrying the potential for variation.

In the case of Song Dong's *Waste Not*, I would say that the minor gesture was more palpable at the Sydney Biennale, where his work extended beyond the walls of the gallery into the outdoor space. At the Moscow Biennale, where his work felt contained by a wall of cardboard boxes that served to mark the edge of the collection, the effect was less operative. Even though in Sydney the participant saw the same objects and was similarly kept from handling them or altering their taxonomy, the space itself seemed to activate a pull from object to object, and from object to the empty frame of Song Dong's mother's house. This pull activated the in-

---

(OPPOSITE) FIGURES 3.1–3.3 Song Dong, *Waste Not* (details), 2013, installation at Carriageworks, Sydney. Exhibition presented with 4A Centre for Contemporary Asian Art in association with Sydney Festival. Courtesy of the artist & Tokyo Gallery + BTAP. Photographs by Vin Rathod, *Through Vin's Lens*.

terval of objectness, opening the multiple to multiplicity and thus making felt the uncountability of the excess at the heart of the project. In Moscow, however, the minor gesture seemed to lay more dormant. This may have been because the boundary created around the work kept the participant firmly within the work's maze, and kept the work itself from engaging relationally with the other works in the exhibition.

To activate its artfulness, the object must be capable of more than its initial transduction from the everyday into the gallery. It must continue to vary and its variation must be serial, in the sense that each object-variation must remain lively with the incipient memory and the imperceptible traces of its passage from one site to another, the sites not only physical, but also conceptual, sites of memory, of anticipation, of attunement. Across the series, in the iteration that tunes from the multiple to multiplicity, a tension appears that makes felt the complexity not of number but of multiplicity as a variation on itself. All becoming, as Deleuze and Guattari write, is minoritarian, and all becoming is rife with the tension that comes with variation. How can the gallery setting imbue the object with the same kind of internal variability?

A minor gesture is a living variation. For the object to become artful, conditions must be created that open the event to variability. What matters is not what the object represents, but what it can do. To foreground what an object can do involves activating its ecology of practices, opening it to its differential. To do so, it is imperative, it seems to me, to include, to make participatory, the ecology of which it is part. This ecology is as much at the heart of the object "itself" as in its seriality. Too often, the art exhibition holds the object to itself as though it were internally bound. In a similar gesture, it foregrounds individual work instead of activating the environment, or foregrounding the relational force between works. Organizing an exhibition according to the emergent ecologies it might call forth as a mobile environment might be one way of making operative immanent minor gestures, in return encouraging the participant, the spectator, the visitor to the gallery, to see art not as a denotative, individual statement, but as an emergent collective articulation that includes what an object can do.

Australian-based Malaysian artist Simryn Gill's work *Pearls* (1999–) is a strong example of how the minor gesture can operate in contemporary art. This work is based on the gift. The gift, in *Pearls*, involves much more than a simple exchange: Gill asks us for a book that we are moved to give her. While it seems clear that the book should hold meaning for us, Gill does not make this a spoken demand. She simply invites a friend, an acquaintance, a fellow artist, to give her a book. This book is then carefully and meticulously torn and pasted to create a string of pearls, which the original owner of the book receives as a gift. Gill keeps the spine. The exchange may seem simple—an object into an object, an object for an object. But try to give away a book, to be ripped, that has followed you, stayed with you, that includes margin notes, that has made you think in ways you couldn't otherwise have thought, that you've returned to either in fact or in spirit over the years, that has become a true friend. This is not an easy task. For three years I've wondered about giving up my first copy of *Le petit prince* with my childhood drawings in the margins, and I still haven't been able to let go of it. Gill knows that the exchange is complex. She is aware that what is moving across is not simply a book for a necklace. What is moving is at once book and the force of memory as it is awakened and created anew in the act of considering the giving-over. The object will not return. What will return will be variation itself.

Proposing variation not on the object per se but on the very quality of its potentializing materiality is what is at stake in *Pearls*. With the passage from one to the other, what is foregrounded is the quality of the object's material-forces rather than its matter-form. Like a shaman in a ritual process, Gill is aware of the power of the act of taking that which cannot be returned in the same way as it was given. This is the work of *Pearls*. What Gill does with the act of variation is make felt the inevitable transformation that always occurs in the sharing. What is given becomes entwined with the belief that the object is always more-than itself. We give the very transformation that is already at the heart of the object. The Benjaminian aura is given and given back, transformed, this in the realm, as Benjamin would say, of both voluntary and involuntary recollection. "Where there is experience in the strict sense of the word, certain contents of the individual past combine with material of the collective past. The rituals with their ceremonies, their festivals . . . [keep] producing the amalgamation of these two elements of memory over and over again. They [trigger] recollection at certain times and [remain] handles of memory for a lifetime. In this way, voluntary and unvoluntary recollection lose their mutual exclusiveness" (1973: 113).

Simryn Gill works with the ethos of care this passage of the aura entails, careful and caring in the act of taking care of the book's variation in transformation. The minor gesture here is the activation of a relational field that includes the book and the beads but also exceeds both of them, opening them up to the vectorization of their incipient tendencies, tendencies that now include, with the memories of the past in the present, the words and

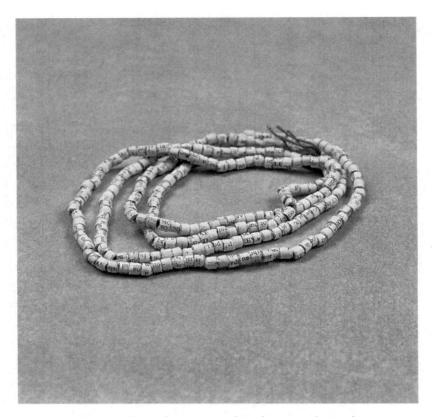

FIGURE 3.4 Simryn Gill, *Pearls*, 2005: *Lenin's Predictions on the Revolutionary Storms in the East* (Peking Foreign Languages Press, 1967), paper, silk, 1 strand 134 cm. Photograph by Jenni Carter. Courtesy of the artist.

pages coming-into-variation as beads and the felt weight of that labor in the form of the necklace.

It is interesting to note that in *A Thousand Plateaus* one of the few mentions of "minor art" is related to jewelry. Deleuze and Guattari write:

Jewelry has undergone so many secondary adaptations that we no longer have a clear understanding of what it is. But something lights up in our mind when we are told that metalworking was the "barbarian," or nomad, art par excellence, and when we see these masterpieces of minor art. These fibulas, these gold or silver plaques, these pieces of jewelry, are attached to small movable objects; they are not only easy to transport, but pertain to the object only as object in motion. These plaques constitute traits of expression of pure speed, carried on objects that are themselves mobile and moving. The relation between them is not that of form-matter but of motif-support, where the earth is no longer anything more than ground (*sol*), where there is no longer even any ground at all because the support is as mobile as the motif. . . . Regardless of the effort or toil they imply, they are of the order of free action, related to pure mobility, and not of the order of work with its conditions of gravity, resistance, and expenditure. (1987: 401)

The pearls are jewels in this sense: their value alive in the transduction they embolden. For they are mobile in their dynamism. Their decorative quality does not reduce them (as the art world often suggests as regards art that can be worn) but brings to them a mobility that can move them beyond the institution back into the everyday. As objects-in-variation, they open the field of contemporary art to its uneasy outside, to that uncertain interstice between art and craft, between what is displayed and what is worn, between what is seen and what is felt. The aura they carry over is subtle, an aura that would probably be neutralized should the beads simply be hung on the gallery wall in multiples, as contemporary art is wont to do. For these beads are for wearing, for moving, for giving, for becoming-with the multiplicity that is occasioned in the act of fashioning the body, fashioning the world. This fashioning is key to their variation-on-potential.

Minor gestures trouble institutional frameworks in the same way they trouble existing forms of value. This is their potential: they open the artistic process beyond the matter-form of its object, beyond the prestige value that comes with all of the artistic conclusions that surround us.[5] The minor gesture is the felt experience of potential, the force that makes felt how a process is never about an externally situated individual, but about the ecology it calls forth.

When speaking of minor literature, Deleuze and Guattari begin with the proposition that what characterizes minor literatures is that "everything in them is political" (1986: 17). What they mean by this is that the minor gesture is always already a collective expression, collective in the sense that it emboldens the art of participation. Against the major tendency of seeking mastery, the minor gesture pulls the potential at the heart of a process into a mobile field replete with force-imbued-material that is capable of making felt not only what the process can do but how the ecology of which it is part resonates through and across it. Always alive with a certain quality of transduction, the process clinched by a minor gesture is one that makes the threshold between process and object/effect felt.

In 2006, I began work on a piece entitled *Weather Patterns: Entertaining the Environment*. This artwork, which is still evolving, is less about creating a finished work than about putting into play a proposition: how to work with different technologies to activate a field of relation that, while it includes the human, does not depend on the human. When I began the work, I hadn't considered the concept of a minor gesture, but now I can see that it was indeed the question of the minor gesture that was at work from the very outset: what would a work be like that was capable of opening up the question of interaction and, ideally, of emergent relation, toward a more-than-human perspective? What would a work look like that was capable of making felt something akin to the reddening of time of a summer tending to autumn? How would a work work whose main concern was how the field of relation itself touches the limit of the sensible? What would a work be that was capable of awakening and keeping alive the intensive variability of the artful?

This is not to dismiss the human's role in the field of artistic participation, but to recognize that the weather pattern does not primarily express itself in or via the human. Weather patterns move across experience in the making in a field of relation activated in the register of the more-than human in the ecology of practices generated by the variational field itself. What would a work feel like whose mandate it was not to entertain us, but to entertain the already entertaining environment? To attend to this question is to open up the issue not only of where the human is situated in the process of emergent fieldings activated by weather patterns, but to inquire into the very limits of interactivity. For there remains a tendency, within the very concept of art-based interaction, to place the human in the center as the arbiter of process. To conceive of a work that resisted this tendency, to emphasize the transindividual share foregrounded in the art of participation, would necessitate a focus directed toward the environment's *own* capacity to make felt the complex ecologies at work. Such an inquiry, it seemed to me, would not only open up the question of how an artwork can create the conditions for a participation generated as much by the environment itself as by human engagement, but would also provide a stronger sense of how, even when the participatory component of a work is led by human intervention, much more than human agency is at work.

Weather Patterns began with a textile collection entitled *Volumetrics*. Conceived in relation to my other textile collection, *Folds to Infinity*, *Vol-*

umetrics is a series of sixty large rectangular black pieces of fabric, each of which has rare earth magnets sewn into its surface. These magnets, as in the *Folds to Infinity* collection, encourage connection across pieces as well as enabling intuitive practices of folding (a folding that occurs despite the participant as the magnets connect to each other across a single piece of fabric or between two or more pieces). In addition to the magnets, elastic cord is woven through buttonholes with toggles to stop the cord. With the magnets, this allows for the creation of complex shapes. Snaps and zippers are also sewn into several of the pieces, as well as a few buttons. All of these connective propositions work together as an invitation for a hands-on participation that can lead to the creation of both garments and, in the best-case scenario, mobile architectures.[6]

Initially conceived as a way to open the *Folds to Infinity* collection to a more volumetric composition (the fabrics used in *Folds to Infinity* are diaphanous and smaller and tend to be used in superposition), *Volumetrics* was exhibited in its first iteration as a complement to *Folds to Infinity*. What I soon found, however, was that *Volumetrics* was incapable of doing the complex work I had come to expect from the *Folds to Infinity* collection. In the context of a participatory proposition, *Folds to Infinity*, in both its iterations as *Slow Clothes* and *Stitching Time*, was easily approachable, mostly due, I think, to its brilliant color, enticing fabrics, and beautiful buttons. All kinds of people gravitated toward it and generally seemed open to exploration, either creating garments or moving the fabric to activate the architecture of the environment. This participation was also activated perceptually through the field effect created by color and light, an effect that made felt the shifting affective tonality of the environment. This emboldened the work to become a choreographic object: with participation, both perceptual and physical, the work became capable, in several of its iterations, of tuning movement to shifting spacetimes of composition.[7] Becoming choreographic, the work was capable of making felt its own art of participation, its transindividual share, while co-composing with actual participants in the space.

Volumetrics, on the other hand, seemed to read more as a stable object, its black volumes deadening participation. Perhaps it was its blackness, perhaps it was the large size of the individual pieces or their weight, or perhaps it was how the pieces read in the context of contemporary art's interest in the minimal (often untouchable) object, for the black volumes do on their own give off a sense of elusiveness that the *Folds to Infinity* collection does not. Whatever the reason, it was noteworthy that on the few occa-

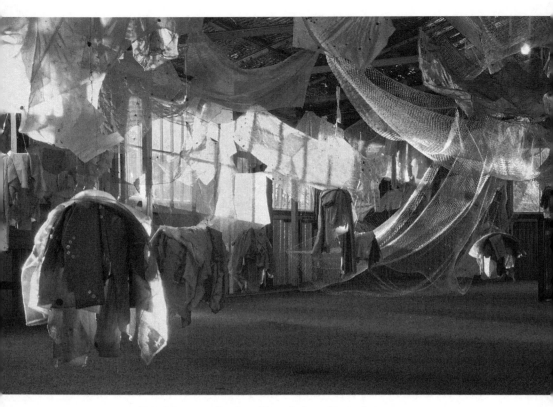

FIGURE 3.5 Erin Manning, *Stitching Time*, Sydney Biennale 2012. Photograph © Leslie Plumb.

sions when the two collections were exhibited together, the black volumes tended to be left untouched. This led to the slow incubation of the problem of how to generate a weather pattern with *Volumetrics*, one that included the human but didn't depend on human participation.

Weather Patterns is a work in progress precisely because such events that are ecological at their core and resonant in excess of human participation are extremely difficult to actualize. The past five years have been a time of continuous experimentation in this regard. The first stage involved sewing conductive fabric into a third of the pieces of the *Volumetrics* collection and connecting the conductive fabric to wireless proximity sensors also sewn into the fabric. This was done to make the fabric responsive to its environment without needing to be directly handled. The idea was that movement in the proximity of the conductive fabric would generate a data stream that could be transduced into sound, activating an emergent sound-scape in conversation with the incipient mobility of the environment itself. With the collaboration of artists Nathaniel Stern, Bryan Cera, Mazi Javidiani, and Andrew Goodman, this allowed us to extend the notion of participation beyond human tactile exploration of the fabric to how field effects (air movements, electromagnetic current) might tune the environment. The performance of the work would be measured according to its capacity to field subtle changes generated by the work over time.

In the second iteration of this process of experimentation (of which there have been five so far), fifty analog speakers were connected to a MAX MSP patch and distributed in the space, activated in relay. In a third iteration, light and movement sensors were placed in the environment, multi-plying the conditions through which sound data was transduced from the environment into the software. Tiny computer fans were also mobilized in this iteration, though never successfully connected to the system. Nonetheless, they provided a complexity to the field through the background sound and subtle air currents their movements produced. A future proposition would be to link the air current to the responsive environment.

FIGURE 3.6 Erin Manning, *Stitching Time*, Sydney Biennale 2012. Photograph by Brian Massumi.

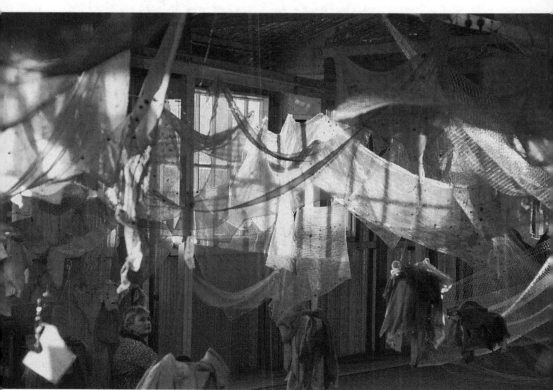

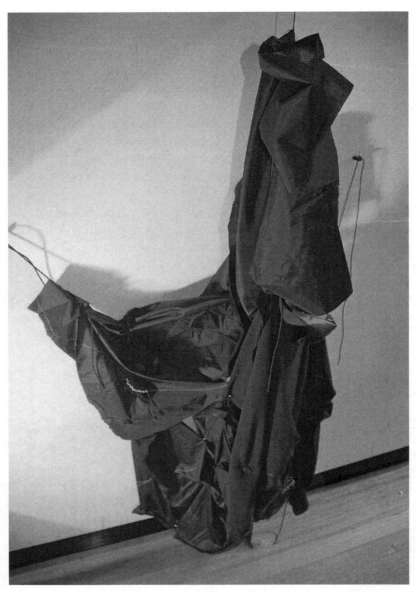

FIGURE 3.7 Erin Manning, *Volumetrics*, 2006. Photograph by Brian Massumi.

The mobilization of *Weather Patterns* over a series of gallery exhibitions, first in Milwaukee (with Nathaniel Stern and Bryan Cera), then in Melbourne (with Andrew Goodman), and finally in Philadelphia, where artists Megan Bridge and Peter Price experimented with it choreographically, allowed us to experience how data—as produced not only by human movement but by all movement—might enable us to experience a quality of environmental relationality that was otherwise imperceptible. This is what I am calling "entertaining the environment," entertainment here linked strongly to Whitehead's notion of "presentational immediacy," the experience of qualitatively felt effects in a relational field.[8]

When artwork entertains the environment, the proposition is that there is an awareness in the field of relation to how the environment is attuned to the gestures active within its ecology. From these exhibitions, a number of questions emerged: How do we make felt, for the human participant, a minor gesture that remains largely imperceptible? Does the work do its work if it cannot be readily experienced as such by the human?

When a minor gesture opens the way for an experiential variation on the object, what emerges is artful. Artfulness is the expression, in a time of its own making, of the processual force of what art can do. It takes seriously the how of the object's variability, taking as art's measure not how it fits within the matrix of what is currently on exhibition in art circles, but how a process's minor gestures generate the more-than of art-as-object or effect.

The artful is not about a form, or a content—it is the capacity to make felt, in the event-time of a work's composition, how an object is already a field of relation, a differential variability. For the artful, alive with minor gestures, and engaged in the rituality of the crossing of the threshold in more than one direction, is always already collective in the sense that the how of its process is an uncountable, unparsable multiplicity. The artful celebrates the art of participation, making felt how an ecology can become expressive, and tuning that making-expressive toward the generation of an aesthetic yield, aesthetic in its original definition of making sensible, making felt.

Weather Patterns is in progress because it fails more often than it succeeds. Glimpses of the artful have been generated in each of the exhibitions of the work, but as an artistic experience, it remains tentative. This is also what keeps it alive. For the tentative is replete with tendency, open to vectors that activate the differential from which the minor gesture can

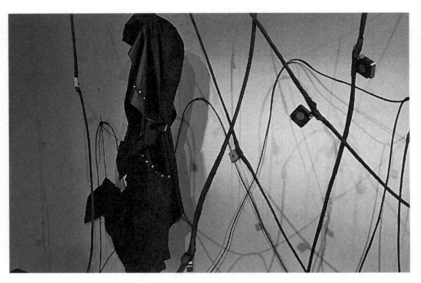

FIGURES 3.8–3.9 *Weather Patterns, Entertaining the Environment*
(Phoenix Gallery, Melbourne, 2012). Photographs by Brian Massumi.

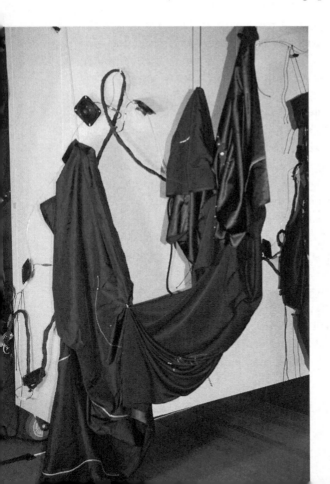

be crafted. Amplifying tendency in the spirit of the tentative, what is most interesting to me about *Weather Patterns* as it has evolved is its capacity to open itself to problems that invite the process to linger. What has become key to the work is not so much the outcome (though how the work individuates in various exhibitions is central to how it continues to resolve its conditions of emergence), but what kinds of minor gestures are generated in the process. This is why, in 2012, I decided to begin to send the work (as a proposition-on-variation more than as an object or a set of objects) to different artists—including, so far, choreographer Megan Bridge, sound artist Peter Price, and designer/scholar Samantha Spurr. The work, in its current iteration, has also returned to Nathaniel Stern and Bryan Cera, who will mount it in the context of their own collaborative work, thereby giving it a different inflection. Creating in a crowd, all of us taking as points of departure our own differing approaches to making a work work, makes even more apparent the inherent variability at the heart of the process of creating a weather pattern.

I outline this messy and nonlinear process of making a work work to suggest that many of us who are intuitive to art's problems are in fact engaged in the making of weather patterns and the activating of their minor gestures. For works that emerge out of an intuition that seeks to activate the art of time are works that trouble, complicate, nuance, embolden how experience is felt both for the human and beyond the human in the more-than human realm, the realm that connects to and composes with the human but is not limited to it. Such works, it seems to me, are especially strong when they take as their governing mandate the problematization of the interactive gesture itself, asking how it might be possible to make felt threshold transitions occasioned not only by the human participant, but by the wider environmental ecology, hence making the move from interaction to relation. How to make felt the relational field that is embodied in the shifting of light, the rhythm of tone, how to make felt the field effect of color? How to move the participant beyond volition to the experiential realm, both nonsensuous (alive in the fielding of involuntary memory) and sensuous (transducing into the now of event-time), where the conscious meets the nonconscious and new nonvoluntary, unpredictable, generative movements can be crafted?

A weather pattern is brought into experience through a minor gesture. When the artwork exceeds its status as an object, when the work becomes relational rather than simply interactive, when there really is a sense that what is at stake is more-than the sum of the artwork's parts, a minor gesture has been generated. This minor gesture, present in each of the fields of action the work emboldens, is not the work as such: it is how the work works. Here, where entertainment exceeds human-centered narratives of consumption so aligned with capitalism, something else is at stake: entertainment is distributed across the ecology of experience. The major language of matter-form, the object, the gallery itself, is tampered with, and what emerges is the force of a gesture that opens art to the artful.[9]

Weather patterns are serial processes. Their beginnings and ends are difficult to ascertain. They are less directional than ecological. Their effects are distributed. None of these qualities make them ideal for the scene of contemporary art, a scene too often constrained by the bounds of what is already recognizable, what is already imaginable.[10] Like the academic institution, the scene of contemporary art has much experience in generating false problems and in posing badly stated questions. Weather patterns, like the minor gestures that inform them, invent both modes of thought and modes of perception. In this sense, they are what Deleuze and Guattari call "collective assemblages of enunciation" (1986: 18). They are field expressions that intensify experience without reducing it to a single point in time or space. They are not metaphors but metamorphoses, active transducers of the everyday in the everyday.

When a technological process is used to activate a weather pattern, as in the most recent iterations of the work entitled *Weather Patterns*, what is necessary, it seems to me, is a sense of how the technological itself can operate as a minor gesture. How can technology activate a field effect without making the field effect about the technology itself? How can technology be used to make mobile the sense of time in the event, the time of the event? How can technology be mobilized to open the event to both its individuation and its transduction? How can technology activate something akin to the aura of the ritual event in the artistic setting, an aura capable of opening the event to its involuntary memory. For, as Michael Taussig writes, "it is involuntary memory which composes, no less than it is composed by, correspondences, and provides the home for aura" (1995: 381). How can technology get beyond "mechanical reproduction" to activate the artful that is process-in-variation?

Weather patterns are everywhere present in our everyday. Some of these presentnesses are artful, and some not. Those that are artful are ones that make felt the intensity of material-forces. Not all art is relegated to the human realm, and not all art is artful. The artful makes felt the art of time, the event-time of the threshold, of the weather pattern. The artful is more-than-human. It is ecological at heart, multiple, serial. Minor gestures couple the artful and art, "wresting from one's own language" a minor art (Deleuze and Guattari 1986: 19). And here, in the midst of variation, in the differential, the environment is entertained.

DRESS BECOMES BODY

Fashioning the Force of Form

> My intention is not to make clothes.
> —Rei Kawakubo, November 2012 interview with Miles Socha

> Some shapes hold things apart.
> —Madeline Gins, *Helen Keller or Arakawa*

"Cut to invent anew," proposes Rei Kawakubo, owner and designer of the fashion label Comme des Garçons. "Make an abstract image." "Break the idea of clothes."

"Break the idea of clothes" has been Rei Kawakubo's call for over forty years, a call that has motivated the creation of some of the most intriguing clothing of the late twentieth and early twenty-first century, opening up the field of fashion to an architectural potential perhaps unprecedented. With Rei Kawakubo's insistence that clothes are not a predetermined category, but a proposition according to which a body is invited to continuously re-invent itself, she has led the way toward a textile-based architecting of experience. In this regard, Kawakubo has pushed and continues to push the Spinozist mantra "we know not what a body can do" to its limit, recasting not only the realm of fashion but the way fashion situates itself in relation to other practices, especially that of architecture.

That Kawakubo's creations are sculptural is well known, but they are also more than that. They are what Madeline Gins and Arakawa would call *procedural* architectures. Procedural architectures are propositional: it is what they can do that is foregrounded. To say that fashion is architectural is often to speak of it in representational terms. Despite the visible architectonics of Kawakubo's designs, to focus solely on their form would be re-ductive: Kawakubo's textile creations function architecturally in ways that

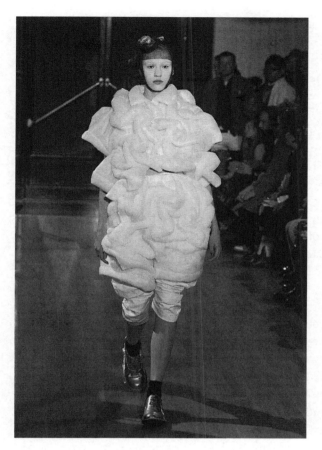

FIGURE 4.1 Comme des Garçons, SS 1997.
Photograph courtesy FirstView.

far exceed representation. They are productive. It is in this sense that they are procedural.

Arakawa and Gins define procedural architectures as "overlapping tissues of density" (Gins 1994: 2). Architecture understood this way must be considered beyond the built environment. Procedural architecture is "a world-constituting procedure."[1] It builds worlds more than buildings, its mandate to directly cleave the biosphere, or, in Arakawa and Gins's vocabulary, "to biocleave." The biocleave procedural architecture fashions never stops cleaving. It is an active, procedural milieu that remains in-act as a persistent reminder that what sites life also cleaves the environment, opening it to its differential. Cleaving cuts open the field of experience. This cut has the effect of reorienting the field: the cleave, like decision in Whitehead, is the decisional force that activates, that tweaks the in-act toward the punctual creation of life-living.

A procedural approach depends on the rigor of the proposition that sets it in motion. An architecture is procedural if it is capable of opening up a field of relation or an emergent ecology such that it can activate the conditions for the continued interplay that keeps life in the process of self-invention. Most architectures, Arakawa and Gins argue, do anything but, deintensifying life rather than opening it to its potential difference. We follow their routes, we embrace their limits, and in so doing our lives become predictably oriented by them. What if instead we built toward the density of experience, beginning not with form but with textures of life-living, embracing the force of form that is the lively interstice of environment and body? What if, instead of assuming that the built environment contained the preconstituted body, we interested ourselves in the amalgam of their co-constitution?

The challenge is that the procedures of a procedural architecture must continuously be reinvented to stay apace with the architecting of experience. No procedure is failsafe, nor does one procedure work in all similar circumstances. A procedure must be crafted with care, must be relevant to the conditions already at hand, must be capable of activating the ecology of which it is part, must have enough longevity to leave a trace. More procedures fail than succeed. But this is part of their necessity, that they put us in the way of experimentation.

A procedure is always connected to a constraint. At its best, this constraint is enabling. It asks of habit that it activate its conditions of possibility. From here, the procedure pushes possibility to its limit, excavating at the edges where possibility and potential meet. This is where the procedure most often fails: habits die hard, including our habits of reconstructing the already-known. A procedural architecting will not be capable of opening up the field of experience if the manner of opening contains the habit fully formed. What is essential is to work from the habit's edging into experience, experimenting with the ways a habit's repetition activates minor departures from the norm, keeping in mind that the only habit which holds on absolutely to its form is the habit of reducing experience to the *what was*.

With the work of Rei Kawakubo, I want to explore how procedural architecture activates minor gestures within fashion. Where the proposition, following Whitehead, is the lure that gets a process on its way, and the minor gesture is the activating force in the field of relation of the work's working, the procedural is the following-through of a set of conditions toward repeatable difference. The procedural, as Arakawa and Gins define it, is what gives the minor gesture consistency without allying it to precomposed models of formation. For the procedural is not a set of instructions. While instructions are usually organized according to a linear set, the procedure is more diagrammatic, in the Deleuzo-Guattarian sense: it activates zones of intensity in fields of relation and directs a follow-through that reintensifies at every turn. Where instructions are reiterable in their form and content, producing not difference but repetition of the same, the procedure does quite the opposite: it sets a path in motion that asks to be returned to, toward different results. "Let the word 'procedure' stand for that which baffles us as to what it is even as it brings us world" (Arakawa and Gins 2011).

ENABLING CONSTRAINTS

In the everyday, habit operates as a choreographic tool. It directs our movement, organizes our time, makes experience predictable, framing it in ways that are usually associated with comfort and well-being, two concepts that make Arakawa and Gins highly suspicious. For well-being and comfort too often keep us in the same place, a place we return to daily without much thought, a place that doesn't encourage experimentation. This place, framed as it is by the architectures that surround us, is anything but procedural, they argue.

Despite the focus in Arakawa and Gins's work on the necessity to break habit, to open experience to invention and surprise, there is nonetheless in their work an attentiveness to *what else* habit can do. For habit, as both Arakawa and Gins and Kawakubo recognize, is a mutable force. Habit directs our movements, constraining other tendencies. These other tendencies, constrained as they are, can be said to still be operative in germ at the heart of habit. The challenge is to make these minor tendencies operational, thereby opening habit to its subtle multiplicity and exposing the fact that habit was never quite as stable as it seemed.

In creating conditions for new modes of existence, in the crafting of a procedural architecture, habit should therefore not be fully discarded. A procedural architecting must look at habit's repetitive pathways to see how they subtly diverge from what is perceived as their assigned choreography, finding within repetition the difference that keeps habit inventive. This difference, alive as it is with minor tendencies that keep habit from ever fully reproducing itself, is what procedural architectures make operative. As a world-constituting procedure, procedural architecture works from these minor tendencies to extend experience to its full potential.

This is another way of saying that what procedural architecture does, before creating architectures, is create modes of existence. Modes of existence, as Étienne Souriau defines them, are not states but passages. They are the transitory and fragile interstices of experience in the making.

Modes of existence neither emerge from nor belong to a subject. They do not define existence: they propose it. On a continuum with the White-headian actual occasion, modes of existence are ecologies that activate a field of concern. This concern is active in the event itself, a concern for the world in its unfolding.

Modes of existence are less species than speciations, where speciation is understood as an emergent field of relation.[2] They are speciations because they don't fit into existence preformed but activate the minor gestures of its most potentializing edgings into experience, pushing existence to its intensive limit. They are speciations because they don't name a state, but activate ecologies that in turn activate differential tendencies in the milieu of their co-composition. Modes of existence act, cut, reorient: they are world-constituting procedures.

Modes of existence are precarious. They emerge as they are needed and then, like actual occasions, they perish. It is not their stability that defines them, but the persuasiveness with which they affect all that comes into contact with them. This persuasiveness is what makes them compelling. Their persuasiveness is an active participant in the event of their coming-to-be.

Modes of existence come into being through enabling constraints. They emerge out of a necessity that has a procedural tending. This necessity is enabling in the sense that it provokes new forms of process, but constrained in the sense that it occurs according to the limits of this or that singular junction. Each time a mode of existence comes into being, it does so "just this way," in direct accordance with how the constraint was enabling in this singular set of conditions.

For Rei Kawakubo, crafting enabling constraints for each new process is key to the techniques that make up her procedural architecting of experience. Her practice involves continuously experimenting with constraints she sets in place to see where else the process can lead, not only as regards the potential of the fabric she works with, but also with respect to the very tissues of density she takes as her matter of concern. For Kawakubo as for Arakawa and Gins, what is at stake is not simply the form the product takes.

What matters is how the constraint embedded in the procedure becomes enabling of new processes.

Body and environment are, for Kawakubo, complicit partners in the re-orientation of what textile can do. They are her palette. But neither is pre-defined, and importantly, she does not pretend to know, from one process to another, where the details of their co-composition will lead her: each new process requires a new inquiry into the body-environment constellation. With this as the directive that drives her practice, Kawakubo invests in the field of relation, the orientation of her practice always transdisciplinary. In the ecology of practices, she requires that her process be invented each time anew through an emergent activation situated in the event of creation itself.

Kawakubo emphasizes that the intuitive problem, the problem that opens experience, cannot be searched out from beyond the bounds of a given process, cannot be found in a world preconstituted. She writes: "Going around museums and galleries, seeing films, talking to people, seeing new shops, looking at silly magazines, taking an interest in the activities of people in the street, looking at art, travelling: all these things are not useful, all these things do not help me, do not give me any direct stimulation to help my search for something new. And neither does [the] fashion history. The reason for that is that all these things above already exist."[3] Kawakubo is not inspired by the already existent configurations that make up our worlds. She wants to create at their interstice, in their coming-to-be: "In order to make this SS14 collection, I wanted to change the usual route within my head. I tried to look at everything I look at in a different way. I thought a way to do this was to start out with the intention of not even trying to make clothes. I tried to think and feel and see as if I wasn't making clothes."[4] The enabling constraint here is clear: to work from the perspective of a new way of seeing, in the event. The intuition will emerge in the process, creating the problem in the art of time if Kawakubo doesn't assume she already knows what fashion can do.

For Kawakubo, what is at stake is making itself, not the making of the object. The object does not define the purpose and cannot be subsumed to it. What she strives toward is the creation of a series of enabling constraints for each process, constraints that, in the best-case scenario, are procedural enough to create new modes of existence. Hers is a procedural fashioning: each new process invents procedures that push the very idea of what a garment can be to its limit. Kawakubo seeks not the final form, not the production of a neutral layer for a preexisting body, but the creation of a propositional field that activates what a body can do in its co-constitution with an emergent environment.

This process of engaging with the working of the work is what Souriau calls *"faire oeuvre."* Like the mode of existence, which composes in the between of existence's necessity, or existence's persuasiveness, the *oeuvre à faire* is the force of making that only knows itself as such after the fact, in the tense of "Oh! This is what I was looking for!" (Souriau 2009: 109).

The not-knowing-in-advance is part of the procedure. For knowing is always to some degree reducible to the already-known. Habit will play a part in the process, but it must be procedurally tweaked. What emerges from the process must push habit to its limit.

The habitual carries within itself a certain degree of belief. The ecology of practices that is fashion believes, for instance, that it makes sense that a dress follow the shape of what we perceive as our body-envelope. This, we have come to learn, is how to clothe a body. We know, of course, that there have been other habits within fashion that have involved cutting cloth to accentuate parts of the body in ways that are today unimaginable.[5] We know that historically the body-envelope has shifted in its proportions and emphases. We know that, despite the growing homogeneity of fashion across cultures, there remain cultural differences in regard to cuts, fabrics, and habits of dressing. But nonetheless, we tend to dwell within the realm of the already imaginable.

Certainly a quota of the unimaginable does grace the seasonal fashion runways. But this is the crux: the unimaginable is only to be paraded, not really to be worn—note that the bustle has not yet come back into fashion despite Yamamoto's and Kawakubo's best efforts! This is not to deny that each season does bring something new and that we as consumers tend to welcome seasonal shifts in fashion. Sure, we say: *Lengthen and accentuate the leg with low-waisted skinny jeans!* Or, *Let's put everyone in maternity clothes for a summer!* And then, the next year: *Widen the pant to accentuate the waist!* Despite the normative directions of fashion's operations—retain the proportion between waist, breast, and hip!—mutability does have its place.

But these are not examples of the unimaginable. They are simply small deviations from the norm. Within most contemporary fashion, difference remains relative to what came before. While change is an option, the commitment to difference tends to be constrained to possibility: difference rarely engages with true potential, with the unimaginable not-yet. This allows fashion to plan itself long in advance (designers tend to work up to two seasons ahead), holding creativity within a relatively predictable frame.

We might see a change in color, or a change in cut, but we will rarely be introduced to a completely different paradigm. The tweaking of the habit thus still remains within the realm of the habitual—it is more of a lateral stretch than a recomposition.

Kawakubo does not operate this way. Against the parsing of fashion into seasons, she works procedurally, her attention not focused on the already-existent. This is the force of her procedural fashionings, that she understands that the edgings into existence of habit's mutability are composed of the more-than of form, the more-than of the existent shapings of garment-imagination. In this regard, her work proceeds at the pace of a world-constituting procedure.

World-constituting never means world-*constituted*. To craft a procedure that is world-constituting, the fine-tuning must occur *in the event*—it must be immanent to the event's coming-into-itself. Fashion that follows habit fully formed is not doing this. It is created according to an externally imposed normative framework. Kawakubo's practice departs from this approach: she is very much engaged in the constitutive tendencies that open habit to its more-than.

In this regard, her fashionings actively produce what Deleuze calls "a belief in the world" (1989: 172). Like the world-constituting procedure, a belief in the world refuses to follow the world as given. A belief in the world is about crafting the conditions to encounter the world differently each time. Procedural architecture takes this as its mantra. To become procedural, a practice has to directly connect to habit's mutation and, from there, create not new habits, but new incipient directionalities. These incipient directionalities will have the tendency, over time, to morph into habit. A procedural architecture must therefore be capable of activating minor gestures that continuously direct incipiency toward new modes of existence. Much tweaking is necessary to find the right balance between the static and the chaotic.

When incipiency tunes toward new modes of existence, it is because the emergent event has been mobilized in the differential of the in-act and the acting. Arakawa and Gins define this differential as "a tentative constructing toward a holding in place." Scales and speeds coexist in this tentative fragility, reminding us that the procedural must work at differing degrees of intensity. "Everything is tentative, but some things or events have a tentativeness with a faster-running clock than others. So that there can at least be a keeping pace with bioscleave's tentativeness, it becomes necessary to divine how best to join events into an event-fabric, which surely involves learning to vary this speed at which one fabricates tentative constructings toward holding in place" (Arakawa and Gins 2002: 48).

To become procedural, scales and speeds must be taken up from the perspective of the event. This approach ensures that we do not fall prey to building world-constituting procedures that are simply sized and timed for human benefit. Procedures must be crafted that are capable not only of creating the conditions for an event that is perceptible to the human, that engages the human (within the scales and speeds of our own emergent bodyings), but that are also capable of fielding difference and creating openings in the continuously speciating arena of the more-than human.

In Arakawa and Gins's writings, as in Kawakubo's, there is sometimes the sense that the human body rears up as the starting point rather than one of many potential fields of activation within the relational milieu. Yet a closer look at the workings of their work (including their writing, in the case of Arakawa and Gins) makes it amply apparent that it is the *event* of the work's workings that matters. In their *faire oeuvre*, in terms of what they can *do*, both Arakawa and Gins's architectings and Kawakubo's fashionings challenge the view that the human subject is at the stable center of experience and that the body can be abstracted out from the complexity of the milieu. Arakawa and Gins write: "We do not mean to suggest that architecture exists only for the one who beholds or inhabits it, but rather that the body-in-action and the architectural surround should not be defined apart from each other, or apart from bioscleave. Architectural works can direct the body's tentative constructing toward a holding in place, its forming in place. But it is also the case that how the body moves determines what turns out to hold together as architecture for it" (2002: 50). The tentativeness is of the body as mobile concept. A body is not a definitive form, but a tentative construction toward a holding in place. The tentativeness of all bodyings must be attended to in the creation of procedural architectures, for this is what keeps the event open to speciating potential.

The minor gesture makes ingression into the procedure at just this intersection: the minor gesture lands onto tentativeness. In landing onto tentativeness, the minor gesture opens up the field of relation, making felt how the field is, by its very nature, co-compositional. In this tentative field of relation made felt by the minor gesture, "how the body moves determines what turns out to hold together as architecture for it." The action does not belong to a preconstituted body. Body is "tentative constructing toward holding in place."

Similarly, Kawakubo does not design for a preexisting form. She designs in the event-fabric of a reorienting of what fashioning can be. "I put parts of patterns where they don't usually go. I break the idea of 'clothes.' I think about using for everything what one would normally use for one thing. Give myself limitations."[6] In Kawakubo's practice, even the fabric, the materiality of the proposition that moves her work, becomes procedural, oriented toward a tentative encounter with emergent modes of existence that activate a bodying not yet defined. Procedurality moves materiality to its limit.

That Kawakubo's experiments are not constrained to a focus on the garment is key: otherwise she would not be capable of pushing the material beyond its attachment to the forms vividly associated with current habits within the fashion industry. "The main pillar of my activity is making clothes, but this can never be the perfect and only vehicle of expression. I am always thinking of the total idea, and the context of everything. Fashion alone is so far from being the whole story."[7] The "total idea" Kawakubo composes with includes the totality of what a material can do, the material here never abstracted from the question of bodying: when Kawakubo asks what the textile is capable of, she is necessarily also asking how a bodying exceeds its putative limits. Creativity is at work, but a creativity not restricted to the creation of either a subject or an object. When Kawakubo says "One cannot fight the battle without freedom. I think the best way to fight that battle, which equals the unyielding spirit, is in the realm of creation. That's exactly why freedom and the spirit of defiance is the source (fountainhead) of my energy," what is at stake is not a capitalist creation of the newest new, a new body, a new object, but the activation of the force of relation that has as its goal the fashioning of a new mode of existence.[8] Freedom here, as in Bergson, is allied to the in-act, activated in the field of experimentation. Linked to the concept of creativity, which in Whitehead is defined as the "actualization of potentiality," Kawakubo's work creates sites of freedom for fashion. As procedural fashionings, her work invites us to reinvent what constitutes value at that lively interstice between bodyings and worldings.[9]

Speaking of modes of existence, Souriau writes: "It's a matter of invention (like you 'invent' a treasure)" (2009: 142). There is no predetermined existence (just like the treasure only takes form "as treasure" when it is considered one). Since existence is only ever invented from within the field of relation and no two events activate the same field in the same way, modes of existence as Souriau defines them are by necessity interstitial. This interstitiality is what gives modes of existence their differential force and protects them from becoming restricted by habitual forms of life. At the same time, to "become a treasure," a mode of existence needs a push toward a degree of consistency. The minor gesture is what gives the mode of existence the consistency it needs to become itself. How the minor gesture courses through and punctuates a mode of existence will define how the mode's interstitial nature lands as event-time. A procedural fashioning is harnessed in the now of a potentializing architecture.

BEYOND SITE

Kawakubo resists being cornered into ethnicity. Where she comes from is an accident of birth, her husband, Adrian Joffe, reminds a journalist.[10] This is not to say that the country of her birth has no effect on her practice. What it means is that with the creation of new modes of existence come new tentative ways of siting oneself. Historical memory crosses over, of course, but Kawakubo is firm: her practice is never a replaying of history as a simple score. What matters for her is not the cradle of inheritance, but the force of form that pushes experience to its limit.

This is not to underestimate the importance of what came before. As Whitehead would say, nonsensuous perception, the way pastness folds into presentness to tweak the in-act, makes a difference in the coming-to-be of what experience can do. The key is to understand that nonsensuous perception is not analogous to the carrying-over of a history fully formed. Nonsensuous perception is an inheritance of the past in the present, an inheritance always in the midst of reinvention, of recomposition. The past is in this way always a futurity in the making. In Kawakubo's case, one of the areas of inheritance, I believe, is a specific cultural encounter with two singular forms of spatial patterning: the kimono and the tatami. These two patternings have orientations in common: both tend toward a complexity of potential form-takings; both are minimal in their cut, preferring the simplicity of a straight edge that refuses to mold to a predefined shape; and, as a result, both are open to various interpretations of what a fashioning (of the environment, of the body) can do.

In the kimono, a garment used across genders that is cut in a way that does not conform to a given idea of preexisting body-contours (cut beyond the length of the body, for instance, refusing to use body-dimension as a point of departure, preferring instead to foreground texture, color, the artistry of the textile itself), there is the inheritance of a different way of thinking the pattern: there is a sense of the infinite in the cut of the kimono, of the infinite line. For the kimono is not made to fit, its lines are not contouring, its cut is not first and foremost gendering (though its textures can be). How it is worn is what makes the difference, and there of course contouring and gendering both occur. But that this happens in a second stage means that the garment retains an openness to invention: as emergent patterning, the kimono evokes not shape as aligned to preexisting form, but a processual unfolding that changes in each singular instance of dressing.

This history of an openness to the line—think the kimono as an assemblage of straight lines—an openness that at all stages of the process inquires not into the fit of the garment according to preestablished body-constraints but into its material potential, is perhaps what gives Kawakubo the confidence to ask her pattern-makers to work collaboratively with materials before even thinking of the form they can create. She mentions, for instance, giving her pattern-makers a crumpled piece of paper with an invitation to create something beyond a form, something that is not yet clothing, not yet architecture, but a mode of existence that brings both into tentative appearance (Rissanen 2007: 3).

The tatami, as I mentioned above, is another example of an inheritance that may have an effect on the kinds of constraints Kawakubo develops in her procedural approach. The tatami as it is used architecturally can be seen as an activator of space's malleability: the tatami room, in a traditional Japanese context, keeps the environment bare enough that the space can become the conduit for more than one kind of activity. Furniture is kept to an absolute minimum, the space itself open to continuous reorganization. In this regard, the tatami room can be seen as an architecting of mobility for a tentative holding in place, for an experience of spacing or bodying wherein "the design process never starts and finishes."[11]

Both these inheritances encourage us not to delimit Kawakubo's creations to a superficial definition of "Japaneseness," but to emphasize that inheritance as a nonsensuous operation has procedural potential. These inheritances, if they make a difference, do so in the way they energize a procedure yet to be invented, opening experience in its unfolding to the discovery of the oeuvre à faire, not the work as it has been historically pre-oriented, but the work's working in the now of its evolution.

Take the Comme des Garçons collection "Dress Becomes Body." The public's response when this collection came out was to see the clothing only with respect to what it did to the preexisting body and how it aligned

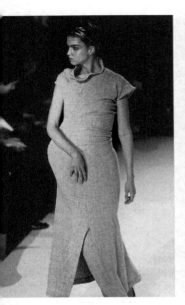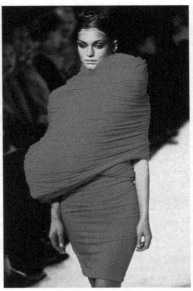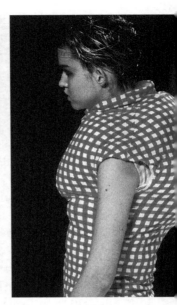

FIGURES 4.2–4.4 Comme des Garçons, SS 1997. Photographs courtesy FirstView.

with or diverged from the history of fashion design. Within this contingent of responses came the unsettled gaze that wondered whether this was a collection that idealized deformity or disability, whether it was an affront to the body itself.

Such responses to the collection depend on preexisting categories not only as regards the fashion, but also as regards the body. What if we look further, taking Kawakubo's procedural fashioning at its word? What if instead of beginning from what we know, from the habits of fashion, we began in an encounter with tentativeness? "Persons need to be rescued from self-certainty, but they also need to put their tentativeness in precise order in relation to works of architecture" (Arakawa and Gins 2002: 50).

In the "Dress Becomes Body" collection, a shaping occurs. Why must we assume that this shaping hides a body? Why not instead take this shaping for what it is, as the event in itself, an event that includes a body-world co-composition? What if instead of assuming that the person is not the shape, we were open to a different concept of personing that included its architecting? Arakawa and Gins speak of "organism that persons." Could this be what is at stake in "Dress Becomes Body"?

Look again, this time refusing to abstract body from shape. See the personing as the architecting and refrain from selecting out from the emergent shaping the contours of the body's skin-envelope. See the shape for what it is: a new contouring. Acknowledge this tendency to see textile as that which covers and not as a materiality in its own right. Then see textile in the moving, as an active shaping of what a body can do. See textile as an ecology of practices that is not separate from the body it clothes. And now wonder at the ways you have become capable of abstracting the one from the other (and then wonder about how you abstract the sitting body from the desk, the walking body from the street, the sleeping body from the bed).

Look again. This time see the shaping not as a still body covered with material, but as mobile architecture. Can you see the bodying beyond an image of what you consider a deformation of a preexisting shape? Can you see that the humpback, the strange shoulder-hip tumor, may not prefigure the grotesque body of your horrified imagination, but might instead remind you of what you see every day as you walk around the wintry city of Montreal?

Look again. Now see the tentative architectures. See the movement that was made invisible by the tendency to abstract textile from body. See the backpack, see the cross-body purse. See the puffy coat with the baby underneath, collar slightly open for its head. See what you see every day from November to March in your cold climate and wonder again why when you saw it in the subway, on the street, in the café, you didn't see it as a disfigurement. Wonder at how quickly just yesterday you were able to see this body-dressed-for-winter as a body separate from its fashioning, at how quickly you unburdened the skin-envelope from its Michelin Man coat. And note in surprise what Kawakubo's work has given you: a new mode of perception. Now look again and see not the clothing that *masks* a moving body, but a shape in the making that includes movement, that includes textile, that includes body, the three together an ecology that is an emergent bodying, a procedural fashioning. Note with some awe that the "Dress Becomes Body" collection is not the high and inaccessible fashion you may have assumed it was, but a lively encounter with the everyday.

The envelope has been ruptured. We are accustomed to the act of excision, of subtraction. Parsing is what we neurotypicals are best at. We see the winter-clad body with its thick coat, the knapsack, the heavy bag, and we simply excise them from existence. We assume that the body is the shape underneath instead of the force taking form of an ecology, instead of a speciation. What else does that mean we don't see?

The "Dress Becomes Body" collection is a world-constituting procedure for autistic perception: Kawakubo has created a shaping that refuses

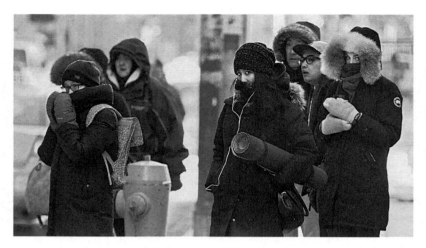

FIGURE 4.5 *Cold Weather* (2015). Photograph by Richard Lautens/getstock.com.

to celebrate the parsings that make reflective consciousness the order of the day, and she has made it available to all of us. With "Dress Becomes Body" she has introduced us to a modality of perception not so far from our everyday experience that we can't account for it once it's made available for perception, and yet far enough that we perhaps realize how we've become distanced from the operative interstitiality of modes of existence in-forming.

Souriau has a word for the cleaving that makes operational a mode of existence: *instauration*. This untranslatable word, which means "to constitute, to create, to found, to inaugurate," is defined in Souriau as the capacity of the mode of existence to settle itself into the world as procedural. "A philosophy of *instauration* will bring together at once the modes of the in-act and those of being, studying by which path they can be combined" (2009: 164). *Instauration* directs the mode of existence toward what Whitehead calls the becoming of continuity. *Instauration* is the inflection that makes felt the difference in the event. Allied to the punctuating force of the minor gesture, *instauration* marks the decisional cut in experience. It is here, in the activation of difference, that new modes of existence are redirected toward new forms of life-living.

The "Dress Becomes Body" collection invents a mode of existence that is in alliance with what Arakawa and Gins call "a site of sited awareness" (2002: 51). It makes felt the double articulation of the in-act and the acting at the very level of perception itself. To articulate the concept of sited awareness, Arakawa and Gins develop the concept of the landing site. The landing site seeks to articulate how a perception, a movement, a tendency, extracts itself from the wider field of experience to land *just this way*. For Arakawa and Gins, this landing can be said to be an "apportioning out": "That which is being apportioned out is in the process of landing. To be apportioned out involves being cognizant of sites. To be cognizant of a site amounts to having greeted it in some manner or to having in some way landed on it" (2002: 5). It is important to understand that the landing is not first and foremost spatial, nor is it oriented by a preexisting subject or object. The siting is a bringing into relation. This bringing into relation has the capacity to dimensionalize, and when this happens, architectural tendencies in the environment are brought to the fore. But the landing site can also have other functions, working more at the level of perception, of attention, or even making felt edgings of experience that are still in germ. Arakawa and Gins write of "dancing attendance on the perceptual landing site," of "landing sites dissolv[ing] into each other, or abut[ting], or overlap[ing], or nest[ing] within one another," of "distributing sentience" (2002: 7–9). The landing site is not a location, not a point, but the tending, the abutting, the segmenting that selects out what is most persuasive at this eventful conjuncture.

"Dress Becomes Body" sites awareness by creating the potential for a perceptual landing to occur differently. How perception lands has an effect on how a tentative architecting toward a holding in place *bodies*. In the event of "Dress Becomes Body," the emergent shaping procedure invites perception to reorient: perception lands differently. The landing site activated by the collection is operational; it makes felt perception's processual nature. Siting awareness in the field of relation opens perception to its neurodiverse potential. This challenges our tendency to assume that what we perceive is simply preconstituted form, opening perception to what for neurotypicals has tended to become latent. With "Dress Becomes Body," we directly perceive the activity of shaping. Because perception lands differently, the work gives the neurotypical the rare opportunity to participate in the ecology that is autistic perception, an ecology where morphogenesis trumps form and body becomes bodying.

In the siting of awareness activated by this and other Comme des Garçons collections, as with Arakawa and Gins's built procedural architectures such as Bioscleave House in Long Island and the Reversible Destiny Lofts in Tokyo, what is at stake is the process of shaping that lands awareness differently. To land awareness is a way of working the work, of *faire oeuvre*: it brings into focus not the work as such but the very procedural-

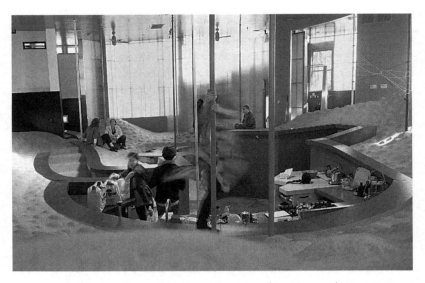

FIGURE 4.6 Bioscleave House with Madeline Gins (October 2011), New York. Photograph by Léopold Lambert for *The Funambulist*.

ity of the work's workings. This is not to say that all work by Kawakubo and Arakawa and Gins does this to the same degree. Different procedures produce different ecologies, and vice versa. While for me, for instance, Arakawa and Gins's Tokyo lofts are capable of activating a procedural architecture that remains vital and reorienting at each juncture, I find myself less certain about Bioscleave House in Long Island. Similar materials were used in these two architectures, yet what they do is divergent, it seems to me. This is likely because the fields of relation (cultural, social, environmental) are profoundly different in the two cases. Whereas in Tokyo the architectural inheritance of the tatami room brings a certain continuity to the work of Arakawa and Gins, opening habit to its mutation in a way that makes the everyday operational in new ways, in New York the house feels strangely deactivating, its hard, bumpy floor sometimes more of an affront to movement than an activator. Perhaps in New York, the house is simply too excised from the everyday, out of context and therefore procedurally not quite ready yet. This is not to say that the house has no potential, but simply to emphasize that each ecology of practices will emerge to different effect, opening up different fields of potential that will themselves always to some degree have to connect with the inheritances that come with the act of life-living.[12]

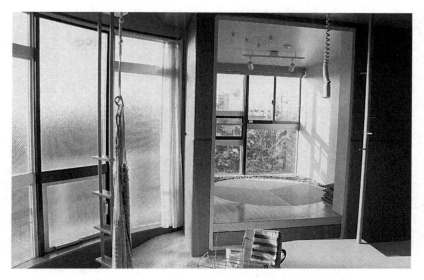

FIGURE 4.7 Mitaka Lofts, Tokyo (October 2014). Photograph by Léopold Lambert for *The Funambulist*.

What is most interesting about a procedural approach, it should be clear by now, is not the final form a process might take. What is at stake is the shaping itself—how a form might be capable of remaining procedural, and, even more so, how its procedurality is capable of keeping minor gestures alive. In the case above, both architectures remain procedural, but they do so to different degrees. What matters is how these degrees are taken up in experience. What matters is what new processes they enable: what new modes of existence they solicit, what minor tendencies they call forth. What matters is how the work is attended to in the modality of sited awareness, how its *instauration* is felt and how the work's *faire oeuvre* persists, persuasively. What matters is how the event continues to be procedurally capable of carrying the untimeliness of event-time—"Oh! That's what it was!"—while operatively attending to the singularity of the event in *this* iteration of its coming-to-be. For work that works does take a stand. It stands in the time in which it lands, and it makes demands on that time. It marks it. A procedural architecting, a procedural fashioning, always involves an encounter with a work that persists even as it stands, that engages with the openings of potential even as it takes its place, here and now.

This is the strangeness of the procedural as world-constituting, that it must at once be taken up in the absoluteness of its self-determination in the here and now and that it must at the same time remain open to the differential of times not yet invented. How to create conditions whereby the here and now and the necessity of time's unfolding coexist? This might produce some anxiety. "What can I do so as not to be paced out of existence?" ask Arakawa and Gins (2011). The only way not to be paced out of existence is to remain steadfastly in the act. For to be paced out of existence suggests being on existence's edge and watching it go by. This only happens when there is an assumption that what matters is outside of the event, this event of life-living. If we consider our being to always be in the midst, if we consider that the body is never one, never outside, never enveloped, but always a singular speciation of an emergent ecology, there is no danger that we will be paced out of existence. But this does not mean that the immortality Arakawa and Gins make the beacon of their work will be attained.[13] What will remain immortal is not the human body, but the procedural force that bodies, that architects, that fashions, the procedural force that sites awareness in the field of relation. What will persist, in shifting ecologies that include us but are not limited to us, is the more-than, the body as a society of molecules, a tentative construction toward a holding in place.

Modes of existence as they are crafted out of ecologies of practices are never primarily human. They are ecological, active at the interstices of what life is becoming, life understood not only in terms of the vital, but as an active vector that passes through the organic and the inorganic. Life as life-living, as force of form invented in the cut that cleaves experience, opening it to new modes of existence.

CHOREOGRAPHIC ARCHITECTURE

In addition to siting awareness, "Dress Becomes Body" architects mobility. Architecting mobility does not mean creating a site for mobility. It refers instead to a way of understanding the siting of awareness through a focus on the force of form. A choreographic architecture dances attention, siting an event in the midst of its potentiality. When a choreographic architecture comes to the fore, what is perceived, what is lived, is not the siting of the body but the fielding of its mobility.

It is here, in the differential folding of the choreographic potential of mobile architectings, that fashion and architecture most readily meet. For when fashion becomes procedural, what it does is assist us in attending to how a bodying is already an architecting of mobility at a different scale.

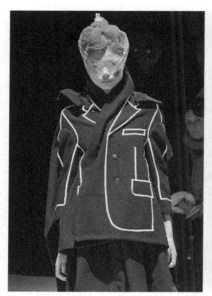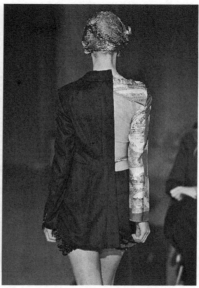

FIGURE 4.8 Comme des Garçons, AW 2009. Photograph courtesy FirstView.
FIGURE 4.9 Comme des Garçons, AW 2011. Photograph courtesy FirstView.

Kawakubo's work embodies such choreographic tendencies, bringing to awareness the dance of attention active in the materiality of her textile creations. This is very apparent in her early work, often termed "deconstructive." I draw attention to the work of the so-called deconstructive period for two reasons: to challenge the usage of the term "deconstruction" in fashion, and to suggest that deconstruction, taken as an engaged rethinking of what textile can do, is still very much at work in the current collections produced by Comme des Garçons.[14]

When deconstruction is theorized in relation to Kawakubo's work (as well as other Japanese designers, such as Yohji Yamamoto), it tends to denote the making apparent of the seams of a garment in a way that creates a conversation about the garment's form. It foregrounds the unfinished seams, for instance, and tends to make a statement about counterculture (emphasizing, for instance, the way a given designer refuses to conform to haute couture's norms). Derrida's definition of the term takes it much further. For Derrida, deconstruction is never a method, but rather a way to return again to the act of reading or making in order to see how it stages its alliances to form, to history, to epistemology.[15] This approach encourages an account of how the work moves, and what it can do in its incipient activity. In the case of fashion, this encourages a turn not to the form itself but to the materiality of construction itself, to the ways in which the deconstructive gesture activates the force of form.

In the context of the choreographic in its relation to dance, it is always compelling, I find, to explore the share of movement that "remains," that is "left over" in the passage from force to form. This is particularly perceptible in the work of choreographer William Forsythe. In rehearsal, Forsythe repeatedly encourages his dancers to "leave behind" the form of the movement in order to explore what exceeds its form, its representational stature. I have written about this in terms of the "what else," asking what else movement can do in its fielding of relation. It seems to me that the *what else* is of central importance in Kawakubo's so-called deconstructive work, a gesture that once again brings architecture and fashion together, not in terms of scale or form, but in terms of what is left behind. How, for instance, has what takes shape altered, refigured, reoriented past ecologies of fashion in the making? How has its operation incited a reengagement with inheritance? The garments portrayed in the images from the spring–summer 2011 collection (figs. 4.10–4.11) are particularly interesting in this regard. What is at stake here is not simply the making apparent of the seams of the garment's production but a foregrounding of the immanent potentiality in the seams, at the edges, in the linings of the garment. The infinite line returns here, but where it goes is not toward the kimono. The kimono is perhaps what the form could have been. The garment pictured is what was left behind.

What was left behind is the "what else" of Kawakubo's procedural fashionings. This leftover share of movement-moving, the share that has not quite taken form, opens up future processes. Like the *what else* in Forsythe that activates the more-than of form, the *what else* of fashioning is what opens material to the potential of its infinite line.

It is important to emphasize that these garments (like many others), placed on display for the runways of that 2011 season, are not for direct consumption. They take the season's garments (the works that will be sold in boutiques around the world) and emphasize their procedurality, making felt not only the tentativeness of their propositions, but the more-than, the *what else*, of their constructedness.

Kawakubo states repeatedly that fashion is neither the starting nor the endpoint of her research. Fashion for her is not limited to the idea of a holding-in-place of a body as pre-formed. Nor is it about deconstructing the past in the linear sense often attributed to both her work and that of

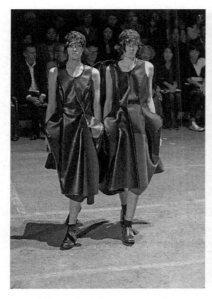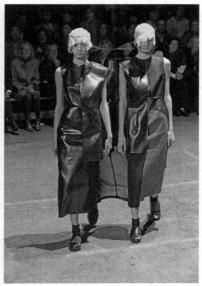

FIGURES 4.10–4.11 Comme des Garçons, SS 2011.
Photographs courtesy FirstView.

other Japanese designers, such as Yohji Yamamoto, nor simply, as the deconstructive vocabulary within fashion would have it, of revealing tradition
and pulling it apart at the seams. It is, rather, about constructing toward a
tentative holding in place, thereby cleaving the body-concept toward an
architecting that sculpts mobility more than form. That this work reveals
its seams is of course necessary at times, and among my favorite pieces of
Comme des Garçons are these early works, not simply because they shed
and fade and show their fragility, but because they open the act of dressing
to the fragile articulations of fashion's very composition, allowing the garment to function as a lively interstice. That the garments feel alive is key to
their artfulness.

Kawakubo does not work from a desk. She does not use fabric swatches.
She does not sketch. She seeks no ultimate experience, no precise moment
of revelation. As she says, "There is no eureka moment, there is no end to
the search for something new." Instead, she works, intuitively, problemati-
cally, to create conditions for the activating of connections heretofore un-
available to her. She constructs to make felt a relation that has not yet come
to the fore. But she does not stop there. "Often in each collection, there are
three or so seeds of things that come together accidentally to form what

appears to everyone else as a final product, but for me it is never ending." Kawakubo continues, she persists in a serial manner, working in the interstices of what is on the way, in the art of time. "There is never a moment when I think, 'This is working, this is clear.' If for one second I think something is finished, the next thing would be impossible to do."[16]

In a procedural fashioning there can be no end to the process. This is a serial adventure with pinnacles of form that emerge along the way. The middle, the milieu of the in-act, is what is at stake. In this milieu, architectings of mobility produce tentative bodyings. Fabric shapes. But metamorphosis is what is most sought-after. Kawakubo designs in interstitial seriality, always toward that which "can and cannot be found." "Boundaries for an architectural body can only be suggested, never determined" (Arakawa and Gins 2002: 68).

In the middling, everything is at stake. Remember: this is not pure process. It is replete with the becoming of continuity, with the cleavings, the enabling constraints that make of process a practice. A collection must emerge, for it is from here, from the materiality of a form-taking, that the next procedure, the next dress, coat, pair of pants will invent itself.

But are these really still dresses, pants, coats? Ideally we would need a processual concept for these incipient forms. A dressing? A coating? A trousering? The same would need to be said of the procedural architectures—not a house but a housing, a lofting, a rooming, a thresholding. For procedural processes to make a difference, they must be created such that they can perform, reshape, constrain in ways unforeseeable. This is a difficult call, and often it fails. When this happens, the potentializing "dressing" returns to the habitual "dress," the "thresholding" becomes reduced to "entryway." In such cases the modes of existence the procedural fashioning sought to create lost the sense of their potential trajectory, becoming less a pathway than a finite project, as Souriau might say, losing the force of their incipient directionality.

The complicity here between a procedural fashioning and a procedural architecting is as speculative as it is pragmatic. In either case it cannot be about the product. It has to be about how the procedure does its work, and keeps working. This is hit and miss. It requires a long and rigorous process of experimentation, of study, and a willingness to begin anew without pretending to know the starting point. Recall Kawakubo's constraint: begin with the belief that we don't know what clothing can be.

In a procedural approach nothing can be taken for granted. It is always a question of the ecology at hand, of the architecting toward mobility of an emergent bodying. "Landing site configurations articulate at least this

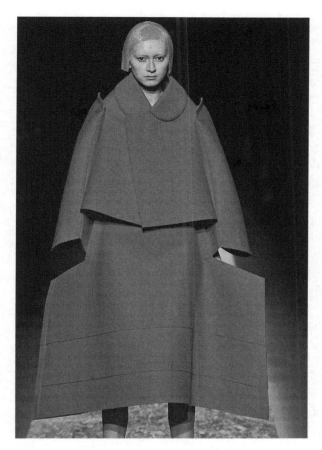

FIGURE 4.12 Comme des Garçons, AW 2012.
Photograph courtesy FirstView.

many positions; nearnearground, nearmiddleground, nearfarground, middlenearground, middlemiddleground, middlefarground, farnearground, farmiddleground, farfarground; nearmiddlefarground, nearfarmiddleground, middlenearmiddleground, middlenearfarground, farnearmiddleground" (Arakawa and Gins 2002: 71). But take care, Arakawa and Gins remind us, not to think of these shifting grounds as positions, for they are also "areas of an architectural body, which takes its ubiquitous cue and command from the form and features of an architectural surround, subtending all positions within the surround's confines" (2002: 71).

The environmental surround in a procedural fashioning is infinitely productive, for the starting point is topological: the body is that which folds.[17]

Without articulating it as such, I believe Kawakubo's procedural fashioning takes this notion of the body as its starting point. The fold is where it always begins—the fold of the tissue paper she gives her pattern-cutter as an inspiration, the fold of the texture that constrains the scissors when she cuts, the fold that resists, that reshapes, that escapes finite form. Hers is a lifetime of research into the fold, the fold produced by the body's bending, its kneeling, its touching, the fold of the texturing of a given piece of fabric, of the pleating so often part of her designs, the fold of the inside-out that brings the back to the fore in a garment, turning the seam on itself, the fold that resists becoming a seam, the imperceptible fold, even, of the infinite line.[18] For it is a fold, imperceptible as it may be, that I see as the inspiration of her autumn–winter 2012 two-dimensional collection, a collection that strangely accentuates the body's n-dimensionality.

A procedural architecture, in its siting of awareness at the scale of the middlenearmiddlefarground, takes the fold at its point of inflection, making apparent how the fold is the force of form the Euclidean architecture of our most normative surrounds must always build against: the fold of the hill within the landscape, of the air as it rushes against cement, creating a vortex that bends and twists, the fold of the body that moves with the building's capacity to make space for it. To commit to a procedural approach is to commit to this fold, imperceptible as it might be, and of course to commit to how it cleaves, and then to persuasively include it, to architect at its limit, inventing new ways of colluding with it, all the while attending to the dance of attention active within the force of the event's own procedural unfolding. For what the fold does first and foremost is remind us that the body is never one, is never outside the ecology of its environmental architecting, its nearfarmiddleground never a question of bare ontology. The body is that which folds into the architectural surround, that which folds into the architecting of mobility that sites awareness, that which folds into its own activity, that which remains infinitely serial, that which cannot but procedurally unfold. What a procedural fashioning can do is bring this tendency to its limit. Kawakubo's procedural fashionings begin here, at this point of inflection, architecting toward the creation of fragile modes of existence. Here, in the edging into itself of world-constituting procedures, Kawakubo designs not for the body but for a belief in the world.

CHOREOGRAPHING THE POLITICAL

Like many classical autistics, Ido Kedar came to language late. Coordinating his fingers to be able to type was a long process, and because his body often went against his wishes, moving in directions contrary to those he thought of as aligned to his conscious intentions, it was incredibly difficult for him to demonstrate to his aides that he was indeed capable of understanding their directives. This condition, which affects all classical autistics to differing degrees, is defined most aptly in the current literature as "autistic movement disturbance." Following older neuroscientific literature, Kedar calls it "motor apraxia."[1] Through his writing in *Ido in Autismland: Climbing Out of Autism's Silent Prison*, Kedar hopes to educate neurotypical readers and parents of autistics about movement disturbances in autism.[2] His outspoken desire is that parents and specialists no longer rely on the outward appearance of autistic movement to determine what autistics can do. Just because autistics have challenges with movement and communication, Kedar argues, does not mean that they cannot understand what is going on around them. Referring to the period before Kedar could express himself in writing, Kedar's mother explains: "Ido was bored out of his mind, trapped in a paralyzing silence and frustrated beyond belief. He tried hard to show that he was smart but his hands and his body did not cooperate with his mind, so everyone assumed that he just didn't understand the concepts. I cannot imagine a greater exercise in frustration." "The experts," Kedar says, "have no clue" (2012: 24).

Opening with Kedar's experience of his own type of neurodiversity, what I would like to do here is to take autistic motor disturbance as the starting point for a discussion of a body-world split I feel is endemic to the neurotypical account of experience. While it would be impossible to generalize across any group of people, and any autistic will reiterate that there are as many autistic experiences as there are autistics, I will take autistic perception as the starting point to this exploration. Autistic perception, as I underscored in several of the preceding chapters, is not meant to describe a group of autistics. It is, rather, a tendency in perception shared by all that privileges complexity of experience over category. Autistic Anne Corwin describes it as a slowness of chunking: the autistic's entry into an environment begins not with a perception of objects (chairs, tables) or of subjects (people) but with an edging into form, a tending of light and shadow and color. While this does eventually lead to the taking-shape of the environment, to its parsing, autistics benefit from the direct perception of the active ecologies of experience in-forming. Corwin, as well as autistics Tito Mukhopadhyay, DJ Savarese, Amelia Baggs, Ido Kedar, and many others, describe a field perception that foregrounds the heterogeneity of a welling experience before it succumbs to the categorization of its parts. While, as with neurotypicals, the environment does eventually chunk, there is an important time-lapse between the direct perception of the emergent ecology and the actual taking-form of the objects and subjects in its midst. Neurotypicals will not tend to be aware of this direct perception of experience except in extreme circumstances—shock, drug use, exhaustion—or perhaps in mindfulness exercises such as meditation.[3]

My purpose in starting with Kedar's experience is not to suggest that the extreme forms of body disturbance—the partial loss of the ability to coordinate and perform skilled, purposeful movements and gestures with accuracy—associated with autism are easy to live with, nor do I want to suggest that autistic perception is ideal in our neurotypically oriented worlds. There is no question that the world we live in is aligned to chunking, and that the quicker we get to perceiving objects and subjects, the easier the everyday is to manage. What I do want to argue is that were we to consider the connection between body disturbance and autistic perception, we might develop a stronger sense of how the neurotypical alignments of experience are limiting as regards the complexity of the body-world ecology.

Neurotypical experience is built on a few key beliefs. First, able-bodiedness is taken for granted as the ideal starting point for existence. Second, independence is put forward based on the idea that self-sufficiency is the goal. A self-sufficient body is regarded as a body that can consciously make decisions based on a strong sense of where the body ends and the world begins. Freedom is defined according to this notion of self-sufficiency. As I suggested in the introduction, these beliefs frame the prevalent and seemingly unshakable triad intentionality-volition-agency.

Starting with neurodiversity shakes the very foundation these beliefs are built on. Instead of beginning with the self-sustaining individual and a strong belief in selfhood/independence, I therefore begin here. I start with relation, proposing that autistic perception gives us a direct account of relation in-forming, an account that challenges the notion that the world comes parsed. Taking neurodiversity as the point of departure, I suggest that a body is a field-effect in a complex relational milieu that includes the sense of its limits—a body-envelope—but in no way stops there. What if instead of seeing the nonconscious unaligned body-world continuum Kedar describes as something to be overcome, we began the conversation from the perspective of *what else a body can do,* creating a robust account of the role of nonvolitional or preintentional (nonconscious) expression in the event of life-living? Kedar laments: "It's that my body finds its own route when my mind can't find it" (2012: 47). This neurodiverse misalignment with what is defined as conscious intentionality is no doubt frustrating. I don't want to underestimate that. But what if we took a different perspective on it? What if the path to neurotypical functioning were not the ideal one, the belief that *we* are the absolute directors of our movements? What if a different account led Kedar to find his motor disturbance helpful in the complex aligning of experience in the making? Are we certain that our "able-bodied" approaches are as ideal as we say they are?

Reading of Kedar's trauma as regards his experience of not being able to demonstrate his understanding of the world around him, it might be tempting to say, as Kedar himself does, that the rift between body and world, which translates to a body/mind dichotomy in his work, is really what is at stake. After all, it is a relief, as we read his book, to see him more and more capable of aligning his experience to that of neurotypicals— holding back his stims, writing, coordinating his body to his intentions— finally being taken seriously and considered intelligent by those around him.[4] But is the body-world, body-mind distinction he articulates as needing to be overcome not a measure of neurotypical, able-bodied reasoning? What if instead we approached this question of how body and world co-compose from the perspective that "finding" the body in time and space is a learned experience? What if we followed Bergson's account, outlined in the introduction, concerning the functioning of "continuous movement," thereby questioning our presuppositions about what is voluntary? What if we suggested that the relational experience of bodying described by so many autistics—where body is a field of sensation more than a locus—is closer to the complex reality of experience's formation than the neurotypical account we are fed from our earliest acquisition of motor skills?

It is not my wish, once again, to underestimate the frustration Kedar feels when he writes: "I am sure a lot of autistic people are smart like me, but they have no means to show it. It's not just speech. It's fine motor. It's body awareness. It's insurmountable obstacles that prevent the reply, so the autistic kid is treated like an unintelligent kid" (2012: 48). The neurotypically oriented world we live in privileges consciousness as aligned to instrumentality over nonconscious, nonvolitional tendings. It is this very neurotypical perspective that teaches us that a body begins and ends in a skin envelope we can readily perceive. Again and again in young childhood we are given instructions that assist us in differentiating our skin from that of the world. Think, for instance, of the young child's difficulty in assigning hurt when they fall, and their tendency to point to the ground instead of their knee. These teachings, which also tend to foreground the normatively rational over the emergently creative or intuitive, the individual over the relational, tune our existence toward a very simple notion of what a body can do. This, over time, convinces the child that singling out objects and subjects by categorizing experience is a necessary part of growing up. That this approach backgrounds the animism of their childhood beliefs is simply taken as a necessary rite of passage toward the agency that comes with adulthood. This invariably results in the backgrounding in experience of the lively continuity and co-composition between body and world.

Growing up means contending with a neurotypically oriented world, which in turn means dealing with the importance given to intentionality. "I don't know why initiating is so hard," writes Kedar, voicing what I am certain is one of the most discouraging aspects of autism. Autistic motor disturbance is certainly the main reason many autistics are not perceived to be capable of thinking for themselves. And yet it is likely this very difficulty that makes autistic perception prevalent and that allows autistics to dwell longer in the still-composing precategorized field of relation.[5] It is also this openness to experience in-forming at the edges where body and environment are not yet two that explains the fact that most if not all autistics are synesthetic. As Kedar describes: "If I hear some music I get hot or cold. It's like a full sensory experience of sound, sight and temperature. . . . It's interesting to experience things on more than one sensory level. . . . To see music takes music to another level, however it is also possible for me to get overwhelmed because my senses bombard me with so much information" (2012: 73).

I want to begin here, in the midst of a paradoxical experience where on the one hand there is difficulty as regards initiation and follow-through, where there are real challenges with communication and body-movement alignment, and on the other hand there is an acute richness of relational intensity that facilitates a perhaps more complex encounter with the world in-forming. From this perspective, where bodies are often not yet—"If I have my eyes closed I don't know where my hands are" (Kedar 2012: 81)— it would be easy to simply suggest, as Kedar often does, that there is something profoundly lacking that must be rectified. Kedar certainly thinks so: "My exercising is helping me to feel [my body] more. My body is beginning to connect more to my brain. I'm determined to overcome this challenge" (2012: 81). But as the above paradox makes apparent, this is not an all-or-nothing proposition. Certainly, I fully support and understand the importance for Kedar and other autistics to design techniques that make neurotypically inclined existence easier to navigate. But this does not preclude valuing aspects of autistic experience that tend to be undervalued (even by autistics). And so this is where I start, in the midst of the uneasy body-world relation Kedar describes.

FROM BODY TO BODYING

If the body is a dynamic constellation in co-composition with the environment, if it is an ecology of practices, and if thought is an active contributor to the feltness of experience, it seems to me that the starting point in challenging the body-world split is *putting thought in the world*. Thought as Kedar experiences it is not "in" his body. It is across experience, in the synesthetic sensations that refute the absolute locatedness of body and world. That he has such difficulty aligning body to conscious will does not mean that the activity is not full of thought, nor does it mean that he is not in awareness. It likely means quite the opposite—that the thought is so full, so complexly aligned across a relational field that includes body and world in their co-composition that the thought's subtraction into one conscious task ("point at that") is extremely difficult.

There is an important difference between conscious thought and thought that moves with experience in the making. Conscious thought is but the pinnacle of a much more complex thinking, one that aligns to field perception but does not yet single itself out for conscious discrimination. Nonconscious thought is everywhere active in experience. It moves at differential speeds. It cuts across. It opens up. It shifts. It is not *in* the body or *in* the mind, but *across* the bodying where world and body co-compose in a welling ecology.

In Kedar's case the movement of thought is not the problem. The problem is in the making-conscious of this movement, in the subtraction from the field of relation to the actual occasion. The field is simply too complex to easily pull out of it one single thought-activity. What makes it so complex is the movement in it. A body trained to subtract, to parse, is a body that has learned to find a certain stillness in, and believes it can differentiate itself from, the commotion of the ecologies that compose experience.

A movement of thought is elastic. It always begins in the milieu, in the midst of experience. This is another way of saying that it begins in movement. For the world is nothing if not in continuous movement. In Kedar's narration of experience, this kind of thinking is of no use-value. It simply doesn't add up to anything. But that's because so much is at stake in his need to convince those around him that he can think. This urgency is partly due to his long history of being treated with Applied Behavioral Analysis (ABA), still a far too common therapy for autistics. The interventionist model of ABA assumes that the autistic's way of moving must be eradicated, thereby denying the complexity of thought-movement that takes place in the movement-dance of autistic perception. Kedar writes: "Each day the experts denied me hand-flapping but I had no other outlet for my feelings. . . . In the ABA years I lost hope. . . . I longed so badly to be able to make my ideas known. I got flashcards instead. 'Touch your nose.' 'Touch tree.' 'Touch your head.' 'Do this.' 'Sit quiet.' 'Touch red.' 'Good job.' 'Hands quiet.' 'No.' 'Great.' 'No.' 'Great' 'No.' 'All right!' 'No'" (2012: 58).[6] Further along in the book he continues: "Some people prefer not to see the truth. If I'm doing what I do it means others can too. If they refuse to see it, they don't have to change how they teach kids. . . . I guess that watching the films [of me communicating] and asking my therapist questions would be too risky. Someone might get convinced that a retarded autistic kid was really intact in thinking. That would mean that they would need to see autism in a new way. Can't let that happen. Suppressing alternative viewpoints is better" (2012: 79). This history of not being believed, of having to prove his intelligence over and over again, leads Kedar to privilege cognition over autistic perception, situating his native way of thinking-feeling on the lower rungs of worthwhile ways to live. But all of this doesn't deny the complexity at work in his movements of thought:

Nature isn't neat or orderly. The grass is waving this way or that. The branches are crooked and gray and gnarled. The path is lopsided from rivers of rain and erosion. The plants grow in random places. I see no pattern, unlike a landscaped lawn. I fit in so well. I am so at home in the messy beauty of nature. I see the system is messy, but it works and it is wow. I see my illness this way. It's not pretty. It is messy. It has erosion and rivers of mud too. But it is part of nature in the same way. (2012: 119)

AN ECOLOGY OF PRACTICES

What makes *this* experience come into itself just *this* way? A neurotypical account would say that volition is at the heart of it. *I* want to focus my attention, *I* want to move. Volition, intentionality, and agency co-compose to create the free individual. But is this really how we move through the world?

I want to propose, as I have done throughout, that experience cannot be reduced to individual volition. It is collective—ecological—at its very core. The concept I want to foreground here for the selecting-out of experience is inflection. Inflection is a concept close to the idea of the differential as theorized by Leibniz and then Deleuze. In differential calculus, a point of inflection is defined as "a point on a curve at which the curvature or concavity changes sign from plus to minus or from minus to plus. The curve changes from being concave upwards (positive curvature) to concave downwards (negative curvature), or vice versa."[7]

Within the complexity of movement-moving, there is movement not yet actualized for experience—Jose Gil calls this *total movement*—and there is actual movement.[8] Similar to Bergson's theory of duration, where time actualized in experience is always co-composing with the durational field from which it has emerged, a field that is virtual but real, movement actualized does not neutrally detach itself from total movement. Like duration, total movement is a field of relation that is always actively co-composing with the actual in its emergence: the virtual, felt in its effects, is always active in the actual—this is what makes it real. When this or that experience differentiates itself from the field, when it becomes this or that, it has therefore altered the wider field of experience. The field, as I argued in the introduction, has changed in nature.

What occurs to activate the pulling of a movement in a new direction if human intentionality or agency is not the core activator? What I want to suggest here is that every experience of movement felt is the result of a point of inflection in experience, an inflection activated not simply by the individual but by the tending of the field itself.

The inflection is the point at which a tending breaks off, the point where a vague incipiency becomes a directionality. This directionality need not be a trajectory. It is less a point in space than an intensity that morphs the line that has formed in the moving. Perceiving the inflection does not mean being aware of it as though you could be outside it. It means moving in its tending. It means attending, in the event, to how movement diverges from its flow, attending to how movement moves.

The extraction from the field of total movement initiated by the point of inflection results in a co-composition—virtual and actual movement compose to create the durational movement-field experienced in the moving. This calls for a complex relational attunement, in the event. Speeds and slownesses and scales of action must attune as the field changes in nature. If the shift in scale or speed is acute, the attunement in its difference is felt as the *what else* of the movement's coming into itself, as I described in the last chapter. This occurs thousands of times a day, though it is rarely noticed consciously.

The inflection occurs in the midst even as it marks the event's divergence from itself. It is the force of difference that cues a transition. This transition dephases movement-moving. There may be a change in direction, or the movement may seem roughly continuous, but what is certain is that there will be a change in quality. The change in quality shifts the field of movement, altering not only how you move, but how the emergent movement moves you. The ecological effect of the inflection is felt as the sharpening, the lengthening, the deepening, the closing or opening of the field. What is felt is the uneasy twitching of movement-conditions. This attunement to the field in its divergence calls the field to attention. This makes the field lively with attention, an attention that affects the you you are becoming. The field feels poised.[9]

The poised field is alive with tendencies. Not each tendency will inflect. Many will simply perish, active only as potentiality. This means that their microinflections, while they may have affected the field in minor ways, are not active enough to cause a remarkable transition. There will not have been a transduction, but the tendency for a microdephasing will have been alive for that split second of their contribution to the field in-forming. This will likely only be realized after the fact when the felt effects of the inflection have been consciously absorbed.

Whitehead talks about this as negative prehension. In the actual occasion, in the event of activity realizing itself as event, there is a taking-up of experience through prehension. Prehension is what culls this or that from the field of movement-moving. When the prehension actualizes as occasion, the world has appeared in its singularity and created this or that felt experience. But what of the almost-felt in its push-pull elasticity? Hasn't this too made a difference, even if it wasn't aligned to in the event?

The *almost* makes a difference. It is the more-than of experience in the making. This more-than is alive in the productive schism between the act and the in-act. It is what remains, but also what exceeds the event. Every event is made up of this surplus. This surplus is elastic. It has no form as such, it has no tense, it cannot be categorized. It is neither of the present, of the past nor of the future. It is pulled across times in the making, felt in its resonance. The *almost* shapes the present-passing without inflecting it, yet it contributes to the ways the inflection can create new directionalities.

It is important to not place the inflection in the realm of human intentionality. Movement inflects due to movement's own processes. This does not mean that the human has no role to play. Of course how the body moves has effects, and there is no end to inflections activated by tendings that include the human. It's just that the intention is not where we usually assume it is. It is *in the event*, in the ecology. Perhaps one way of thinking inflection as more-than human is through gravity. Gravity acts on the body. It activates vertical movements, moving organs, limbs toward the earth. It also activates lateral movements, widening, pulling toward depth of field. Gravity can be defined as directional activity in the event's coming to be.

Gravity does not create the inflection. It is part of the conditions through which certain tendential inflections become more typical than others. For instance, gravitational movement tends to move toward the earth rather than away from it. But gravity does not always body the same way. What it can do is dependent on the ecology that is co-activated in the bodying. Gravity is a field, after all, not simply a directionality. The potential of the field cannot be understood apart from what it does, from what it can do, in relation to the fieldings it co-activates.

Attending to the more-than is a way of saying that the field itself is attentive to its potential shifts, that the field has within its potential the capacity to create the conditions for difference. The more-than is everywhere present in different constellations—in and across the human, the animal, the vegetal, the mineral. In this emergent speciating field of experience, I propose to explore the workings, nonintentional and yet free, as Bergson would say, of nonvolitional movement. Urgent questions frame the analysis: How can we articulate in language the *agencements* at the heart of the event's dance of attention in a way that doesn't simply take us back to the neurotypical account of experience and its alignment to subject-centered agency? Can we imagine not being the masters of our acts without falling prey to the idea that if we are not master, someone or something else must be? Is it possible to create an account of immanent movement and autistic perception that convinces us that there are other ways to be free?

ATTUNING TO THE INTERVAL

The how of movement-moving is a question of the interval. Intervals are qualitative holes of movement-moving opened up by inflections. Relational movement generates and is generated by intervals.[10] Imagine a busy subway station. There are many coimplicated directionalities, your movement always cueing in the complexity of the speeds and slownesses around you, a score that moves more than just you.

Consider this scenario: You feel the subway coming toward the platform before you see it, its sound and its vibrations preceding it. This movement tunes the whole platform, qualitatively altering the posture of those waiting. You may not yet see movement, but it is welling, its incipiency felt across the multitude. If this is rush hour at the Lionel Groulx station in Montreal, hundreds of people are poised. Some are stiller than others, waiting quietly for the subway doors to open, some are shifting impatiently between those standing in line, others are walking down the platform, their rhythms a mix of hurried and languid, some are talking on the phone, some are reading.

As the subway doors open, a subtle anticipatory shift in posture and tonality can be felt across the platform. Where before there seemed to be a relatively simple directionality, most of it tuned toward the subway doors, now a bidirectional tendency begins to form. These two movements can be quite frantic in their co-composition, especially when in addition people are running from the just-arrived train on the other side of the platform, hoping to make it onto the one you've been patiently waiting for. Yet very few collisions occur. And this is with many distractions—people listening to music with their earphones, friends talking, people running to get in before the doors slam. How do we all move together so seamlessly?

The choreography of collective movement is made possible by the interrelation between the intervals the movement creates and the collective capacity to cue and align to them, in the moving. Cueing is an important activity in the relational field. It is not directly tied to volition or intentionality. It happens in the moving. Although it may feel like it is individuals cueing to one another, what is actually happening is that movement is cueing to a relational ecology in the making.[11]

The cueing to conditions of change cannot happen in the real-time where these shifts reach conscious perception. That would be too slow. The cues are moving you before you consciously realize the need to make a minor shift, to tend in a certain direction, to alter the quality of your movement. The nonconscious movement of thought moves you, a thinking *in the field* that cannot be separated from the moving, alerting you to the fact that you have moved only in the event of attention becoming conscious. It is only now, and barely so, since conscious and nonconscious perception are continuously realigning, that you realize you have made way for a change in the relational field. This choreographic impulse is distributed, the movement attuning to cues that are themselves shifting in the mobile ecology that is the subway platform.

I suspect that cueing to movement in its co-composition is more intuitive across the spectrum of neurodiversity than cueing to movement-position. How counterintuitive, then, to approach autistic movement—or any movement instruction, for that matter—from the perspective that there is a definable frame as regards where movement begins and ends? Why, knowing about autistic movement disturbance, would we ask autistics to measure their capacity to move on the accomplishment of a pre-choreographed task instead of investing in modes of cueing and aligning that celebrate incipient movement? Why, when for all of us a relational movement-moving is more intuitive than a staged movement-task, do we still tend to privilege the neurotypical account that movement begins with stopping (think of the typical dance class that begins every movement from stillness, as opposed to those fantastic choreographers who "find" the movement in the middle of its self-expression), that movement is organized through frames imposed from the outside (think of the typical way of teaching a danced movement sequence from the perspective of an 8-count that begins with 1 and ends with 8 as opposed to the more fluid rhythms of a volleyball game, where it is the movement of the ball that choreographs movements already moving)? Clearly both tendencies are well and alive—so why do we still persist in privileging so-called "volitional" movement?

About the difficulty of initiating movement, Kedar writes: "I have been thinking a lot about my nonresponsiveness. It's almost like a form of paralysis [yet] I'm not paralyzed to wave ribbons, or to pace, or things like that.

Then I'm the opposite of paralyzed. I can't get my body to stop moving around, though I want it to" (2012: 101). Autistic Naoki Higashida concurs: "When I'm jumping, I can feel my body parts really well . . .—my bounding legs and my clapping hands—and that makes me feel so, so good. . . . So by jumping up and down, it's as if I'm shaking loose the ropes that are tying up my body" (2013: location [hereafter "loc."] 435). Cueing to movement-moving is clearly not the challenge: it's starting from stilled movement that is so difficult.

Most of our education systems are based on starting from stillness. We learn in chairs. We associate concentration with being quiet. We discourage the movement of thought we call daydreaming, particularly in the context of "learning." We consider the immanent movements of doodling to be a distraction.[12] We are told not to fidget. Reason is aligned with keeping the body still. What if instead we invested in movement-moving, asking children not to stop moving but to become increasingly aware of the share of creativity in the incipient directions of the movements that move them? What if we taught them that the ideal posture for learning or listening or "paying attention" was not standing still (or sitting still), but attuning to cues active in the field of relation?[13] What if we directly allied the movement of thought to movement-moving? If we took the common event of cueing to movement-moving outlined above as the ground of experience, what else would we become capable of perceiving? What else could learning (and listening and attending) become?

What else we would perceive, were we to invest in relational movement instead of stopping movement in the midst, are movement-intervals. Intervals invite and steer movement. They also open the movement to its own time, event-time. Think of event-time as the time, in the event, of cueing and aligning to the futurity of experience in the making.

Honing the interval is a technique that is capable of altering the flow of movement-moving. I call this choreographic thinking. Choreography at its best is not about aligning bodies to precomposed shapes. It is about generating modes of moving that make felt the complex ecology of incipient movement, to make felt what I have elsewhere called movement's preacceleration and its elasticity of the almost.[14] It is about composing techniques for experiencing the more-than of form. To choreograph the interval is to attend, in the event, to how movement's force-form is elastic, to sense the shift activated by the inflection and to fashion ways of cueing and aligning that keep the field of activity alive to the virtual effects of total movement.

Think the interval not only as the force of form in the context of a simple movement. Think it also in its potential as an opening onto *agencement*, as opposed to agency.

Agency begins in a category. It is used to place the action of volition in a subject or a group. That said, I recognize that agency is often used in academic discourse to give voice to an underrepresented group. We talk about the agency of the disabled, the agency of the autistic, the agency of women of color. We speak of the need for the disenfranchised to have agency.

The last thing I want to do is to deny the complexity of power and the ways in which it sidelines populations. Indeed, what is important here is precisely the question of how an emphasis on the in-act of event-time opens the way for a rethinking of power and the politics that accompanies it. Focusing on *agencement* instead of agency, I want to argue, allows us not only to value modes of experience backgrounded in the account of agency, it also shakes the powerful foundations of neurotypicality, a mode of existence that profoundly devalues accounts of experience that cannot be reduced to the volition-intentionality-agency triad.

My proposal is that an approach that begins in the field of relation is precisely political because it does *not* begin with the agency of a preconceived group or solitary identity. Rather than beginning with subject-based identity, this approach begins in the ecology of practices where there is still room for new modes of existence to be invented. New modes of existence call forth an articulation of the political that is not reducible to preexisting constituencies, and thus is open to creating and celebrating modes of life-living as yet uncharted.[15]

Where agency returns to the identity of a precomposed category, *agencement* speaks to the interstitial arena of experience of the interval, an interval not of the category but in the pre of categorization where the field is still in formation. In Deleuze and Guattari's *A Thousand Plateaus*, Brian Massumi translates the untranslatable *agencement* with "assemblage."[16] Unfortunately, assemblage has too often been read as an object or existent configuration, rather than in its potentializing directionality. This is why I return to the French term here. *Agencement*, which carries within itself a sense of movement and connectibility, of processual agency, is used first in *A Thousand Plateaus* with relation to the book. A book, Deleuze and Guattari argue, is an *agencement*. They write:

There is no difference between what a book talks about and how it is made. Therefore a book also has no object. As an assemblage [*agencement*], a book has only itself, in connection with other assemblages [*agencements*] and in relation to other bodies without organs. We will never ask what a book means, as signified or signifier; we will not look for anything to understand in it. We will ask what it functions with, in connection with what other things it does or does not transmit intensities, in which other multiplicities its own are inserted and metamorphosed, and with what bodies without organs it makes its own converge. (1987: 4)

This is another way of saying that a book can activate a movement of thought. A book is an *agencement* in its capacity to create linkages not yet assembled, to produce ways of becoming, to invent new modes of existence.

It seems to me that there is more agency in *agencement* than there is in its usual alignment to an identity category. If we take the field of movement in its capacity for differentiation as the motor for change, there are a lot more openings for difference. The difficulty is in harnessing this potential without backgrounding its co-compositional nature. This is where technique comes in.

Techniques are associated with both habit and skill. For those of us who have practices honed over time, such as playing an instrument, dancing, painting, we have a strong sense of what technique might be, usually associating it to repetitive gestures and, in the case of skill, with virtuosity. At the other end of the spectrum, where technique is more tied to habit, technique might be associated with ways of keeping house, ways of bringing up our children, ways of being in a relationship, ways of teaching. We also have techniques for walking in the snow, for interacting with strangers, for dealing with fear.

The difference between a technique and a habit is a question of degree. Like habit and procedure, in the last chapter, or habit and rituality in the one before, they exist on a continuum as limit concepts. Whereas habit's technique is backgrounded and often lingers on the edge of the nonconscious, technique's habit is often consciously honed. Do you call the way your feet take you to the coffee machine in the morning a technique or a habit? I would say that with the early-morning coffee, or the walk to the toilet, these are more habitual because their techniques are so backgrounded. But if you're dealing with an onset of Parkinson's, the old habit may require new techniques. Now that you are less sure on your feet and your energy wavers from day to day, or even hour to hour, you will likely find yourself seeking out new techniques to hone the habit. Habit's techniques will thus foreground themselves, and you might begin to think of your movements less in terms of habit and more in terms of technique. New techniques might include holding on to the piece of furniture on the way to the bathroom with your stronger left arm, or making sure there are no obstacles in the way that you might inadvertently trip over, or, in the case of making coffee, setting up the coffee machine where you can sit to prepare your morning coffee, or even changing your espresso-machine coffee habit to the simpler technique of making instant coffee. Techniques open habit to its potential undoing as much as they make apparent habit's stubborn place in our life.

With regard to the potential of *agencement* in the intervals of existence-in-the-making, technique makes all the difference. This is why techniques are so central to the work done at the SenseLab, the laboratory for thought in motion where much of my thinking and making around choreographic thinking takes place. Here we ask ourselves what kinds of techniques would best create the conditions for the opening of a field of experience to a different way of functioning. If we are working toward creating an event, for instance, we will work to make sure that the event's thresholds (the ways people initially enter the event) will be capable of creating emergent attunements. Previous to the event, in weekly SenseLab gatherings, we will invent movement exercises, for instance, that explore how a relational milieu opens itself to modes of encounter. We will then explore how the openings created might allow for a qualitatively different entry as regards ordinary habits of self-presentation.[17] We also work to create techniques that open the event to its more-than human ecology. Usually we will spend a full year on these techniques with the hope that one or two will actually make a difference in the event.

But technique on its own is not enough. The technique will only open the field, altering the conditions of its emergence. What is also needed is a minor gesture that is capable of tuning technique to what I call its technicity. Think of ballet, for instance. Through repetitive techniques—including practicing for hours at the barre, honing flexibility in the joints through daily stretching, practicing jumps over and over again to create better balance, repeating particular forms daily—a body will begin to become a ballet-body. Hips will open in a way that will allow for a diversity of movement quite unusual for most standing bodies, toes and feet will become accustomed to the pain of pointe shoes if they are used, the extension of limbs in the predictable orientations of a ballet-aesthetic will become second nature. But these shifts in the dancing body won't by themselves be enough to make a dancer really dance. What will make the dancer dance is technicity, the outdoing of technique, the capacity to take technique to its limit, and then to go elsewhere.

Technique and technicity coexist. Where technique is defined by the repetitive practices that tune a process, technicity is a set of enabling conditions that exact from technique the potential for the process to exceed its form. Where technique paves the way for a degree of complexity within a given field of experience, technicity opens the event to its *agencement*. Activated by the minor gesture that bridges technique and its more-than, technicity moves the process toward a practice still to be defined. This is the potential we sometimes see in that one dancer in the *corps de ballet* who stands out even though the form of her movements doesn't necessarily depart from those of the dancers around her. What makes this one dancer stand out is the quality not of the form of her movements themselves but of the *what else* within her movement-moving, the tenor, the intensity, the color of what the form leaves behind. Think technicity as the *agencement* that stretches out from technique, creating brief interludes for the more-than of technique, gathering from the implicit the force of form. Think technicity as the art of the event.

CHOREOGRAPHIC THINKING

"Choreography starts from any point," writes William Forsythe (in Casperson 2000: 33). Choreography co-composes with the event's point of inflection. It cleaves an occasion, activating its relational potential. It makes time, beginning its process anew always from the midst of the event. Choreography is thus a proposition *to* the event. It asks the event how its ecology might best generate and organize the force of movement-moving.

Choreographic *agencement* is a complex of experience that in itself cannot be mapped. What emerges choreographically is less an organization of bodies than a cartography of incipient tendencies, of force of form. In this sense, choreography is less about a body than about an ecology. This ecology is more-than-human, composed as much of the force of atmosphere, of duration, of rhythm, than it is of something we might call the body-envelope. This more-than is not activated by decisions in the standard sense of being willed by the individual, but by the immanent creation, in the event, of points of inflection that affect the very tenor of movement-moving. How we cue and align to these inflections, how we move with intervals in the making, is spurred by an activating cut immanent to the process that cleaves the event, creating a vectoring into contrast. Decision in the moving—like thought in the moving—is the event of tendencies colliding such that they coalesce in the time-slip of the new, spurred into invention by the ecology of the dance itself.

I want to think this immanent editing of decision in a choreographic practice as the activator of an *agencement* that occurs in event-time. Event-time is not linear, metric time. It is a making-felt of the interval, a making-apparent of how time tunes with the inflection of movement-moving. Event-time makes felt the rhythmic differential in the passage from minor gestures to technicity. Event-time cannot be abstracted from the event's coming into itself. It is not a time framed, but a time without measure. Event-time, the art of time, is time in relation, time actively co-composing in an emergent ecology.

Choreographic thinking is a proposition to movement-moving that asks how the plane of experience composes, how it remembers, how it becomes, and how it takes form, all in the register of the more-than-human. It is an everyday activity that tunes habits and invents techniques. At its best, it is an operative technicity that opens experience to emergent collectivity. For its focus is never on the body per se. What moves it choreographically is not first and foremost a body. It is rhythm, a cut in duration, a field of resonance, an interval.

To move the interval, the more-than, rather than "the body," or "the subject," is to create an opening for a politics that doesn't begin with or settle into form, a politics that invents with the inframodality of a making-thinking that refuses to know in advance what it can become. Traditionally, political philosophy does not make space for the interval within the vocabulary of the political subject (or its adjacent concept, the body-politic), yet the interval has nonetheless leaked into the complex iterations of experience we call the political.[18] What a focus on movement can do is bring to the fore the potential of a different perspective, one that leads away from a humanist bias that builds on intention and volition toward the complex intervals of an ecological world in motion.[19]

This has effects for political thought. The *agencements* of event-time open the way for what Guattari calls an ecosophy, a politics both ethico-political and aesthetic. Such a politics is as far as one can get from a politics of individual or group identity. It begins instead directly with the *agencement* active in movement-moving, gathering not around the individual but around what Guattari calls a group-subject, the collective momentum of a field of relation cueing and aligning to modes of thought in the making. This is not to entirely background the individual. Of course the individual reemerges at key moments, but always as transindividual: the force of form activated in the ecology of practices is tuned here such that what makes a difference does so at the level of the collective rather than through what are perceived as individual acts. Following Simondon, think the individual in this context less as an initiator of experience than as one of the ways in which the field inflection comes to determinate expression.

In his work at La Borde, a psychiatric clinic founded by Jean Oury, Guattari's focus was on the schizoanalytic encounter with group-subjectivity. For Guattari, creating and defining new forms of subjectivity was urgent, for it was only in the practice of rethinking the subject in the analytical context that the dominant paradigm of the psychoanalytic, where the subject is very much predefined, could be sidestepped, creating a platform for neurodiversity. La Borde was an ideal site for this kind of research. Peter Pál Pelbart explains: "La Borde was a polyphonic laboratory. And it's true: someone who suffers from psychosis is completely deterritorialized from the subject, immediately. In other words, the subjectivities and the subjectivations have absolutely nothing to do with the identity of the subject before us. All of this allows all sorts of entities from elsewhere to proliferate."[20]

It is worth repeating that a group-subject as Guattari defines it is not simply a group of individuals. The group-subject is defined by the group as it is formed in the encounter, not organized around the self-presentation of its members, but directed by the ways the group attunes to the necessity of its coming-into-formation. The group is never the sum of its parts, but rather an emergent collectivity which, for Guattari, always co-composes across the overlapping fields of the environment, the social, and the psychic. At La Borde, the focus on the group-subject serves to reorient the very question of mental illness, placing the burden not directly on the individual, but asking, as the movement for neurodiversity does, that difference be seen as a conduit for the crafting of transindividual modes of existence, modes of existence capable of integrating complex notions of interdependence and care. The goal is not to deny the needs of each person, but to recognize that it is impossible to abstract conditions of well-being from the relational field.

A politics in movement is a politics in the making allied to an activist philosophy. As Brian Massumi defines it, activist philosophy is concerned with "coincident differences in manner of activity *between* which things happen [where] the coming-together of the differences *as such*—with no equalization or erasure of their differential—constitutes a formative force" (2011: 5). The activist philosophy I am proposing here is neurodiverse. This means that it cannot be contained within the limits of neurotypical experience. Neurotypicality, as I argued in the introduction, is as much a construct as any other identity politics, and yet it is perhaps even more insidious, for, in most cases, it remains almost completely backgrounded in experience. We learn so early that body and world are separate, that intentionality trumps mutual determination, that intelligence is defined by rationality, that thought is conscious and ideally linguistically articulated, that sitting still is necessary for learning, that daydreaming is a waste of time, that the edgings into perception that distract us (or, more likely, attract us) are hallucinations, that the act belongs to a subject, that we often don't realize to what degree neurotypicality works as the very definition of human existence.[21] Nonspeaking autistic Amelia Baggs writes:

> If we were real people, killing us would be bad, and killing ourselves would be unfortunate rather than something people build special laws to enable.
>
> If we were real people, the world would be designed in a way that allowed us to move through it without extra obstacles thrown in our way.
>
> If we were real people, people would see us as individuals, rather than heroes, tragedies, inspirations, or representatives of our entire impairment group.
>
> If we were real people, then giving us proper medical care would never be seen as pointless.
>
> If we were real people, the whole myriad range of disability stereotypes would look flimsy and silly because people would see us as we are.
>
> Of course we're already real people. But the problem is that so few people have noticed.[22]

Choreographing the political means devising techniques, in the moving, for an activist philosophy that is ecological and neurodiverse at its very core. An activist philosophy born of a commitment to neurodiversity means refusing to situate movement in a preconstituted subject; questioning the place of volition in experience; resisting normopathy as a point of departure; embracing autistic perception.

As I will outline in the next chapter, to continue down the road of activist philosophy, it is necessary to go to the heart of why volition does not define experience, and to explore further how agency, as tied to intention and will, has served not to bestow power but to parse the world into subjects and objects, thereby startlingly disempowering difference. An activist philosophy involves diverging from the intentionality-volition-agency triad to become attuned instead to the art of participation that is life-living.

An activist philosophy begins from the perspective of the more-than, where the as-yet-uncharted movements of *agencement* are at their most operational. Here, in the midst, an important task of an activist philosophy is to attune to the ways in which ecologies settle into (trans)individuals. These individuals, these speciations, mark how an event has resolved into an act. Speciations are not created to last. But their passage makes a difference. An activist philosophy is interested in how their appearance into existence alters the quality of the event's coming-to-be. For, how an event comes to be, how it occasions, *is its value*. This is not about value-added in any capitalist sense. For what speciations bring to experience is a valuation of process in the event, not an external evaluation of form. Inasmuch as an activist philosophy directly engages with neurodiverse forms of life in their emergence, with speciations in-act, it is a philosophy of value.[23]

Speciations are rhythmic activations of an ecological body that never precede the event of their coming-into-relation. They give rhythm, give tone, to the how of the event's in-forming, cutting across the idea of species fully formed. Speciations are never one thing—think of them instead as complex tendings, as conglomerates of activity. They are not categories, and their taking-form cannot be separated out from the event of their coming-to-be. In their taking-place, in their chunking as this or that, speciations nonetheless never quite resolve into an identity. This is because the collectivity at the heart of the ecology that defines them remains active, participatory, even in the occasion that settles the act.

Choreographing the political begins here, in the midst of shapeshifting speciations. Allied to activist philosophy, allied to the kind of study that happens in the undercommons, a choreographing of the political sees minor gestures everywhere at work, and it seizes them. Choreographing the political is a call not only for the collective crafting of minor gestures, but for the attunement, in perception, to how minor gestures do their work.

CARRYING THE FEELING

> Remember that my body and its "orbit" include my thoughts, my real
> emotions, and what I call my "feelings." These are not the same as what
> you people, i.e. neurotypicals, call "feelings" but are my carrying . . .
> vibrations, flashes, visual-blocks, touch-horrors, smell-tickles and the
> cross-over that comes from them.
> —Lucy Blackman, *Carrying Autism, Feeling Language*

In autistic Lucy Blackman's writing, carrying attaches itself to nouns.
"When I refer to something within myself," she writes,

> I often use the word "carrying" as an adjective just before the word
> for the emotion or whatever. So when I draft what I want to say, the
> word "carrying" frequently appears but I usually edit it out so it doesn't
> confuse or distract other people. . . . What do I mean by "carrying my
> world"? I think that most people see themselves as moving between
> the things and the space on each side of them, so that the area in front
> comes up and parts before their faces, because that is how the television
> camera shows "reality." Somehow I use space differently. My space envel-
> opes me as if I were in a cocoon, and the items and other aspects of my
> environment enter and leave that cocoon. (2013: 6)

Carrying moves the noun. With this motor attached to it, the noun becomes a field of sensation, making felt the ineffable more-than of perception, the welling nonconscious activity of experience in the making. As an
autistic writing herself into neurotypical experience, Blackman feels the
carrying needs to be edited out—not experientially, of course, but linguistically. The more-than of experience in the making must be left unspoken.
And yet this more-than cannot so easily be excised. It remains active, despite her desire to background it. We hear it in her descriptions of neuro-

diversity—it lurks in her prose, it enlivens her metaphors. It is there when she talks about her experience of a body, articulating the difficulty she has in defining where the body ends and the world begins. It is there when she speaks of the challenge of moving in a world that refuses to settle itself into a stable locus where objects and subjects are clearly differentiated. It is there when she writes of memory, articulating the difference between a kind of experiential memory felt in the moving and a linguistic memory activated for the telling. Everywhere, Blackman's experience is one of carrying, one that privileges the felt experience of emergent relation. For her, a body is a carrying-across, a relational field that incorporates the environment in its infinite metamorphosis. It is an orbit that includes even as it creates, an orbit that cannot be abstracted from the vibrations, flashes, triggers that cross over into the world in-forming, an orbit that is less a body as such than the activity of crossing, the activity of aligning. An orbit is not a site, Blackman emphasizes again and again, but a region, an opening onto experience, a co-composition with a world in the making. A worlding.

Carrying is always tied to movement. As I outlined in the last chapter, to move as an autistic is to live in paradox. On the one hand, there is nothing but movement, most of it nonvoluntary, which, for neurotypically inflected existence, translates as strange, unpredictable, disturbing—the autistic body simply moves too much. On the other hand, it is this same overabundance of movement-moving that keeps the autistic singularly open to perception in its most complex iterations, making directly felt the world's edgings into itself. "Sometimes I pity you for not being able to see the beauty of the world in the same way we do. Really, our vision of the world can be incredible, just incredible," writes Naoki Higashida. "When you see an object, it seems that you see it as an entire thing first, and only afterward do its details follow on. But for people with autism, the details jump straight out at us first of all, and then only gradually, detail by detail, does the whole image sort of float up into focus" (2013: loc. 513).

This capacity to directly perceive experience in-forming, what I am calling autistic perception, involves a continuous carrying, a moving-with of experience in the making. What if we took this carrying that Blackman feels she has to background for neurotypical consumption and made it the motor of experience? What if we said that carrying is precisely what motivates an experience to become what it can do? What would this approach alter in terms of accounts of agency? How would such an approach give credence to this most lively of modes of perception that is autistic perception?

Following the work of the last chapter, which explored the role of inflection, relation, and the interval in movement in order to foreground the nonconscious share of movement-moving, linking it to an activist philosophy that is neurodiverse at its core, I want to expand the account of volition here to ask how carrying takes us further outside of the model of the neurotypical. I want to suggest that there is, in Blackman's account of orbital subjectivity, and in many other accounts of autistic perception, a kind of carrying of mobility that resituates experience beyond the reigning body/world dichotomy.[1]

FROM AGENCY TO *AGENCEMENT*

What Blackman calls "carrying the feeling" is all about the movement of a subjectivity very much in flux. Feeling here, as in Whitehead, is not to be understood as an external response to an existing event. Feeling is what defines the quality of the event *in the event*. There is no external subjectivity here: the subject, as in Whitehead, is not the activator of the act but what emerges in the act. Whitehead calls this emergent individual "the subjective form" *of* the event. How the event coalesces into itself is its subjective form. This subjective form, the subject *of the event*, the event's speciation, does not necessarily resemble a human subject. The subjective form is *how* the assemblage of the event's composition comes into itself. "There are many species of subjective forms, such as emotions, valuations, purposes, adversions, aversions, consciousness, etc." (Whitehead 1978: 24). These subjective forms are oriented by what Whitehead calls the event's "subjective aim." The subjective aim, the event's minor gesture, orients the event toward its actualization.[2] Whitehead calls the process toward actualization concrescence, emphasizing the sense of a growing *in the event* (1978: 25).

Each occasion of experience, once it has achieved its subjective form, is absolutely what it is. It is how this event came into itself *just this way*. But of course each event is influenced by how other occasions of experience have come to concrescence, and it carries those concrescences with it in germ.[3] To create a continuity of experience, there has to be a way that occasions of experience continue to affect one another. One way this happens in Whitehead is through nonsensuous perception, a concept that describes the folding of past tonalities into present events. Nonsensuous perception does not mean that the past fully formed fits into present occasions. It means that the tendencies of pastness contribute to how the current event unfolds. Subjective aim is key here, as a lure for feeling (1978: 85). Feeling here is the force, in the event, that lures experience into a tendency-to-form. This tendency-to-form is not back-traceable to something that could be easily encapsulated as "the past" fully formed: pastness is a current that runs through it. Whitehead writes: "The breath of feeling which creates a new individual fact has an origination not wholly traceable to the mere data. It conforms to the data, in that it feels the data. But the how of feeling, though it is germane to the data, is not fully determined by the data. The relevant feeling is not settled, as to its inclusions or exclusions of 'subjective form,' by the data about which the feeling is concerned" (1978: 85). An occasion of experience is the fullness of what a feeling has felt as actualized through a singular subjective form. This subjective form carries both the feeling in its operative fullness as virtual force and the in-act of what that feeling has felt in this singular instance. The feeling, like Blackman's carrying-feeling, is that which moves the event toward what Whitehead calls its satisfaction. It is the event's agency.

With carrying as a motif, I will continue to use *agencement* as the concept best capable of carrying agency. *Agencement*, whose synonyms include "accommodation," "adjustment," "arrangement," "composition," "contexture," carries with it a sense of a mobilizing—its movement-toward has an undeniable effect on the conditions of experience in their unfolding. Often read in conjunction with Foucault's concept of the *dispositif* (translated as "apparatus"), it has also come to have political connotations in the French, linking it to micropolitics and regimes of power. *Agencement*: the directed intensity of a compositional movement that alters the field of experience.

Agencement directs how the event comes to subjective form. This subjective form is not stable across regions of time and space. It is emergent and co-compositional. It is how the event actualizes as event. But as I have mentioned before, this actualization is brief, always already on the cusp of perishing. What is left over, the fullness of its feelings as yet unactualized, is the conduit for new occasions of experience. When Blackman writes that her feelings "are my carrying . . . vibrations, flashes, visual-blocks, touch-horrors, smell-tickles and the cross-over that comes from them," what she is saying, it seems to me, is that experience doesn't easily resolve for her. Subjective forms are elusive. What is far more current in her experience are carrying-feelings, feelings that do not emerge from a stable place (i.e., a predefined body) or land in any kind of predictable formation. Feelings remain lures.

Autistic perception is the ideal modality for carrying the feeling, since autistic perception does not hurry toward form. While the event of perception does eventually resolve into form, allowing autistics to parse, the fact of living so fully in the act means that the middling of experience is very familiar to them. Blackman can of course move between autistic perception and the chunking of tendencies into subjective forms, and she does. But first, she says, comes the carrying, and so carrying is written into the text before being excised, its excision occurring as though in the real-time of events concrescing. But what of its trace? Can it really be excised? In a gesture geared toward neurotypicals, Blackman attempts to background the carrying to make language more stable, and yet the feeling-full is hard to parse into language-forms: the carrying nonetheless makes itself felt, even in its literal absence, weaving its way through the seams of the writing. For carrying is what language does, particularly when language lets itself feel.

In a neurotypical accounting of experience, there is a tendency to organize feeling-forms into articulations that parse experience into manageable bits. But something else is always also at stake in the operations of expression. Carrying is a conduit in all experience: it is what underlies the mobility of all perception. The main difference between the autistic and the neurotypically inclined is not the modality of perception as such but how perception is fielded. In the neurotypical, because the fielding is more direct in the sense that parsing happens more quickly, the feeling of the subjective-form's inherent multiplicity is not as foregrounded. This is what allows the neurotypical to be so certain that experience begins with them, in the body, in the human. If we view subjectivity from the perspective of autistic perception, on the other hand, the heterogeneity of feeling makes it more palpable that subjectivity is in the making, in the field. Subjectivity is not felt as predetermining: it is connected to the field of experience as it in-forms it.

Subjectivity is a carrying into existence of feeling-forms self-defining. Subjectivities happen. But they are not where experience begins and ends. They exist in the event of their coming-to-be. There is persistence of subjectivities, but not as fully formed entities. Subjectivities persist in germ. This persistence is what we call history. History, from a process philosophy perspective, is the serial activating of a certain degree of continuity. The mistake would be to see this continuity as pure becoming. It is not a continuity of becoming, as Whitehead might say, but a becoming of continuity. Persistence is never persistence of the same, but persistence of a cut that activates the conditions for a seriality in the making.

Serialities in the making rely on the conditions that support their retelling. Neurotypicality is one of those conditions from which the cut of

subjectivity is persistently defined. The idea of the neurotypical as building block of human existence is so pervasive that not only is it rarely recognized as such, but most of us have overlooked the ways neurotypicality
structures our original myths, starting from the idea that humans are dis-
tinctly above all other forms of life and extending all the way to the idea
that certain forms of human life are more worthwhile than others. As I
mention in the introduction, this has had an effect on how we value not
only different forms of organic and inorganic existence, but also forms of
human difference. Think, again, of the general belief that Down syndrome
is not a worthwhile life.[4] Or think of the ways in which disabled people are
infantilized, and often mistreated in institutions. Think also of the high un-
employment of people with disabilities.[5] Or think of the destructive ways
in which the cure-focused Autism Speaks devalues autistic experience.[6] Or
think of the ways women have been segregated out of certain professions
because of norms around intelligence that exclude them.[7] Or think of the
legacy of Indigenous politics and the ways in which Indigenous people are
ignored, abused, excluded.[8] Neurotypicality takes for granted what the
human should be and by extension limits the breadth of what a human
subjectivity might look like. Here, a kind of mutated natural selection is still
at work that believes that the fittest (those we've already given the title to)
are the ones to whose image we must conform. The neurotypical mantra
"I can," based on a very narrow definition of volition, deactivates experience rather than opening it to its potential. If *I* can't, what's the use?

With carrying as the silent refrain that moves experience in the making,
this mantra begins to fall apart. Who is the "I" in the ecological field of experience in the making? How does "I" figure in the crossover Blackman writes
about, the crossover that tickles and triggers, that feels the movement in
its coloring of experience? How does "I" figure in an account such as Higashida's, where "the voice I can't control is different" (2013: loc. 182), or in
autistic Donna Williams's complex account of how humans are less bodies
than edgings: "I knew people by their edges" (1998: loc. 734)? Where does
"I" figure in Ralph Savarese's important account of autie-type as relational
activity—autie-type defined as the persistently poetic coming-to-language
of autistics who use facilitated communication. Where does "I" figure in
Lucy Blackman's assertion that "the most interesting reality in my life is the
relationship between facilitation and autism" (2013: 106)?

Facilitated communication (FC), the organization of a support system around communication used by many classical autistics who cannot communicate with their voice, usually begins with hand support but often persists long after hand support is no longer needed. Normative accounts of individual volition suggest that facilitation must mean a lack of authenticity as regards communication.[9] Indeed, a whole backlash exists which argues that the facilitators are actually doing the writing for the autistics. To be considered properly intelligent, autistics must therefore submit to endless tests that control for individual expression: they must show that their words are really their own. When asked about the importance of independence for communication in an interview, Blackman responds: "That is crazy! Communication is interdependent. It is like asking someone to waltz or foxtrot without a partner" (2013: 113).

The account of facilitation as extra to the autistic, where the "successful" autistic is the one who no longer needs facilitation, is built on a neurotypical identity politics that takes subject-based agency as its driving force. Nowhere in this account is there room to consider how *agencement* works in the *event* of communication, or even how facilitation is also part of neurotypically inflected experience. *Agencement*, it bears repeating, is not an action directed by an existing subject, but a force of distributed directionality in the event. Each event, including the event of facilitated communication, crafts tendencies toward subjectivation, sometimes leaving traces that connect to subjects in the making, sometimes not. What I want to argue is this: in the navigation of experience, no one is ever alone, and no experience ever emerges without the facilitation of a process that carries the event in its coming to formation.

Lucy Blackman's 2013 *Carrying Autism, Feeling Language* (with commentary by Mary Jane "Jay" Blackman) everywhere returns to this question of facilitation. Composed almost two decades after Blackman's first autobiographical account of coming to language through facilitation, this recent account, written after having received an MA in English literature and publishing her own fiction, is less about Blackman's need to prove her intelligence than it is about querying the neurotypical assumption that experience, and specifically its relationship to language, is inherently individual (Blackman 2001). Communication and the art of participation in the world for Blackman clearly includes the carrying of facilitation.

Carrying is everywhere present for Blackman—in the act of writing, in the walking, in the eating, in the sensing, in the perceiving. It is not a value judgment on experience, but an articulation of how experience feels, and how it fields: carrying is the expression of the relational force of movement-moving in terms of how bodies and worlds co-compose. Carrying, as the more-than, is therefore also what makes many tasks difficult. For Blackman, for instance, it comes with seemingly infinite sensory confusion and overstimulation. Most of her experience, after all, is of autistic perception, a term she uses herself. Autistic perception, for all its exquisite opening toward experience in-forming, is also an often prohibitive barrier to a neurotypical world. This is because, as I have mentioned throughout, autistic perception does not parse out or select as easily from the welter of co-composition. Autistic perception foregrounds mobility, and to cut into this mobility is singularly difficult. Techniques are of course created by all autistics to make this possible, but even these techniques do not always suffice, for not only does autistic perception—like all perception—change and morph over time, requiring a continual set of new ways of making the transition to *this* world, *this* time, it is also singularly compelling, enticing the autistic to dwell on the cusp where the world is still in-forming.[10] Recall the beauty Higashida describes. This dwelling in autistic perception can make autistics seem unengaged, distracted, when actually they are lingering in the true fullness of attention, lured by infinite complexity. A philosophy of *agencement*—where the motor of experience is activated by a directional force that facilitates a certain singularization—honors the welter, this singular complexity of a world in-forming. And it honors the lingering. Rather than denying the complexity of autistic perception, *agencement* celebrates its potential, proposing pathways through the more-than that do not reduce it, as though field perceptions were but neutral transitory effects of a solid and finite form-taking.

In neurotypically inflected experience, the more-than also plays an important role. It is simply more backgrounded. Here, the challenge is often the opposite: we neurotypicals, especially the ones interested in processual activities such as artmaking, or those of us engaged in exploring movement, must learn to develop techniques to chunk *less* quickly, and must habituate ourselves to the idea that form is not the concrete and finite structure we have likely been taught it is.[11] Our challenge is to become more attentive to how the more-than is eclipsed in our perceptions of experience and, in so doing, to become more attuned to what James calls pure experience. James writes: "My thesis is that if we start with the supposition that there is only one primal stuff or material in the world, a stuff of which everything is composed, and if we call that stuff 'pure experience,' then knowing can easily be explained as a particular sort of relation towards one another into which portions of pure experience may enter. The relation itself is a part of pure experience; one of its 'terms' becomes the subject or bearer of the knowledge, the knower, the other becomes the object known" (1996: 4). Pure experience suggests that all experience is relational, knower and known defined not in advance of the occasion but in the midst. James continues:

> According to my view, experience as a whole is a process in time, whereby innumerable particular terms lapse and are superseded by others that follow upon them by transitions which, whether disjunctive or conjunctive in content, are themselves experiences, and must in general be accounted at least as real as the terms which they relate. . . . In such a world transitions and arrivals (or terminations) are the only events that happen, though they happen by so many sorts of path. The only function that one experience can perform is to lead into another experience; and the only fulfillment we can speak of is the reaching of a certain experienced end. When one experience leads to (or can lead to) the same end as another, they agree in function. But the whole system of experiences as they are immediately given presents itself as a quasi-chaos through which one can pass out of an initial term in many directions and yet end in the same terminus, moving from next to next by a great many possible paths. (1996: 62–63)

Autistic Thomas McKean describes this well: "I don't think what I see is what you see. That is unless what you see are vague clouds and shadows of substance. . . . I am pretty good at deciphering what I am looking at now after practice but sometimes I do still have troubles, especially with colors" (in Bogdashina 2005: loc. 576). Blackman's orbit is also an account of pure experience. Recall that she describes the orbit as only hers insofar as she moves with it. It is not hers in the sense that it belongs to something predetermined as "I." It is a carrying-feeling, a vibratory moving-with. The world of pure experience orbits as much as it is orbit: it is a world felt in the nonconscious, active in edgings of experience that are more contributory than actual, real but virtual.

To activate pure experience for conscious expression is to move that experience across the carrying toward a vocabulary that stabilizes it, at least to an extent. This is extremely difficult, in no small part because the parsing requires a parsing of sensation into meaning. This challenge is one discussed by all autistics I have come across. It requires a composing-with of perception's edging into experience, a composing-with of the beneath of words.[12] Composing-with always requires a certain reorienting of the experiential. How to articulate in words sensation, rhythm, feeling?

In Blackman's case, this would already be difficult were her movements through the world predictable. But they aren't. Like so many other classical autistics, body and world co-compose to a large degree in ways that are nonlinear and unforeseeable. Higashida writes: "Your vestibular and proprioceptive senses are . . . out of kilter, so the floor keeps tilting like a gerry in heavy seas, and you're no longer sure where your hands and feet are in relation to the rest of you . . . Even your sense of time has gone, rendering you unable to distinguish between a minute and an hour, as if you've been entombed in an Emily Dickinson poem about eternity, or locked into a time-bending Science Fiction film" (2013: loc. 45). "Even before we start interacting," writes Blackman, "we are handicapped. Our eyes and brain don't always process colour and depth very well, and these are the basis of 'reading' faces. And then we have problems with sequencing movement, and this is how most people interpret body language and expression" (2013: 8). Without a clear sense of linear or metric time, without a strong sense of depth perception, with a shifting panoply of edgings of color and texture, how to field experience in a way that enables the kind of parsing necessary for so many neurotypically inclined tasks?

The world of pure experience is for all of us a shape-shifting as-yet-unparsed ecology, but for autistics, because they dwell in autistic perception more than neurotypicals do, the ungainliness of its potential is foregrounded in ways that make more apparent the necessity for *agencement*. *Agencement*, like its sister concept the minor gesture, comes from the field, from the region of experience toward which and through which the event is unfolding. In neurotypical experience, this process of the shift from the as-yet-unparsed to perception is so backgrounded that the *agencement* necessary to bring things into focus seems to occur volitionally, in the subject, in the individual body. As I have argued throughout, this is a mirage supported by the identity politics of neurotypical able-bodiedness, fed to most of us from earliest childhood by our cultural surrounds and bolstered by our education. Because this viewpoint is so pervasive, autistics are made to feel as though their way of functioning is completely off.

If instead of succumbing to the neurotypical account as ground of experience we begin with autistic perception, the focus changes. We move from the idea that the act must be directly allied to an individual's volition toward an account of *agencement*. Donna Williams explains: "Because things that were meant to be tuned out weren't, these things were all competing for processing when they shouldn't have been. I was jumping between processing the white of the page as well as the print, the flicker of light and shadow as well as the objects themselves, the sounds of the people moving about in between syllables of words being said at the same time, the rustle of clothing and the sound of my own voice" (1996: 92). The competition for processing, as Williams calls it, foregrounds the workings of *agencement* emphasizing the nonvolitional share of event-directionality. Event-directionality makes stabilizing difficult, however. Blackman explains: "Eventually as an adult I came to understand that other people could stand still because the world around them was triangulated. That is they could work out distance from something from their own depth perception. They could then feel their feet (or their bottom if they were sitting down) as another point in this metaphorical triangle" (2013: 9). Autistic perception, because of its direct engagement with the field in-forming, does not privilege the kind of triangulation Blackman believes facilitates standing still in the neurotypical population. Because parsing comes more slowly, stability remains evasive. The irony is that triangulation is not actually how neurotypicals move — it is simply how they account for their movement in the backgrounding that comes through conscious reappraisal. After the fact, in the account that returns volition to the subject, we parse our movements as though planned in advance to operate in this or that specific arrangement. In the event, however, as I outlined in the last chapter, movement has more to do with incipient choreographies of movement-moving than with subject-directed agency. At issue is therefore not simply the question of parsing, but how directionality is allied to incipiency. What might a technique look like that facilitated a kind of movement-moving that privileged the welter of autistic perception?[13]

For Blackman the world is always encountered anew, in the midst, and its infinite mobility just doesn't seem to facilitate the kinds of movement arrangements that would allow her to pass as neurotypical. It's not that there isn't also in autism the capacity for a conscious accounting of experience after the fact. It's just that, even post facto, triangulation doesn't compute. There is no stable surface, no stable ground, no fixed structure, with which she could easily triangulate. When the body-world continuum is not ruptured, an account of where one begins and the other ends simply doesn't make sense. If everything is in motion, if everything is process, feet and ground co-composing, skin and air, vision and wind, sound and depth, how to select one body, one experience, one object?

Also: "Speech grows in one for a number of reasons" (Blackman 2013: 9). What might it mean, in the context of a world that doesn't parse easily, for language to "grow in one"? What would facilitate such a growing of language? What carries language? Can the carrying, the growing of language, of speech, have different rhythms, different sonorities? Can language be in line with autistic perception? And if so, how is this facilitated?

Facilitation is usually understood as anathema to independence. In autism research and education, the term *facilitated communication* has been used, as I mentioned above, to discredit autistics' capacity to think and write. A person who needs facilitation is understood to be incapable, to varying degrees, of directing their own experience. All of these beliefs around facilitation are neurotypical to the core. With an account that begins with pure experience, where predetermined subjectivity is not at the forefront, where the event-orienting *agencement* is what moves experience, facilitation begins to mean something quite different. Is facilitation not everywhere present in experience, all along the spectrum of neurodiversity? What communication could ever happen without *agencement*? If we consider facilitation as the conduit, the *agencement* of a field of forces, what movement does not require it? What movement is not directed by it?

Lucy Blackman makes it clear that for her facilitation cannot be reduced to an active-passive relationship. Nor is facilitation strictly reduced to hands-on assistance. It does not simply mean to "create a path . . . for reaching certain objectives" (2013: 35). Quite the contrary. For Blackman facilitation is about developing a reciprocity in a field of experience that unlocks directed movement in a way that enables communication in and beyond language. "All I know is that some kind of touch or reciprocity makes me calmer, and the greater certainty of success in hitting the key that I visualize means that I can express the visual language which for so many years I had been cherishing" (2013: 35). Facilitation happens in the relation. Facilitation might for instance mean discovering together how to create what Blackman calls a "coactive sensation of touch," how to create a certain contact, hands on or off, that might stabilize vision, how to invent a certain sense of presence that can trigger an activation that in turn can propel a thought into the actualization of words on a keyboard. However it unfolds, what is most important about facilitation is that it evolves in the emergent field of relation not only of autistic and facilitator, but of the wider ecology itself continuously transformed by this collaboration.

In the context of writing, Blackman describes facilitation as regulating an impulse. Her words simply don't transfer to the keyboard easily. She writes: "In my mind I feel as if my hand is moving in the direction of each letter-key, but that impulse doesn't transfer itself to my real hand unless something is triggering the movement. By trigger, I don't mean a jerk or push. If you were to point at something, the trigger would be your intent. However the intention or motivation in my mind somehow gets lost in my body" (2013: 35). For her, touch, even a simple contact on the thigh, "is the conduit that gets some kind of impulse more organized" (2013: 35–36). How to think of this contact, of this relation, in other terms than those of the worn dichotomy of independence/dependence or volition/non-volition?

Perhaps the best place to begin is, once again, with movement. Neuro-typically inflected movement is usually taken to be voluntary. As outlined in the last chapter, the presupposition tends to be that the subject moves the movement. I want an apple, I reach for an apple, I take the apple into my hand, I move the apple to my mouth, I bite the apple. The neurotypi-cal takes this sequence for granted, believing that the motion was unfacili-tated, placing the "I" at the center of each gesture. The autistic, on the other hand, because of sequencing issues and difficulties with activation, may not be capable of "volitionally" grabbing and eating the apple. The apple *may* nonetheless get taken and eaten, but it might just as well end up staying on the counter because for some strange reason the body moved away from the table. Voluntary/nonvoluntary would be an easy dichotomy to use to separate out these two experiences. But if instead of beginning with agency we turn to *agencement*, asking not what the subject did but what the event proposed, another version of the task comes to light.

Let's say that in both cases we are in the same kitchen. The tending toward apple for the neurotypical is likely facilitated first by a sense of hun-ger. In this situation, hunger may seem solely located in the body, but it is actually an effect of the field. Think, for instance, of how often hunger strikes at the *idea* of food, even without a prior conscious sense of being hungry. In these cases the food acts as an *agencement* to hunger, activating the experience of "a body feeling hungry." This is equally the case when the food isn't actually there. When this happens the subjective aim is tuned to a virtual object. In either case, actually or virtually, pulled by the sense of hunger, you find yourself reaching. The apple becomes the facilitator for a gesture that does not strictly belong to you. This gesture is in an ecology of hunger, apple, body, movement. The apple activates it in co-occurrence with the feeling of hunger, and the reaching responds. What is emerging is an event of hunger appeasement.

In the reaching, something else happens as well. Perceptually, a parsing has occurred that singles out the apple from the counter and everything around it. This parsing, with the nonsensuous perception that accompanies it, also brings along a felt impression that the apple has a specific size, depth, weight. You see it as an object, and, in doing so, you unsee the environment with which it co-composes. This allows the reaching to be precise. You grab it, and the apple finds itself in your hand exactly as you had previously seen-felt it, or so it seems. This grabbing, which included a seeing-touch previous to the actual touching, was made possible by the hapticity in the visual perception, which provided, in advance of the actual touching, a sense of what the apple might feel like, a feeling that likely also is starting to include a preconscious tasting. Your mouth is already watering. This doubling of touch-vision mixed with the tripling of touch-taste-vision, which includes a singular parsing for hunger-apple-reaching, allows you to grab the apple and bring it to your mouth. You take a bite of it, most likely unaware of the complex movement just executed.

In the case of the autistic, things may not go so smoothly. First, hunger and impulse-control may be overlaid, leading toward actions that are more confusing than those outlined above. Blackman speaks of her echolalic tendency of saying "McDonald's" whenever she sees the large *M* of the restaurant's "golden arches." This tends to lead people to assume that she wants to eat there, when in fact she doesn't like the food. She writes:

> [In crowded restaurants] I reverted to asking for food that I associated with that kind of interaction, but this was less a request for what I really wanted to eat as a memory process. I had to make do with what I had preprogrammed, much as the way I would ask for a hamburger if I saw a McDonald's. I learned this was involuntary the day we were standing on a pedestrian crossing in sight of the big gold *M*. We were talking about where we would have lunch, and I typed, "PLEASE DON'T LET ME MAKE YOU GO TO MCDONALD'S!" As I got to "the *M* word," my voice cut in and I declaimed "McDonal'!!" while physically tugging at my bewildered companion so forcibly that we ended up through the sliding doors and in the line of surf-crazy youngsters almost before she was aware of it, and certainly before she could begin to analyze her own responses. (2013: 68–69)

Here, the lack of impulse-control becomes its own kind of foothold on experience, fostering as it does an *agencement* not directly allied to the feeling of the event at hand, but to a spectral feeling activated in the repetition of a memory. A kind of short-circuit of nonsensuous perception takes over, the past fielding the present against what the current moment desires. Two event-paths collide. The more-than is here revealed in all of its contradictions as the surplus that should have been excluded. But this is the effect of autistic perception—that exclusion is difficult. Lack of inhibition has its advantages and its disadvantages.

Say McDonalds were nowhere close by, and the impulse controlled itself enough to direct the field of attention toward the apple on the counter in the kitchen. Another challenge might still be in store. The apple might just not resolve itself clearly for perception, backgrounding itself instead in experience. The vase beside it, reflecting the sunlight, might stand out much more. In this case, the hunger *agencement* might be redirected toward a light-reflection *agencement,* thus leading the autistic's movement toward the vase despite what they initially perceived as their actual interest in the apple. This might confuse the onlooker, who might then assume that the autistic wasn't hungry, or, worse, that she couldn't distinguish between vase and apple. If this is the case, other techniques will need to be invented that facilitate the right balance between depth perception, color, tactility, hunger, and movement. This facilitation is likely going to involve another person with whom the environment in its unfolding will be navigated in ways that will morph over time based on the needs of the relation.

Placing "carrying" in front of words is a way of inscribing, for thought and language, this necessity of relation, foregrounding how each act necessitates its own variety of carrying across the field of experience. For Blackman, touch does a lot of this carrying. Speaking of how touch facilitates the process of coming to language, she writes: "What I did not realize then was that when I tried to plan [a] movement, I was unaware of the exact position of my fingertip in time and space, much as I was uncomfortable walking on slopes because my foot and my sight were sufficiently out of sync to make me uncertain as to the exact moment my sole could start to bear my weight" (2013: 23). Facilitation, she continues, was capable of "unlock[ing] purposeful movement" (2013: 21). "A hand on my arm or wrist makes a comfortable control, and a continual challenge by the difficulties of sustaining my concentration makes coherent language overcome the intellectual cascades of my internal thoughts" (2013: 35). Even when Blackman no longer needed hands-on facilitation to write, she continued to feel strongly that the "reciprocity" of facilitation was essential. To repeat: "All I know is that some kind of touch or reciprocity makes me calmer, and the greater certainty of success in hitting the key that I visualize means that I can express the visual language which for so many years I had been cherishing" (2013: 35).

This kind of facilitation, seen as the creation of a relational field for experience in the making, is quite common in the everyday. Think of the university classroom, of the ways in which pedagogical tools are used to activate discussion, to pull thinking out from the group, to generate new movements of thought. This collective act is understood to be a key part of education, and yet the facilitation needed by many autistics is still too often understood as interfering with what is considered the "natural" independence key to learning, as though thinking-with or composing-with were not at the very heart of experience. This is not the only irony, as Blackman rightly points out: where the neurotypical is assumed to be inherently relational in terms of intersubjectivity, the autistic is far too often still wrongly considered to be incapable of relation. This makes the critique of facilitation particularly paradoxical: "It is . . . funny . . . that the principal objection—but I have to say not the only objection—to hands-on support is the possibility of influence, and the likely feeling of close emotional connection, both of which are typically [regarded as] deficits in autistic relationships!" (2013: 39).[14]

For Blackman, another role the facilitator plays involves "standing in" to activate her visual field. Blackman's technique for this is "to make the other person a part of my visual field" (2013: 81). She reasons that the necessity comes from having lived with "real problems knowing exactly where my connectional limbs and trunk were, where they would move to next, and, even more frighteningly, where they had last been positioned" (2013: 81). Facilitation, and specifically the body of the facilitator, is here used as an enabling constraint—it allows the field of vision to settle around a specific area. This kind of "mirror imaging," as Blackman calls it, controls her "visual fluctuations" by setting up a living boundary or an orbit around a certain situation. Blackman does this by borrowing what she perceives as her facilitator's body-space to secure a landing in a more coherent fielding of time and space. Blackman describes it this way:

> [Imagine] a hypothetical little old lady walking in the same direction I am. As she moves, so do I because her body is now mine—that is until her movement is out of kilter with what I project as the future. In that

event I float off, or if really terrified, . . . I scream and then bite my hand on the existing scar below my thumb. . . . I can't see why other people cannot understand that people with autism need the other partner in an interaction to do what my mother describes as "socialize for two." (2013: 81)

If we take Blackman's example and read it from the perspective of a body-world continuum—"[not] knowing exactly where my connectional limbs and trunk were, where they would move to next, and, even more frighteningly, where they had last been positioned"—it seems to me that what is happening in the mirroring is not the taking-over of a body, but a doubling onto a becoming-body. Blackman must do this to land because the dimensions of her existence are still orbiting. In this case, the facilitator acts as the *agencement* for the bodying.

Socializing for two is therefore always less "for two" than about the more-than one. It is the more-than that is sought in the mirror imaging, a more-than that can act as both the activator and the stabilizer of movement-moving. The facilitator acts as a bridge, Blackman suggests. This is not a bridge between two precomposed subjects, but within a field of tendencies that work together to create a momentary boundedness. This boundedness continues to carry a certain mobility, tending in ways that facilitate the production of sense out of welter without negating the fullness of experience. When facilitation tunes toward communication, the bridge similarly allows sense-making to keep its complexity. This is not to suggest, of course, that writing is the only way to communicate. Autistic experience is lively with forms of communication "beneath the words." As Amelia Baggs has shown in her important video *In My Language*, all language cannot be reduced to the spoken/written word. What of the language of movement, of texture, the language of sound merging with color, of edgings vibrating to the rhythm of weather patterns, of thoughts lingering in the prearticulation where words are not yet? Sadly, too often, written communication trumps nonconscious forms of communication: in a largely neurotypically inflected society, written communication continues to be what most strongly demarcates the "intelligent" from the "nonintelligent."[15]

COMPOSING-ACROSS

Facilitated Communication opens up experience, accommodating the *agencements* of the field in its co-composition. And yet because agency and volition are so prized in the neurotypical worldview, it continues to be seen as a counter to "really" individual expression. Many autistics therefore find themselves having to fiercely guard their so-called "independence" from facilitation, not because they don't honor the relation, but because with it they are not perceived to be so-called independent thinkers. Speaking of the relentless focus on the question of independence, Blackman writes: "I find it really difficult to understand why other people are more interested in the process of what I produce than the content. I have sometimes felt that being a demo is not the point of my being a student, and really that this kind of discussion is more about wanting to be 'normal' (which I don't) than about what I am achieving in terms of pure intellectual thought" (2013: 80).

This common belief that facilitation and self-expression are counter to one another is compounded by the fact that studies of autistic language done by neuroscientists, for instance, see it as a necessity to segregate autistics from their facilitators during the experiment, thereby underscoring the accepted belief that true language emerges independently of another person. The result is that autistics tend to grow language always with an overhanging belief imposed from the outside that the language will only truly be theirs if they can write in a vacuum. Not only does this completely undermine the notion of how relation activates the complexity of experience, it also comes with another danger—that autistics may lose the poetic voice that emerges with facilitation. Blackman writes: "I love getting flashes of autistic perception. This is a picture of what my brain makes of what I see, hear and feel from my skin, balance and body-in-space. That is who I am. That is how I felt almost continuously as a child. As an adult I can see and hear much more like typical people, but my underlying brain processes are still quite different" (2013: 117). Forcing herself to write independently has in some senses been a loss for Blackman, who feels that the emphasis on certain ways of coming to cognition has depleted her experience of autistic perception and, with it, affected the poetics of autie-type. Likening language to "a chaotic sludge [which] transforms to clarity in intent" (2013: 106), Blackman mourns her poetic voice:

My inside language had changed completely. Previously my mind and my voice had warbled and cooed in unison, and my typed language and my visual words were positively reinforced by that magical process. . . . In a path to rather more typical language processing, I lost the most precious gift of the poetry of thought, of a dancing and swooping mind and body. . . . Of course, I still had most wonderful control of words and I drew great pleasure from fluent prose writing, but had more thought-work in putting the characters in my brain through my finger and onto a screen. In my mind I had words, but I had not retained the gift of autistic enjoyment to the extent I had before. (2013: 106)

The irony is that the backlash against facilitated communication (the be-lief that the facilitator imposes their voice onto that of autistics) and the re-sulting insistence that autistics prove their ability to write "independently" seems to have been yet another way of segregating autistics from their po-tential. As Blackman argues, it isn't facilitation that backgrounds her sin-gular poetic voice, but precisely the focus on independence and its em-phasis on "more typical language processing." As she became more and more capable of writing beyond the register of facilitation, it seems that her language began to lose the rhythm and tonality of autie-type, the composing-with of autistic perception. For instead of deadening the liveli-ness of perception's complexity, as language is wont to do, autie-type seems to be singularly capable of funneling it, carrying into language its prearti-culations. This is not to say that the force of autie-type is completely absent in Blackman's writing. It is simply to note that it is backgrounded in com-parison to the poetic writings of autie-typers such as Tito Mukhopadhyay, DJ Savarese, Larry Bissonnette.[16] Is it because in their case facilitation con-tinues to be more present, either in the form of direct contact or in a more relational sense? Or is it because Blackman's writing has been influenced by her academic experience? Either way, let there be no question: Lucy Black-man remains not only a poetic thinker, but also a poetic writer. Everywhere in her prose carrying the feeling moves thinking in the act, composing-across the complexity of how to articulate the unsayable in the said.

THE FEELING OF EFFORT

In my attempt to think beyond the neurotypical aligning of volition, in-tentionality, and agency, I am of course not suggesting that no will is pres-ent in movement. Volition always has a role to play in the way expression arises. A shift away from the triad simply suggests that volition is not where we usually assume it is: it is not ahead of experience, but *in* experience, in the between of the conscious and the nonconscious, actively composing in the ecology of practices. This has ethical consequences. What is at stake in the pervasive account of aligning subject-based volition to experience? What happens to our unwavering belief in neurotypicality as the measure of human existence when its central tenets are put into question? Similarly, what happens to the narrative of neurodiversity when we stop speaking of the involuntary—or, better said, the nonvoluntary—as though it were other to "better" ways of moving, of thinking, of speaking?

William James's essay "The Feeling of Effort" is very interesting in this regard. Beginning with an account of neurotypical experience, James explores the place of volition in movement. Here, he proposes a vocabulary for feeling that refuses to be led by a concept of subject-based agency, exploring instead, like Whitehead does, how the aim, active *in the event*, creates the conditions for the act in its unfolding. The concept James will later use to articulate this—terminus—is not yet part of this early piece, and yet its presence is everywhere felt. For this reason, it is useful to become familiar with the sway of the concept of terminus as it plays out in his later *Essays in Radical Empiricism* before turning to how volition is theorized in "The Feeling of Effort."

In *Essays in Radical Empiricism*, James writes: "Knowledge of sensible realities . . . comes to life inside the tissue of experience. *It is made;* and made by relations that unroll themselves in time. Whenever certain intermediaries are given, such that, as they develop toward their terminus, there is experience from point to point of one direction followed, and finally of one process fulfilled, the result is that *their starting-point thereby becomes a knower and their terminus an object meant or known*" (1996: 57). In "The Feeling of Effort," James similarly sees the feeling as occurring "inside the tissue of experience." Yet, and this is where his later work assists in the understanding of the text, while created in the relation—"made by relations that unroll themselves in time"—the feeling (of effort) only comes into itself as such through the motor of a terminus. The terminus is what vectorizes the *agencement*, pulling the force-of-form to singular expression. This motor is not the end point in any direct sense. It is a force that activates the movement. The terminus acts as the pull, setting up the field that becomes the knower-known relation. Here, once again, there is not yet a predetermined subject or object, but rather, as Whitehead might hesitantly say, recipient and provoker.[17]

The field's concern for its parsing cannot be separated out from what is experienced. The pull of the terminus moves the event, but *is not the event*. How the event comes to be, its subjective form, is how the knower-known relations have resolved themselves for this singular occasion, coming together in just this way. The coming-into-itself of the event is therefore simply goal-oriented. The terminus is not the end as seen from a neutralized external perspective. The event, as I have emphasized before, is not pure process: it is actively disjunctive—a becoming of continuity, not a continuity of becoming. "In a world where both the terms and their distinctions are affairs of experience, conjunctions that are experienced must be at least as real as anything else. They will be 'absolutely' real conjunctions" (James 1996: 60). How the conjunction or the disjunction operates is how the event has come to be. Importantly: without disjunction there would be no cut, no cleaving, no inflection, no minor gesture. No event would ever come to be. Terminus is the operative pull of this coming to be, not its predetermining result.

James continues:

> So much for the essentials of the cognitive relation, where the knowledge is conceptual in type, or forms knowledge "about" an object. It consists in intermediary experiences (possible, if not actual) of continuously developing progress, and, finally, of fulfillment, when the sensible percept, which is the object, is reached. The percept here not only *verifies* the concept, proves its function of knowing that percept to be true, but the percept's existence as the terminus of the chain of intermediaries *creates* the function. Whatever terminates that chain was, because it now proves itself to be, what the concept "had in mind." (1996: 60–61)

If the autistic grabs the vase instead of the apple, it is too simple to say that her body didn't go where her mind wanted to. What actually happened is that the apple, as terminus, despite being the motor of the event, was supplanted by the insistence of the light-ray, which monopolized the event in its in-forming to such a degree that it ended up becoming the conduit for the reaching-movement. This, as James might say, was what the event ended up "having in mind." This is not to deny the frustration of the hungry autistic who now has a vase in her hand. It is to emphasize that the voluntary/involuntary dichotomy devalues the complexity of what has actually happened. Neurotypical experience is not so different. Its ends simply look different because what the event had in mind more often seems to cohere with where the movement was initially going. The challenge is to understand the *agencement* of terminus as an activity of the field itself, and to become aware of the backgridding necessary, even on the neurotypical end of the spectrum, to make the terminus conform in its generative pull to the subjective aim.

The feeling of effort can perhaps assist us in understanding this play, in the terminus, between *agencement* and aim. James begins "The Feeling of Effort" by asking where effort comes from in the movement act. Is the effort situated in the body? Can it be consciously aligned to a muscle? Does the effort "come from us"? Or must we think the feeling of effort of a movement more in alignment with the notion of "the effort to remember, . . . the effort to make a decision, or to attend to a disagreeable task" (1969: 154)?

For James, the feeling of effort is less connected to a specific tissue or muscle mass in the body than to the field of experience. The feeling of effort, like the percept above, *creates the function*. "Our motions are the ends of our seeing," writes James. "The marksman thinks only of the exact position of the goal, the singer only of the perfect sound, the balancer only of the point in space whose oscillations he must counteract by movement, . . . each variation in the thought of the end . . . functionally correlated with the one movement fitted to bring the latter about" (1969: 156). It is the terminus that activates the sequencing which, as James underlines above, "now proves itself to be what the concept 'had in mind'" (1969: 61). Movement folds through movement, its parsing activated not by a volition occurring outside the event, but by the very flow of movement-moving nonconsciously coursing through the pull of the terminus.

But what happens when the terminus is a region of incipient activity? Turning to autistic perception, where the terminus is less differentiated, or more mobile, the question is to what degree the reaching for the vase instead of the apple must be read as a movement gone wrong. In this context, how do we understand James's proposition that "the end conceived will, when these associations are formed, always awaken its own proper motor idea" (1969: 157).

Termini—or motor ideas—are infinite and variable. The terminus is not one movement, one object reached-toward, but a region of variation. For the neurotypical, whose ability to parse-in-movement is more available than it is for the autistic, the parsing can seem projective, and therefore voluntary. The apple rests in the hand because there was the intention to take the apple off the counter. But how many times have you landed at the refrigerator with the door open and wondered what you were there for? How many times have you wandered around the bedroom looking for your reading glasses, the ones hanging around your neck? Movement only seems voluntary in the neurotypically inflected reflective consciousness because it connects with what the concept had in mind to the degree that there is a lack of feeling of effort. It all seems straightforward, you think, as you bring the apple to your mouth. The movement comes from me.

And yet there's still the issue of the open fridge. "The end conceived . . . [will] always awaken its own proper motor idea." That a movement will, in conscious reappraisal, be found to have aligned to what the event had in mind is what makes the movement seem subject-directed. This habitual reappraisal of how we've gotten somewhere (I don't know how I got home—I must have walked one step after the other), or how we've brought the food to our mouths (I don't remember eating, but yes, I must have moved my hand to my lips repeatedly), or how we've typed this chapter (I don't remember seeing the keys in their singularity, but since the essay is in front of me, I must have fingered the right keys), is how we develop our sense of intention and volition. Because the frame of the movement for the most part fits our idea of where we needed to go, we align the two and are confident the movement emerged from our personal directives. And when this fails, for instance when we fall on the ice or miss our mouths with our water glass or type the wrong letter, we laugh and say we must have been distracted. But attention is more complex than this, and this is what we learn from autistic perception.

When you missed your lips with your water glass, you weren't unattending. You were likely strongly in attendance, just not to the glass. There was a deviation, unrecognized in the moment, but with consequences for the future. At that moment of what you might like to call distraction, the region of the motor idea expanded, and with that expansion the precision you are accustomed to in your movements was jeopardized. Consider this event of attention fielding to be the common experience of many autistics. If "the end conceived awakens its own proper motor idea" and the motor idea is in the field of relation, it follows that the movement activated may not conform to expectation.

Dancing, I experience this often. Take an example from Argentine tango. The relational movement at the core of an improvisational salon tango practice depends on preacceleration, the virtual force of a movement-moving before it is consciously felt as such.[18] This feeling is shared. If I am leading a movement and I want the other dancer to follow, the movement in its incipiency must be felt in advance of its becoming an actual displacement, for it is into this incipiency that her movement will move. The incipiency cues the movement-moving. What I am leading is not a form, but a force, a tendency, and it is to this tendency that her movement must tune. This tendency is enveloped in a terminus, but a terminus to a large degree activated in the relation. When it happens, as it often does, that a second tendency "distracts" me, my partner will move into the tendency I didn't think I led. She will move into the movement-moving of a deviation-on-terminus. In response to the follower moving to tendency, the leader must reorient, often facilitating an orientation neither could have predicted in advance. This is relational movement at its best.

This is similar to what happens with autistics. When Naoki Higashida writes, "We are outside the normal flow of time, we can't express ourselves, and our bodies are hurtling us through life," what he is suggesting, it seems to me, is that life's pull, the complexity of the field of activity of autistic perception, is so strong that he often has trouble feeling the sense of a single directionality within it (2013: loc. 583). The *agencement* of potential as region is simply too strong, and with it, the motor ideas or termini simply too diverse. And so he jogs and walks "to refresh" his body, and "once refreshed, I kind of feel back home within myself. My sense of gravity is restored, and that calms me down" (2013: loc. 688). Like Blackman's touch, Naoki Higashida's running quiets down the field of sensation, and with this quietening, the pull of the field into a single tendency comes more clearly to attention. Here, momentarily, a sense of agency is felt. But this is not subject-oriented agency. It is agency in the event, agency facilitated by the conditions of this singular field of experience coming into itself just this way. The *agencement* moves the event in a way that makes attention *field* in conformity with it. When we speak of not "paying attention," when we accuse autistics or anyone else of not being attentive, we are often undervaluing the complex modalities attending, in the event, to experience in the making.

HOW THE FIELD ATTENDS

There is often a presumption that volition and attention work together. In this kind of analysis, attention is seen as that which is consciously directed by the subject. But attention, as I've suggested elsewhere, is more distributed than it is situated.[19] It emerges in the event, activated by the force of directionality the event calls forth. This dance of attention — where it is the field that attends and attention is less parsed than environmental — is alive in autistic perception. It is true to say that in the more neurotypically inflected experience, attention does land more easily, but even here it would be a misnomer to suggest that it lands on a predefined subject or object. Attention lands as a vector, activating the subjective form of the event, not a precategorized subject. Like the feeling of effort, attention is culled from the event, its force a pull that organizes the event into the tendency it will follow. Moved by the directedness of the event's force-of-form, attention dances toward the singular experience it has revealed.

In James's "The Feeling of Effort," there is a strong emphasis on how the terminus and attention work together. Again, a subject-oriented approach is critiqued: will is not the *activator* of the pull. Attention is fielded relationally rather than directed by a volitional subject: "Our standing up, walking, talking, all this never demands a distinct impulse of the will, but is adequately brought about by the pure flux of thought" (Lotze in James 1969: 183). Thought, James underlines, is "intercurrent" with action. The movement of thought, which James sometimes calls a "representation," is not representation in any usual sense. The movement of thought is not a precomposed image. It is a virtual event, an activity on the edge of movement, a preacceleration. Attention is in the relation.

In autistic perception, it's not that attention is diluted, as is often assumed.[20] It's that attention is magnified. Higashida writes: "When a color is vivid or a shape is eye-catching, then that's the detail that claims our attention, and then our hearts kind of drown in it, and we can't concentrate on anything else" (2013: loc. 513). The pull of the field is extremely powerful. As Donna Williams writes:

> Most people perceive objects beyond their grainy, sheeny, reflective, flowing, coloured or opaque appearances, beyond their smooth, raspy, cold, textured tactile experience, beyond the sounds of their chinking, thud-thud, tap-tap surfaces when impacted upon, their sweet, or savoury or chemical tastes or smells, their flexibility, solidness or bounce when bitten into or impacted upon. Most people experience the object before the art of it. They whisk over the sensory into the literal and experience themselves not just in the company of glass, wood, metal, paper, plastic derived objects but beyond this to the significant; that these objects are for cooking, decoration, belong to their neighbour, require a good clean etc. (1998: loc. 93)

This overlooking inherent to neurotypical perception, this unattending to the field, leads to a very limited exploration of what the field can do. The attending only to the parsing undermines the potential of the relational field, leading the neurotypical to perceive far less of what appears around them. How can we learn from autistics to become more attuned to the dance of attention? What techniques can we put into place to open the world to its constellations of potential?

Within neurotypical accounts of perception and attention, with the focus on volition, intentionality, and agency, comes a recurrent account of the sensory-motor. James explains:

> The ordinary "voluntary" act results in this way: First, some feeling produces a movement in a reflex, or as we say, accidental way. The movement excites a sensorial tract, causing a feeling which, whenever the sensorial tract functions again, revives as an idea. Now the sensorial and motor tracts, thus associated in their actions, remain associated forever afterwards, and as the motor originarily aroused the sensory, so the sensory may now arouse the motor (provided no outlying ideational tracts in connection with it prevent it from so doing). Voluntary acts are in fact nothing but acts whose motor centres are so constituted that they can be aroused by these sensorial centres, whose excitement was originally their effect. (1969: 189–190)

The sensory-motor is only a small aspect of how perception, attention, and movement work together. A movement felt is a movement-moving. The movement does not flow in a cause-effect scenario that begins with a push from outside itself. Rather, the movement is felt from the middling of its incipient directionality. It is felt because of how it lands, and how it lands is what constitutes its subjective form. Movement does not operate in any absolutely directive sense. It is not linear: it is more recursive—what the feeling has felt, what becomes *this* led and followed movement in the tango example, is how movement-moving has moved into its relational aim, spurred by a terminus that is less its goal than its activator. A movement learns from what it has done, of course—this is where technique comes in—but it is never limited to that learning. Virtuality courses everywhere in movement-moving, its preaccelerations affecting how attention fields and perception settles. Movement therefore cannot be considered as limited to the circuit of the sensory-motor. Movement is by its very nature generative of difference.

Autistics speak of the difficulty of associating one movement-event to another. Whereas a neurotypical might consider every coffee cup to be one and the same in the sense that a coffee cup is anything in which coffee can be drunk, an autistic might be more likely to see the complexity of each cup's difference, challenging the sensory-motor assumption that repetitive tasks easily sort themselves into habits that can then be taken up in a different scenario. Blackman explains: "[As a child] each time I was introduced to [a] practical skill by new baby-sitters, and later by teachers, it was as if it were the very first time, because the concrete movement in my own body was in a completely different universe from the world of chaotic artifacts which I was expected to place in some kind of arbitrary order. In the fullness of time some of these tasks became comprehensible, but this did not mean that I was motivated to perform the jobs that all these people considered important" (2013: 34). The field remains open to potential variation. There is no question that this can be discouraging for autistics, who often mention that they would like the repetition of everyday tasks to come more easily to them.

What autistic perception makes clear is that there is a gap in movement-moving that opens up the sensory-motor to difference. This gap is more about an overfeeling than a lack. It is Forsythe's *what else*, or, in Kawakubo's procedural fashioning, the *remains*—what is left over in the passage from force to form. For the neurotypical, this unparsable share tends to get overlaid by inhibition: it is what we actively *don't* experience. This is why we don't tend to perceive it. James suggests that the feeling of volition is less about volition than about inhibition. This is why we feel it as effort: the feeling of effort comes from actively *not* doing, *not* seeing, *not* moving. The effort is felt because of what *didn't* happen. What we call voluntary is what we have actively *not* done.

The inhibition does not necessarily happen at the level of conscious thought. When I don't pick up the vase instead of the apple, it's not because I am actively resisting it. It's because the apple stands in instead. The vase's presence for perception is being inhibited. In the apple's standing-in, the vase has actually disappeared, or at least unappeared for perception in lieu of the apple-directed hunger-act of reaching-toward. In autistic experience, not only is there, due to issues with impulse control, much less tendency for inhibition, but autistic perception is by its very definition more field-oriented. As a result, field attention is more present and the termini, as I suggested above, are more tuned to their incipient variability. This tends to take movement out of its presuppositional feeling of volition, thereby de-emphasizing the perceived difference between volition and nonvolition, the conscious and the nonconscious. As Donna Williams writes: "When you resonate with an object or surface it is not so much that you have reached out for that object or surface but that it has, somehow, reached into you" (1998: loc. 603). In its effortlessness, autistic perception reaches into the you you are becoming. What isn't asked often enough is: what else, what other kinds of communication, what other potentials for movement, what other fields of encounter are possible from this uninhibited field of relation?

If movement is by nature nonvoluntary, generated to attention by its dance in the between of subjects and objects forming, a new definition of facilitation must be invented. The facilitator is not there to prevent the autistic from wallowing in autistic perception. Facilitation is the force of activation in the relation that allows autistic perception to come to expression. Here, relation must be seen as a relationscape, not as a neutral between of subjects and objects in the model of interaction. How the field parses for experience is always connected to how its relations play themselves out.

To place facilitation in the relation means that the facilitator must become aware of the more-than of experience informing. It is this more-than that the facilitator-autistic relation will field. Carrying is key here. The facilitator must also become active in the carrying that occurs across fields of difference, from edge to language, from intensity to form. Facilitation is therefore something that the autistic and the facilitator must learn together. Theirs is a sociality for two.

A beautiful example of what facilitation can do is seen in the poetic writings of what Ralph Savarese calls autie-type. Autie-type, as mentioned above, is the name Savarese gives to the rhythm and metaphor he sees in autistics who use facilitated communication. Sometimes this poetics weaves through their writings for years after they have come to typing (Larry Bissonnette is a good example of this), other times, as in Blackman's musings on the loss of her poetic voice, the autie-type rhythms can become backgrounded. Either way, certain patterns in the writing are palpable, and this even across cultures and languages.[21]

Autie-type, completely composed by the autistic, relishes the relational pull of facilitation: the writing happens in the between, the between not only of autistic and facilitator, but also of autistic perception and language. In this kind of writing, the facilitator may or may not have direct hands-on contact with the autistic. The direct contact is not the issue. Facilitation is in the milieu: it is a virtual carrier of language, but only in the sense that it activates and nurtures the relation. Care for the field in its unfolding is directly felt, it seems to me, in the writing that ensues.

Listen to the following sentences written by autistics:

Emma Zurcher-Long: Decision to sing while thinking about birds with peek-a-boo tail feathers brings happy feelings. (July 2014)[22]

Larry Bissonnette: Powerfully pushed by climate change, Hurricane Sandy has lapped up on the shores of Mitt Romney's campaign and plopped large loads of wet sand on, looking more shallow now, ideas about privatizing lots of, lending helping hand to less privileged, people assistance. (November 2012)

Larry Bissonnette: The plight of more apples freezing in the orchards of Vermont is what I more immediately worry about but I do peer out beyond our borders and see our connection to the powerful forces of political change. I see the changing of old guards to new patterns of compassionately spread laws to protect our environment and freedoms to be looked on equally regardless of our differences. (January 2013)[23]

DJ Savarese: yes. dearest sad dad you heard fresh self and freshly responded deserting your fears and just freed sad dear saved me. yes. yes. yes. Yes. (November 2007)[24]

Autie-type is a rhythm all its own. Ralph Savarese sees this poetic voice as a starting point for creating a bridge between the autistic and the neurotypical. He writes:

> Poetry might constitute a linguistic meeting point for different neurological types, one that honours both the "unlost instinct" (or pure sensory knowing) of autistics and the symbolic proclivities of neurotypicals. The sensual splendour of the world, to which classical autistics are so attentive, shows up by analogy in poetry. Patterned syntax and sound, pulsating rhythm, emotional prosody as a function of tone — these things might induce non-literate autistics to grapple with poetry's semantic content and, thus, functional language in general. In turn, neurotypicals might be restored to their sensing bodies, and as a result, better understand the sensory world of autistics. Each half of the neurological divide would commit itself to an ethic of neuro-cosmopolitanism. Each would concede the need for repair. (2012: 210)

Ralph Savarese, a poet himself and a committed autism advocate, has worked with emergent autistic poets to assist them in honing this craft, which, while it does seem to come all of its own, deserves the same kind of attention we give to neurotypical writing. "I've already seen significant development in my son's fledgling work," Savarese writes, speaking of DJ Savarese, a young autistic poet who is now the first nonspeaking student in creative writing at Oberlin College, "and together we have vowed to perfect our mutual craft. As [Larry Bissonnette] would say, 'It's past point of personal hobby' or, for that matter, unwitting obsession" (2008: 6). Speaking of poetry as a meeting point between those on the spectrum of neurodiversity, Savarese writes of the necessity of crafting a certain neurocosmopolitanism that might facilitate the carrying of modes of perception across what is too often perceived as an unbridgeable divide. This might in turn create modes of speaking and listening that could weaken neurotypicality as the dominant paradigm of human existence.

In an interview between autistic Tito Mukhopadhyay and Ralph Savarese, Mukhopadhyay explains how poetry figures in his writing practice. "I use verse when I get bored of writing a dragging paragraph. I usually do. Sometimes the topic becomes too thick and intense to write. I get nagged by this boring state that the topic holds for me. Because of that, I seek a way out to recharge my senses. A verse makes me free. A verse recharges my senses. And a verse can distract the eyes and ears of a reader. It is easy to read it that way" (Savarese 2010). Poetry, for Mukhopadhyay, is both a way of coming into language and remaining in the world of words, of growing words alongside perception in the making.

Savarese asks Mukhopadhyay: "What can poetry communicate that prose cannot? You've spoken of your 'love for designs' and 'repetition' when writing? Can you speak more about this love? Beyond the fact that rhyme and repetition seem themselves somehow autistic (in a good way), what do they communicate?" (Savarese 2010). This question is key, it seems to me, in the question of facilitation. How does the movement of rhythm, the tone or taste of words, all of these present in poetry, facilitate the passage from autistic perception to language-based communication? Mukhopadhyay responds: "They make me think about a sound pattern. Designs can be visual and designs can be formed in sound. When I write, 'A rock lay by the stream,' it becomes less of a design than something like . . . A rock lay waiting / By the stream / Ready to step inside, / So that it could begin / An existence—Of a stepping stone! (Whatever be that meaning.) The words make the rock become more than a thing to ignore" (Savarese 2010).

More than a thing to ignore might also be understood as "more than a thing to inhibit." For the neurotypical, might this mean that poetic writing is a facilitator in its own right, activating perception in a way that bypasses the habitual inhibition that occurs in the parsing of the event? For there is no question, it seems to me, that poetry, with its foregrounding of rhythm and sonority over a bald attempt at sense-making, acts as facilitator in autistic writing, and perhaps even autistic experience in general: in the same interview with Savarese, Mukhopadhyay mentions that it was William Blake who helped him learn to tie his shoes![25]

Savarese continues: "I love the phrase 'more than a thing to ignore.' Thinking of my first question, I'm almost tempted to say that the fragments of poetry are prose becoming autistic, if by autistic I mean patterned, musically perseverative. Why shouldn't the things of this world, which neurotypicals often blithely pass over, be keenly, even fiercely, observed? Perhaps the medium of poetry best captures with its interruptive force the rapt attention of autistic engagement. Is there an ethics of seeing implicit in your answer, an injunction to take note, and if so, does it apply to people with autism?" "I cannot speak for other autistic people," Mukhopadhyay responds. "But with my eyes, I may select a fraction of the environment—say 'that shadow of a chair' or 'that door hinge over there'—and grow my opinions and ideas around it. This creates a defense system for my over-stimulated visual sense organ. (Call it keen observation or any other name.) Maybe poetry happens to grow around these things. Sometimes I write them and other times I discard them because there is 'too much to write'" (Savarese 2010).

Poetry facilitates an opening onto the as-yet-unparsed. It moves with the as-yet-uninhibited, finding ways to bring to composition the force-of-form. In this way, it does exactly the opposite of chunking—it hinges back to the field, as Mukhopadhyay might say. Certainly, there is always a certain inhibition that happens in the selection that is language, but poetry remains more open to the rhythm, the tone, the color of autistic perception than do most other kinds of written language. If we see poetry, as Savarese argues through his concept of neurocosmopolitanism, as the "first facilitator" across the spectrum of neurodiversity, might autie-type be an example of the facilitation of facilitation? For the words come best, despite their arrival *just this way*, across communities and cultures, in their singular metaphorical, or, better, metamorphical complexity, with Mukhopadhyay's mother always a few meters away, with DJ Savarese's facilitator by his side, sometimes touching his wrist or sharing in the holding of a pencil, with Larry Bissonnette's facilitator's hand on his shoulder, with the touch that gives Lucy the sense of a body-dimensionality. The words come best *in the relation*.

What I am suggesting is that poetry's inherent capacity to facilitate the creating of bridges between autistic perception and language is multiplied, in autie-type, by a degree of facilitation that explicitly activates the relation necessary in making the transition from perception to words. This second degree of facilitation carries feeling across modes of expression. It facilitates the opening in language of affective tonality, making felt, in the words, what I have elsewhere called the prearticulation of language in the making, the beneath of words.

In neurotypically inflected experience, affective tonality is felt in the minor gestures of the environment's tuning to expression. When affective tonality is most powerful, it becomes difficult to parse experience into words. But a lot of the time, this is not a major issue. Because of the inherent capacity for inhibition, if necessary the affective tonality can be backgrounded, its minor gestures ignored. In autistic perception, however, affective tonality is dominant, active in every aspect of how perception fields. This means that the act of backgrounding necessary to parse words from feelings is more difficult. It also means that the autistic is more aware of the struggle inherent in the task of making intelligible that which is so alive, teeming with the forces of affect. This is where the facilitation of facilitation can make a difference. In the facilitator-autistic relation, the facilitator stands in to modulate the environment so that the affective tonality can co-compose in ways that in turn will facilitate the parsing of experience into language. With this *agencement* the autistic is capable of fielding the environment in a way that attention can momentarily settle. This happens in the relation, which is why Blackman emphasizes that facilitation is much more than simply physically assisting with a task.

The facilitator must therefore be seen as more than a person. They are carriers, conduits for the modulation of an eventful environment. Through a relationship of trust and understanding, autistic and facilitator work together to tune the complexity of communication—both linguistic and nonlinguistic—toward language in ways that do not erase the complexity of the minor gestures at the heart of field attention. Affect is not cast aside, but is conducted in ways that better align with written communication. Facilitation is possible only if the autistic does not feel judged. He must be secure in his intelligence and trust the facilitator to help him create the conditions for communicating his singular way of seeing the world. But even more than that: he must trust the relation's capacity to create pathways for a composing analogous at least in some regard to his lived experience of autistic perception. In this facilitation of facilitation there emerges the capacity for the environment to come to attention in a way that facilitates the invention of new modes of expression.

In the most troubled years of FC, when facilitators were accused of writing in the autistics' stead, the focus tended to be restricted to method.[26] Recall how Blackman, writing about her path to eventually composing on the keyboard without hands-on facilitation, expresses with frustration that over the years people seem to have been more interested in how she typed than in what she typed. She writes: "Most of the next fifteen years [from the onset of typing with facilitation] were really a continual path to typing with minimal physical contact, not because I personally thought it important but because it was essential if I was to establish my own achievement in the eyes of others" (2013: 106). Whitehead's words ring loud: "Some of the major disasters of mankind have been produced by the narrowness of men with a good methodology" (1929: 12). Method is anathema to autistic perception. It is also allergic to relation, for it relies on the ability to stand outside the event and judge it from without. No method will ever embrace the facilitation of facilitation. The *agencements* of attention in its fielding, the contributions of minor gestures, the metamorphical playfulness of poetic writing: these will be resisted by method's desire to orient experience according to the false problems of questions already posed. Against method! screams autie-type, and we should heed this call.

This is a political call. The identity politics of neurotypicality are too dominant and too pervasive for autistics to fight alone. Carrying the feeling is not an individual practice. It is collective at its very core. Carrying the feeling is a relational movement, relational in its capacity to make felt the intercurrent, as James might say, of the in-act and the act. Here, where life is not directed by inhibition, and modes of expression entangle the conscious and the nonconscious, where the nonvoluntary finds its poetic voice, new ways of living become imaginable. What if parsing weren't foregrounded as the method for successful living? What if the nonvoluntary weren't such a threat? What if freedom were more widely understood as the creative force of the in-act? What if the minor gesture, in its poetic force, were not only attended to, but composed with? *What else* would we be capable of thinking-feeling?

Donna Williams writes:

I was deeply mesmerized with all things aesthetic and sensory from at least 6 months of age. Being meaning deaf, I saw musically. Being face blind, I was attuned to movement patterns. Being object blind and context blind, I'd tap everything to make noise, to hear its "voice," flick it to feel its movement, turn it to experience how it caught light, toss and drop and shred and snap and sprinkle grass, sand, twigs, leaves. I'd lick and run my hands and face over surfaces, wrap myself into fabrics. I'd align myself with symmetry and lines, mold myself into forms to feel their shape as them, stare at colors and lights and shapes trying to become one with them.[27]

Facilitation aligns. Recall the proposition from chapter 5 that movement is made possible by the interrelation between the intervals of movement-moving and the collective capacity to align to them, in the event. Note that what facilitates the coming-to-perception in Williams's account above is exactly the same kind of aligning to the interval, an aligning that involves the placing-into-relation not of the objects, but of what they can do, how they sound, how they feel, what they taste like. Facilitation aligns to the field of relation, to its tastes, its feelings, its immanent shapings, and it carries this differential potential across the productive abyss of nonconscious and conscious experience. The alignment to a mobile environment in the making: this is facilitation. Let this be our challenge: to collectively create techniques to carry further the alignment to difference alive in autistic perception.

IN THE ACT

The Shape of Precarity

In a text on Guattari, Deleuze speaks of two Guattaris, a Pierre and a Félix
(he was called Pierre-Félix). According to Deleuze, one was "like a catatonic
head, a blind and hardened body perfused by death, when he takes off
his glasses," the other "a dazzling spark, full of multiple lives as soon as he
acts, laughs, thinks, attacks." These are the two schizophrenic powers of an
anti-I: the petrification and the spark.

—Peter Pál Pelbart, "Un droit au silence" (my translation)

Shortly after Félix Guattari's death, Peter Pál Pelbart—schizoanalyst, philosopher—wrote a text that he ended with an anecdote about Guattari's
inherent doubleness, wanting to get at the complex overlapping, in Guattari, of what Deleuze calls "petrification and spark." The anecdote recalls a
trip taken to La Borde, the clinic where Guattari worked and lived. Pelbart
writes:

> In 1990, passing through France, I went to visit the La Borde clinic with
> Guattari. We left Paris by car. He asked me to drive, and while I was
> driving, he slept, like that, without his glasses, petrified, as Deleuze de-
> scribes it. It is well known that sleep can confer on the sleeper the guise
> of a rock, but the next morning, awake, Guattari hadn't changed. . . .
> I had never seen him this way, even during his many trips to Brazil. To
> escape from a situation that made me a bit uneasy, I decided to go out
> and walk with my partner. Guattari wanted to accompany us. We walked
> in silence. It was late afternoon. We listened to the noise of our steps and
> far-away sounds. Evening was coming. A neighbour greeted us. Every-
> thing was bucolic. And then we found ourselves in front of a pigsty, in
> silence. So I tried to converse with the pigs, using my limited knowledge

of oinking. Slowly, the dialogue became more animated, and Guattari began to participate in the conversation. He laughed a lot, and he oinked a lot. I think that in this day and a half spent at La Borde, this was the only conversation we had—oinked. In front of the pigsty. With a collective of pigs, in a veritable becoming-animal. I left the next morning, troubled. I told myself that a thinker has the right to remain catatonic, to become dead, to oink from time to time, if it please him or her. To tell the truth, since that day, I never stopped envying this catatonic state. Sometimes, of my own accord, I find myself this way, to the distress of those around me. . . .

[Later, in] re-reading some of his texts, I understood that his silence at La Borde was not only a petrification, but also an immersion in a kind of chaosmosis, the mix of chaos and complexity, of dissolution, where what is to come must be engendered. (Pelbart 1994: 10; my translations throughout)

DEPRESSION

In his work on the alignment of depression and capital in neoliberal times, Bifo (Franco Berardi) uses the figure of Guattari—with whom he collaborated when he was also a committed activist—to explore the relationship between depression and the act. Focusing on Guattari's "winter years," Bifo wonders how depression affected Guattari's work as a philosopher and activist. Bifo suggests that Guattari's depression not only left him paralyzed in the face of life, but put him in a situation where he gave himself to causes that he didn't really believe in. Depression, it seems, not only affected Guattari's capacity to be in the act, it transformed his ability to direct his energies in ways that would best move his practice forward. This inability to demonstrate volition with respect to what was most important to him— activism, Bifo argues, is in part tied to Guattari's own reluctance to discuss the relationship between activism and depression. Bifo explains:

I sensed and was convinced that in the final decade of his life, Guattari had at several points undertaken a political commitment in which he did not deeply believe, that is, seeming to him to be his duty to "hold on," that he needed to get past this rather difficult, regressive period, etc. And I perceived a kind of exhaustion in his will to maintain a position. So in this phase of the Guattarian itinerary, what seemed to me to be missing . . . is a reflection about depression. While one would need to enter more fully into this concept, depression basically is a disinvest-ment of libidinal energies in facing the future, in facing the world. Natu-rally it's a question of a pathology, but not only that. Or rather, in short, the pathology is not something to be undervalued. (Berardi 2008: 158)

Bifo, in a move that troubles me, then turns to Guattari's writings to explore the omission of depression. In what seems to me a classic psycho-analytic gesture, Bifo analyzes Guattari's work to see how or why depres-sion was excluded. Turning to Deleuze and Guattari's writing on desire in *Anti-Oedipus*, he writes: "Félix did not pay attention to depression, neither as a philosopher, nor as a psychoanalyst. And we can easily understand why. The methodology [*démarche*] of the *Anti-Oedipus* is not easy to rec-oncile with the possibility of delving into depression. Depression is not just a condition among others, in which a machinic unconscious is assembled, made of existential and chaosmotic fragments proceeding from anywhere to everywhere else. The *Anti-Oedipus* does not know depression; it contin-uously overcomes, leaping with psychedelic energy over any slowing down and any darkness" (Berardi 2008: 11). Personalizing Guattari, and making the dangerous assumption that writing is an act that should somehow mir-ror the writer, Bifo continues his analysis: "Félix knew this, I am sure, but he never said as much, not even to himself, and this is why he went to all these meetings with people who didn't appeal to him, talking about things that distracted him and making lists of deadlines and appointments. And then he would run off, adjusting his glasses to consult his overflowing daily planner. And here again is the root of depression, in this impotence of political will that we haven't had the courage to admit" (Berardi 2008: 13, translation modified).

Using his friendship with Guattari as a guarantor (basing his account of Guattari's mental state on what went on between them as friends), Bifo undertakes a specious project, specious because based on a proposition that uses the personal as the central figure instead of acknowledging, at the very outset, Guattari's lifelong investment in the prepersonal and the group subject. In so doing, Bifo backgrounds the operational nature of Guattari's writing, both alone and with Deleuze. When Bifo suggests, for instance, that their writing on the machinic unconscious is only about "a continuous overcoming," that their writing refuses "any slowing down and any dark-ness" he misinterprets, it seems to me, the machinations of desire as out-lined in *Anti-Oedipus*. *Anti-Oedipus* is not an account of light over darkness, but one of the in-act. The in-act is not positive or negative: it is *productive*.

This is Deleuze and Guattari's definition of the desiring machine. Depression is not missing from *Anti-Oedipus*—the complexity of neurodiversity is everywhere present in the account of what schizoanalysis can do. What's absent is a separating out of depression from neurodiversity as a whole. *Anti-Oedipus* foregrounds transversal operations that propose techniques for creating desiring machines that are capable of cutting through existing systems to create new modes of existence. Psychoanalysis is one of the systems *Anti-Oedipus*'s desiring machines cuts through. *Anti-Oedipus* works against any account that would restratify a neurotypical identity politics or any normative identity structure. For theirs is an exploration, *avant la lettre*, of what neurodiversity can do, not of its failings. To suggest otherwise would be to discredit the force of schizoanalysis so central to Guattari's practice.

Guattari would resist, it seems to me, any normative account of depression that would situate it in the agency-volition-intentionality triad. When Bifo speaks of Guattari's inability to use his time well, he provides exactly this kind of normative account of depression: he proposes that Guattari demonstrates a lack of volition, suggesting that in the best-case scenario, Guattari would have the kind of will, the kind of agency, that would better direct his decision to align himself to projects "that matter." Guattari would also be suspicious of an account of depression that kept it within the bounds of the subject. He would be more likely to align himself, it seems to me, to the following account of depression, which, unlike Bifo's analysis, refuses to situate depression solely in the individual, making it a collective problem for which a group-subject must be invented. This is a story narrated by Andrew Solomon, who has written widely about his struggle with depression. In this story, Solomon recalls a trip to Senegal where he experienced a ritual for depression called *ndeup*.

The *ndeup* is a ritual practice that involves the careful crafting of techniques to create a group-subject. As with all rituals, certain precise procedures have to be followed. Solomon explains: "The first thing we had was a shopping list. We had to buy seven yards of African fabric. We had to get a calabash, which was a large bowl fashioned from a gourd. We had to get three kilos of millet. We had to get sugar and kola beans. And then we had to get two live cockerels, two roosters, and a ram." These effects were purchased at the market, except the ram, which was bought by the side of the road. Then Solomon headed to what would become a full-day ritual. By early afternoon, the ritual really got going.

And the sound of drumming began—the drumming I had been hoping for. And so there was all of this drumming, and it was very exciting. And we went to the central square of the village, where there was a small makeshift wedding bed that I had to get into with the ram. I had been told it would be very, very bad luck if the ram escaped, and that I had to hold on to him, and that the reason we had to be in this wedding bed was that all my depression and all my problems were caused by the fact that I had spirits. In Senegal you have spirits all over you, the way here you have microbes. Some are good for you. Some are bad for you. Some are neutral. My bad spirits were extremely jealous of my real-life sexual partners, and we had to mollify the anger of the spirits. . . .

The entire village had taken the day off from their work in the fields, and they were dancing around us in concentric circles. And as they danced, they were throwing blankets and sheets of cloth over us, and so we were gradually being buried. It was unbelievably hot, and it was completely stifling. And there was the sound of these stamping feet as everyone danced around us, and then these drums, which were getting louder and louder and more and more ecstatic. And I was just about at the point at which I thought I was going to faint or pass out. At that key moment suddenly all of the cloths were pulled off. I was yanked to my feet. The loincloth that was all I was wearing was pulled from me. The poor old ram's throat was slit, as were the throats of the two cockerels. And I was covered in the blood of the freshly slaughtered ram and cockerels.

After a short break, the ritual continued. Solomon was told to place his hands by his side and to stand very straight and erect. They proceeded to tie him up with the intestines of the ram.

In the meanwhile [the ram's] body was hanging from a nearby tree, and someone was doing some butchering of it, and they took various little bits of it out. And then I had to kind of shuffle over . . . and take these little pieces of the ram and dig holes, and put the pieces of the ram in the holes.

And I had to say something. And what I had to say was actually incredibly, strangely touching in the middle of this weird experience. I had to say, "Spirits, leave me alone to complete the business of my life and know that I will never forget you." And I thought, *What a kind thing to say to the evil spirits you're exorcising: "I'll never forget you."* And I haven't.

Solomon continued to speak this mantra. He was then given a package of the millet with which his body had earlier been rubbed and told that he should sleep with it under his pillow that night. He was also instructed to bring it to a beggar "who had good hearing and no deformities" the following morning. Once the millet had exchanged hands, he was told "that would be the end of my troubles."

> And then the women all filled their mouths with water and began spitting water all over me — it was a surround-shower effect — rinsing the blood away from me. It gradually came off, and when I was clean, they gave me back my jeans. And everyone danced, and they barbecued the ram, and we had this dinner. And I felt so up. I felt so up!

Solomon's participation in the ritual places us in a completely different relation to depression's working than does Bifo's account. A Rwandan who encounters Solomon several years later articulates this difference succinctly. After hearing of Solomon's experience in Senegal, this man says:

> You know, we had a lot of trouble with Western mental health workers who came here immediately after the genocide, and we had to ask some of them to leave.
>
> [The problem was that] their practice did not involve being outside in the sun, like you're describing, which is, after all, where you begin to feel better. There was no music or drumming to get your blood flowing again when you're depressed, and you're low, and you need to have your blood flowing. There was no sense that everyone had taken the day off so that the entire community could come together to try to lift you up and bring you back to joy. There was no acknowledgment that the depression is something invasive and external that could actually be cast out of you again. Instead, they would take people one at a time into these dingy little rooms and have them sit around for an hour or so and talk about bad things that had happened to them. We had to get them to leave the country.[1]

This is the key detail Bifo's analysis of Guattari's winter years misses: that all of Guattari's theory and practice emerges from the necessity to bring out the collective resonance of the event, to see illness not as a personal problem to be analyzed outside of the field of relation, but as an event, an ecology, that necessitates the kind of minor gestures that populate the ritual described above, minor gestures that tune the event to its more-than. As outlined so comprehensively in *Anti-Oedipus*, the force of schizoanalysis is that it creates the conditions for opening the event to its productive schism rather than reducing it, as psychoanalysis would do, to a regressive account of a preconstituted past. Time, in schizoanalysis, is of the event, in the group-subject of its co-composition. Any technique created in the name of schizoanalysis needs to be able to craft event-time, to move the event to an operative more-than that persuasively cleaves it with the *instauration* Souriau argues is at the heart of the creation of new modes of existence.

In his years of practice at La Borde, Guattari was everywhere involved in the creation of such techniques that activate the ecological core of experience's more-than. In his writing, where chaosmosis, as Pelbart suggests, is probably the strongest description of the force of petrification and spark, Guattari aligned himself again and again not with pathologizing accounts of neurodiversity, but with the kinds of rituals described above, rituals that involve bringing out the community, rituals that activate the minor gesture, rituals that transform the very ground of experience.

NEOLIBERAL DEPRESSION

Bifo's argument, over the last decade, is that neoliberalism has left the body disempowered, our collective nervous system besieged by the forces of a capitalist takeover. We can, and indeed, we must no longer act. As outlined by Gary Genosko and Nicholas Thoburn in their introduction to Bifo's *After the Future*, Bifo argues that "activism is the narcissistic response of the subject to the infinite and invasive power of capital, a response that can only leave the activist frustrated, humiliated and depressed" (Genosko and Thoburn in Berardi 2011: 7). Activism, Bifo suggests, is a desperate attempt to ward off depression. "But it's doomed to fail and, worse, to convert political innovation and sociality into its opposite, to 'replace desire with duty'" (2011: 7–8).

Bifo sees the current landscape of depression as "a product of the 'panic' induced by the sensory overload of digital capitalism, a condition of withdrawal, a disinvestment of energy from the competitive and narcissistic structures of the enterprise. And it's also a result of the loss of political composition and antagonism" (Genosko and Thoburn in Berardi 2011: 8). Depression is the collective effect of a social tendency, as "born out of the dispersion of the community's immediacy. . . . When the proliferating power is lost, the social becomes the place of depression" (Berardi 2008: 13). In the past, autonomous and desiring politics were actively co-

composing, whereas now, in neoliberal times, such proliferating power is lost, and the act—activism—is incapable of resurrecting it. It's difficult not to see Nietzsche's last men rearing their heads in this dark account that has so completely lost the élan of the in-act. "The earth has become small, and on it hops the Last Man, who makes everything small. His species is ineradicable as the flea; the Last Man lives longest" (1954: 5). This is certainly not Bifo's hope, nor is it what moves his writing, but I wonder whether the account of depression he proposes doesn't end up cementing a reactive nihilism, a cynicism that tends, despite its position "against," to strengthen the status quo. Being out of act, out of service—isn't that the very posture of *ressentiment*?[2]

Despite my respect for Bifo as an activist and thinker, I hope to challenge his account of depression, particularly his account of the relationship between depression and activism. I will do so by paying close attention to the story told by Pelbart of the chaosmosis at the heart of the "not-me" which is inhabited at once by petrification and spark. Taking the act not simply as that which is in the service of the neoliberal economy, but more broadly as the force of the event through which minor gestures course, and taking depression out of the context of an individual sadness, I want to explore the operative passage between petrification and spark.

In doing so, I do not want to discredit the fact that there is extensive turmoil in the face of neoliberalism's excessive takeover of what a body can do. There is no question that these are troubled times. Nor do I want to suggest that depression isn't terrible. It is. What I want to do, always with the ndeup ritual in mind—with its belief that depression carries a more-than that needs to be attended to in its differential force; with its acknowledgment that it is only collectively that new modes of existence can be invented—is propose that depression operates in event-time, not outside the event in a passive relationship to the *what was*. If we start here, the inquiry leads somewhere profoundly different than the path Bifo outlines. Against Bifo's account of the neoliberal takeover of the act, this different path leads us toward a rethinking of the in-act, as I've attempted to do throughout, a rethinking that leads to a neurodiverse exploration of the *what else* at the heart of experience.

In my own struggle with depression, it has become clear to me that what we call depression is nothing if not plural: it expresses itself in an infinity of ways from sadness to hunger, from loss to anguish and anxiety, from a frenetically quiet inner panic to a full-fledged panic attack, from the stillness of a body incapable of moving to an agitated body. For some, all of these tendencies are present, which leads depression to be less about a state that could properly be described than a terrible decalibration that makes it impossible to compose with the world: everything feels out of sync. This is the case for me: the experience is one of not being able to connect to the movements that surround me, not being able to match their rhythms. The best description of this is a sense of misalignment with time. The world moves too quickly or too slowly in ways that are difficult to connect to. It is as though there were multiple speeds and slownesses in continuous unalignable disjunction. Medicated, and with many years of various kinds of treatments, the sense I have is that it has become easier to align and that the field of relation now stabilizes enough to allow a co-composition across worldings. I can participate. But the one who participates is not a personalized "I." It is a schizo-I, like Deleuze's account of "Pierre" and "Félix," a schizo anti-I in the sense that there is no absolute integration, but instead an emergent potential for co-composition across experiential time both quick and slow. Living with depression, and acknowledging the necessity for facilitation in its many relational guises, is an art of participation, and what has emerged through this art of participation is a belief in the world as a mobile site to which alignments are possible.

These alignments are not given. They must be crafted. Opening the way for a co-composition that potentially aligns itself to times in the making requires, I believe, a rethinking of the act of alignment itself. It requires what Guattari would call a group-subjectivity, an account of a collective that exceeds the personal. To connect with this collectivity in the making requires techniques for inventing modes of encounter not simply with the human but in the wider ecology of worlds in their unfolding. For the collective as a mode of existence in its own right is not the multiplication of individuals. It is the way the force of a becoming attunes to a transindividuation that is more-than. To become-collective is to align to a chaosmosis in a way that prolongs the capacity of one body to act.

This is not to underestimate the pain, difficulty, even horror of depression, nor to underplay how complex misalignments make us feel our silence on the one hand, or our anxiety on the other as signs of our decalibration with the world. Nor is it to argue that drugs against depression in its widest definition should be handed out as liberally as they are. It is simply to inquire, across my own experience, and through the moving reading of Peter Pál Pelbart's account of Guattari's petrification, how else we can facilitate emergent collectivities without turning to the neurotypical habit of pathologizing difference, or, in the case of depression, of too quickly aligning the nonvolitional to passivity.

> Neurodiversity is about accepting that there is no normal human brain, that being different is okay, and about working together to discover how we all can participate to the best of our abilities in our lives. We are optimistic that with the proper supports and accommodations, positive attitudes, acceptance, inclusion, and encouragement, that every (autistic) person is able to communicate, interact, and contribute to society while meeting individual needs and respecting one's sense of self and personal rights.[3]

It is very common for autistics to suffer from the disabling anxiety that is on the spectrum of what is treated as depression. It is also very often asserted by autistics that they have a strange sense of time: "Time perception in autism spectrum disorder is a part of the complexity of the condition. Many people with autism experience fragmented or delayed time perception, which can present challenges to social interaction and learning."[4] What I want to do by aligning the autistic's perception of time to the perception of time in the wide array of depressive disorders is not to suggest that we are all autistic, or that all autistics are depressed, but to return to neurodiversity to think about the complexity of experience. In doing so, I want to turn once more to the concept of autistic perception to explore how depression—as the experience of time's differential—is itself on the continuum of autistic perception. This, I hope, will open the way for an alignment between autistic perception and schizoanalysis.

Autistic perception, as I have described throughout, is a direct experience of relation, a worlding that makes felt the edging into itself of experience. This makes it difficult for autistics to have a strong sense, at any given moment, of a time separated out from the event-time of their perception. Metric time, time counted, is often difficult to get a sense of. Of course autistic perception of time varies as much as autistics themselves do, but there are some salient characteristics. For instance, those on the spectrum "experience a delay in how they process certain stimuli, including time. It can sometimes be hard for them to comprehend that hours have passed. For example, a person with autism who has echolalia may hear a phrase in the morning and repeat the phrase hours later out of context." "Anecdotal reports suggest that individuals with autism have trouble gauging how much time has passed, and parsing the order of events."[5] Speaking of her autistic son with ADHD (and wondering where the two conditions meet), Emily Willingham similarly emphasizes a strange sense of time: "One area of overlap is their sense (or lack thereof) of time and timing. They both show delays in responding to spoken questions or requests. When their peers learned to tell time in elementary school, they were completely at sea, unable to instinctively comprehend the passage of time. Even now, in their adolescence, the question 'What day is it?' is frequent, as is 'What are we having for lunch?' within an hour of having had lunch."[6]

Within depression, a similar sense of the untimely is at work. Steve Connor writes: "People with severe depression have a disrupted 'biological clock' that makes it seem as if they are living in a different time zone to the rest of the healthy population living alongside them, a study has found."[7] Personal accounts support this research: "When I am depressed I feel like time goes slowly, yet at the same time I feel like I—or anyone else—has hardly any time to live at all. It feels as if time is running out."[8] "Yes, days go past slower and more boring feeling like everything's going to drag on. On the other hand I can feel like life going too fast and the years are flying by and start getting depressed thinking not long to live now etc."[9] "You cannot remember a time when you felt better, at least not clearly; and you certainly cannot imagine a future time when you will feel better. Being upset, even profoundly upset, is a temporal experience, while depression is atemporal" (Solomon 2001: 55).

If autistic perception is the direct perception of experience in-forming, it is also, as I suggested above, a direct perception of time, but not metric or measured time. It is the direct experience of the time of the event. Event-time is experiential time, time felt rather than abstracted. It is the time of the oinking in Pelbart's story. It is the moment in its alignment to itself, to its enfolding. It is not time in the sense of a pastness that can be recorded on the present. It is the now felt in its entirety, in its untimely infinity. And so it passes too slowly, or it moves too fast, oscillating in a time always of its own uneasy making.

LANGUAGE

When experience resists external organization according to a metrics of time, the linearity of language's enunciation is invariably affected. The experience is that of words blurring, of the impossibility of composing a thought that will survive articulation. As I discussed in the last chapter in relation to autie-type, for the autistic, especially one on the classical end of the spectrum, where motricity is affected such that vocal cords cannot be properly located to permit speech, or where impulse control makes it difficult to direct speech toward what the autistic wants to say, language comes slowly, finger by finger, on the keyboard. But it also comes slowly experientially, moving around images that are closer to metaphors (metamorphoses) than direct statements. As autistic Larry Bissonnette writes: "Typing is like letting your finger hit keys with accuracy. Leniency on that is not tolerated. Am easily language impaired. Artmaking is like alliance people develop with their muscles after deep massage. You can move freely without effort" (in Savarese 2012: 184).

Shifting in and out of autistic perception, language comes in fits and starts, in a time all its own. Watching Chammi communicating in the film *Wretches and Jabberers* (dir. Geraldine Wurzburg, 2010), a film that follows two autistics, Tracy Threscher and Larry Bissonnette, in their travels to meet autistics in India, Japan, and Finland, we see a familiar scene: Chammi types, one letter at a time, while his mother facilitates not only by touching him but also, as is often necessary with facilitated communication, by vocally encouraging him to continue when he becomes anxious. One sentence is typed. And then Chammi pushes the chair away, runs into the next room, waves his fingers in front of his face, vocalizes. For someone unfamiliar with autism, it would seem he has completely lost interest in the conversation. But soon he returns to his chair, where, out of the frenzy of the movement, another sentence is typed. When asked about why he needs to move around like this, Chammi types: "Killingly hard to figure out, the pattern of movement I need to type my thoughts."

Movement makes time, makes time felt. It activates the field in its emergence, making felt how spacetime composes with the time of the body, in the bodying, and, in this case, with the time of language. But let us not forget that the time of the body is doubled, petrification and spark, on a spectrum that is precarious at both ends. As I did elsewhere, I'd like to think of the time of the body in the moving as the shape of enthusiasm.[10] Think the shape of enthusiasm not as a personalized body that is enthusiastic, but as the experience of bodying that shapes the event and is shaped by it.

The shape of enthusiasm is itself a spectrum that swings in an oscillation that moves from the potential energy or the energy-in-waiting of petrification, to the expressive, potentialized energy of the spark. The shape of enthusiasm gestures toward the more-than in the event at both ends of the spectrum, foregrounding how the in-act is operational both in its initial activation and in its coming-to-be as this or that. This is an enthusiasm, a chaosmosis, not with life already engendered, but in the very act of engendering. At the petrified limit, an enthusiasm held in abeyance, absolute movement, energized potential. At the exuberant limit, an enthusiasm fully expressive, in the moving.

Chammi's frenetic movement between sentences foregrounds a bodying that takes the shape of enthusiasm, a bodying here attuned to and in excess of, the articulation of words. This is shaping that defies description, at once anguished and exuberant, frenzied and ineffable. Movement here is itself expressibility, not a deviation from language, but its extension, in co-composition.

Amelia Baggs writes of this experience of the movement of thought in terms of patterns. Through a focus on body language, she proposes that we rethink the neurotypical stance of placing linguistic articulation as primary in the act of communication. For her, the shape of enthusiasm is always before and between language.

> There are entire groups of autistic people out there who communicate with each other using our own unique forms of body language that are different from nonautistic body language, different from other autistic people's body language, specific to ourselves, specific to each other. Who communicate best reading each others' writing, looking for the patterns that exist between the words, rather than inside the words themselves. Who communicate best by exchanging objects, by arranging objects and other things around ourselves in ways that each other can read easier than we can read any form of words. Who share the most intimate forms of communication, outside of words, outside of anything that can be described easily, in between everything, seeing each other to the core of our awareness. Who see layers upon layers of meaning outside of any form of words.[11]

Baggs also speaks of *feeling* patterns: "But I can see the patterns of movement in other people, including cats, whether or not I see them well in the usual forms of visual perception. And those patterns of movement tell me more than any word ever could."[12] These feeling patterns are felt expressions of a language in the making that has not yet expressed itself in words, a language closer to Bissonette's statement above regarding painting: "Artmaking is like alliance people develop with their muscles after deep massage. You can move freely without effort." This is nonverbal communication, but it is also more than that. It is a shape of enthusiasm in the sense that it creates a bodying, a feeling of experience in the moving that invents its own time and takes that time, operating mostly at the nonconscious level. Baggs emphasizes this when she says that "forms of nonverbal communication I understand best are unintentional, in fact. That's one reason tests using actors don't work on me. I know an autistic woman who failed a test of nonverbal communication because it used actors and she kept describing their real feelings instead of their acted ones."[13]

Patterns emerge, and in their emergence they create new kinds of expression in the making, new shapes of enthusiasm in the bodying. As Chammi's coming-to-words through movement makes clear, language is in the moving. Language moves in the shape of an enthusiasm that lingers precariously at once on the side of anxiety, where there is always worry that communication will prove impossible, and on the side of a kind of overpowering Spinozist joy that undoes language of any pretense of linear representation, redefining what communication can be. In a post titled "The Obsessive Joy of Autism" Julia Bascom writes:

> One of the things about autism is that a lot of things can make you terribly unhappy while barely affecting others. A lot of things are harder.
>
> But some things? Some things are so much easier. Sometimes being autistic means that you get to be incredibly happy. And then you get to flap. You get to perseverate. You get to have just about the coolest obsessions. . . .
>
> It's that the experience is so rich. It's textured, vibrant, and layered. It exudes joy. It is a hug machine for my brain. It makes my heart pump faster and my mouth twitch back into a smile every few minutes. I feel like I'm sparkling. Every inch of me is totally engaged in and powered up by the obsession. Things are clear.
>
> It is beautiful. It is perfect.
>
> Being autistic, to me, means a lot of different things, but one of the best things is that I can be so happy, so enraptured about things no one else understands and so wrapped up in my own joy that, not only does it not matter that no one else shares it, but it can become contagious.
>
> This is the part about autism I can never explain. This is the part I never want to lose. Without this part autism is not worth having.[14]

The words just can't do it on their own: the feeling, the carrying feeling, is so excessive, the quality of its shaping too exuberant to be formulated. Hence the rhythm of autie-type, its force of the metaphorical, a mobility that dances before it signifies.

Depression in its alignment to anxiety petrified is not without vitality affect. Nor is it without movement. It is as uncontainable as the spark of its opposite. But its quality is different, and with this difference come different effects. For its shape is always closing in on itself. Direct perception of movement-moving is hampered. It's like walking in molasses. If the shape of enthusiasm is the tremulous field of expression itself, its exuberance, depression is the field's calcification at the limit where expressibility is closest to foundering, especially when called on to order itself into a linguistic articulation. There is simply nothing to say. But there is something to oink. Within the register of uneasy communication, the opportunity to body, to sound, to express in a collective voicing is nonetheless available, and it is this that Pelbart hears that afternoon at La Borde, and it is also this, I believe, that we often hear in the words that align to autistic perception. For the spectrum that precariously balances between petrification and spark is extraordinarily mobile in its tending to one or the other extreme, and perhaps especially so in autistic conversations where each word, each letter typed, is a reactivation that must relocate the otherwise dislocated, multiplying body.

Citing Anne Donnellan, Ralph Savarese writes about the challenge autistics experience in "staging the customary relation of the senses and body parts, which must subtly cooperate to produce the seamless integrity of neurotypical functioning. The tricks that autistics employ to compensate—touching something to make sight useable, for example—reveal the necessary relation: there are no discrete faculties. As the drive to pattern links distinct entities through a process of visual or auditory comparison, the equivalent shows up in language through the practice of touch-based typing. Touch literally coordinates thought, and not just any kind of thought: rather, sensuous, relational thought" (Savarese 2012: 188). Language comes relationally and remains relational: the process of facilitated communication, as suggested in the last chapter, only emphasizes what is everywhere the case: to act is never to act alone. Facilitation takes many guises. For those whose body refuses to organize itself, it acts as an organizing force, it "coordinates thought, and not just any kind of thought: rather, sensuous, relational thought." For there is nothing more frustrating, I'm certain, than when "ladle of doing language meaningfully is lost in the soup of disabled map of autism." Facilitation opens this "disabled map of autism," thanks to a "potholder of touch" (Bissonnette in Savarese 2012: 189). And in the mix of the thinking-feeling-become-writing, the poetic voice of autie-type emerges, caught, always, between petrification and the spark.

The schism between expression and enunciation, the intense passage between petrification and spark, the shape of enthusiasm that bodies, these are schizoanalytic tendencies. Or, to put it differently, the schizoanalytic, the "non-I" of the double which expresses itself as the schizo-flux in *Anti-Oedipus*, can be felt in the bodying-forth that composes at the edges of language where the movement of thought is most active. Schizoanalysis composes with autistic perception.

Autistic perception, as I have suggested before, emphasizes a modality of perception shared by all, but felt directly by so-called neurotypicals only under certain conditions. Depression is one of those conditions. Exuberance is another. In these conditions, what is felt is the precarious edge of existence where experience is under transformation, where the field of expression still resonates with its own becoming. Falling in love is an example of an event where the shape of enthusiasm overtakes what is thought of as the boundedness of the subject to foreground the opening the field of relation provokes. The deep silence of depression, where the world seems to be infolding, or the inner anguish of anxiety, where speeds and slownesses seem to be out of sync with the world at large: these are also events where the relational field vibrates and the sense of a preconstituted self falls away.

This state of vibratory composition, where self and other are not yet, and where the categorical does not take precedence, is very much what Deleuze and Guattari describe as the eventful field of potential. This field of potential is not embodied by the personalized schizophrenic. As they repeat throughout *Anti-Oedipus*, their interest is not in this or that schizophrenic—"someone asked us if we had ever seen a schizophrenic, no, no, we have never seen one"—but of a schizoid pole in the social field. Over and over, they emphasize that schizoanalysis is not about the production of a schizophrenic, but about the schizophrenic process (Deleuze and Guattari 1983: 380). Of course, Guattari worked daily with schizophrenics, but not with "the" schizophrenic, not with schizophrenia as a general idea. Indeed, all of the therapeutic techniques at La Borde emphasized the singularity of a given therapeutic event: there was no generalized therapeutic matrix. This is what Deleuze and Guattari emphasize throughout *Anti-Oedipus*: schizoanalysis reinvents itself through each of its desiring operations. It cannot be contained or described: it is always in the act.

This attention to the difference between the schizoid pole and the production of the schizophrenic as an individual is similar to the distinction

I make between autism as a medical category and autistic perception. I am not making a value judgment on autism when I describe autistic perception, nor am I suggesting that all of autism can be subsumed under its mantle. Rather, I am drawing attention to a perceptual tendency that seems to be extremely pronounced within the autistic community, and also present in each of us who figure elsewhere on the spectrum of neurodiversity. This perceptual tendency reminds us that there is no preconstituted body that stands outside the act of perception, and that objects and subjects are eventful emergences of a relational field in emergence.

Schizoanalysis, as Guattari emphasizes in an interview after the publication of *Anti-Oedipus*, "introduces into analytic research a dimension of finitude, of singularity, of existential delimitation, of precariousness in relation to time and values" (in Genosko 1996: 136). Unlike psychoanalysis, it does not seek to "discover" the unconscious, but asks it instead to "produce its own lines of singularity, its own cartography, in fact, its own existence" (1996: 137). And it does so not through the individual, but through the prepersonal force of the group-subject, a collectivity through which experience becomes multiple. To bring to it the language of autistic perception is to emphasize how the schizoanalytic process foregrounds the becoming-multiple, in an emergent ecology, of the shape of enthusiasm. Not this body, this experience, this identity, but a collective field-effect of relationscapes that map themselves out according to emergent cartographies that exceed this or that subject or object. Experience makes itself felt as multiple, and it is out of this multiplicity that an account of its effects can be expressed. Like the conversation with the pigs, where the force of the oinking exceeds one person's voice, or even one person's idea of what constitutes a conversation, the becoming-multiple of experience through the group-subject allows a fractured, complex, and expressive field of enunciation to emerge. This field resists interpretation: it cannot be explained away. In Guattari's words: "The term 'collective' should be understood here in the sense of a multiplicity that develops beyond the individual, on the side of the socius, as well as on this side (so to speak) of the person, that is, on the side of pre-verbal intensities that arise more from a logic of the affects than from a well-circumscribed, comprehensive logic" (in Genosko 1996: 196).

Schizoanalysis is a practice that reorients itself continuously around the intuition of a problem, in the Bergsonian sense. Its mantra is "What can a body do?" "We cannot, we must not attempt to describe the schizophrenic object without relating it to the process of production" (Deleuze and Guattari 1983: 6). Always linked to desire (also in the mode of production), schizoanalysis taps into the force of a bodying that shapes experience into its exuberant potential, exuberant not in its attachment to a subject, but exuberant in its chaosmosis, in the force of its expression across the precarious chasm of petrification and spark. A productive, material intervention emerges that takes the site of expression as exemplary of *what it does*, not what it fantasizes. The goal is not to locate the symptom. What happens, as Whitehead might say, happens, and it is how its effects resonate that makes the difference. Speculative pragmatism. Not what you think you see, but how the seeing materializes, and what it does. So you don't perceive chairs? Sit on the ground instead. The face doesn't form? Follow the light effects. Writing refuses to come linearly? Mobilize the words in the moving. Stand! Run! Jump! Wave your arms! Huddle, vocalize: whatever it takes. Because this is where the thinking happens, this is where language resides, a language that does not need to come out in words, a language in the bodying.

A language in the bodying takes the shape of enthusiasm: it shapes desire in the moving. "A truly materialist psychiatry can be defined . . . by a double operation: introducing desire into the mechanism, and introducing production into desire" (Deleuze and Guattari 1983: 22, translation modified).

DESIRE

This is where Bifo gets it wrong, it seems to me, positing as he does desire as a counterpoint to depression or panic. He writes:

> The process of subjectivation is based on conditions that have dramatically changed in the forty years since the publication of Deleuze and Guattari's *Anti-Oedipus: Capitalism and Schizophrenia*. Reading that book was a defining moment in my intellectual and political experience, in the first years of the 1970s, when students and workers were fighting and organizing spaces of autonomy and separation from capitalist exploitation. Forty years after the publication of that book the landscape has changed so deeply that the very concept of desire has to be re-thought, as it is marking the field of subjectivation in a very different way.[15]

According to Bifo, Deleuze and Guattari's concept of desire "is in itself a force of liberation, and thus we did not see the pathogenic effects of the acceleration and intensification of the info-stimuli, that are linked to the formation of the electronic infosphere and to precarization of work."[16] And yet Deleuze and Guattari are at pains throughout *Anti-Oedipus* to emphasize that desire is *not* reducible to a force of liberation. As Guattari explains in an interview after the book's publication: "Our conception of desire was completely contrary to some ode to spontaneity or a eulogy to some unruly liberation. It was precisely in order to underline the artificial, 'constructivist' nature of desire that we defined it as 'machinic': which is to say articulated with the most actual, the most 'urgent' machinic types. . . . Desire appears to me as a process of singularization, as a point of proliferation and of possible creation at the heart of a constituted system" (in Genosko 1996: 128). No mode of existence is outside the workings of desire, Deleuze and Guattari argue. "In truth, social production is desiring production itself under determinate conditions. We maintain that the social field is immediately traversed by desire, that it is the historically determined product of desire, and that libido has no need of any mediation or sublimation, any psychic operation, any transformation in order to invest the productive forces and the relations of production. There is only desire and the social and nothing else" (1983: 29, translation modified). To think the shape of enthusiasm in its precarity is to emphasize the materiality of Deleuze and Guattari's argument in *Anti-Oedipus*: "Desire produces the real, or stated another way, desiring production is nothing else than social production" (Deleuze and Guattari 1983: 30, translation modified).

Desire produces not the social preformed, but sociality, "sociality for two." Always more-than, desire is what passes between, what reorients. Activated by the minor gesture, desire is machinic: it co-composes with experience in the making to tune it to what it can do. Nothing mechanistic here: only *agencements*.

Autistic perception sees-feels the workings of desire, its machining, its facilitating. It feels the workings of desire in the patterns Baggs writes about, in the mobility in Bissonnette's metaphors, in the "killingly difficult" of Chammi's description of coming to language. What is perceived at this desiring interstice is the field itself in all its complexity, where, to quote Deleuze and Guattari again, "everything functions at the same time but amid hiatuses and ruptures, breakdowns and failures, stalling and short-circuits, distances and fragmentations, a sum that never succeeds in bringing its various parts together to form a whole" (1983: 42, translation modified). Productive disjunction, or, in Deleuze and Guattari's vocabulary, inclusive disjunction; a panoply of indecipherable effects, directly felt, actively desiring in the rhythm of a collective oinking.

Undoing experience of its reordering through the figure of the stable "I," schizoanalysis is concerned first and foremost with opening experience to its prepersonal singularities. This enables it to compose well with autistic perception and to design techniques that honor its precarity. For schizoanalysis is allergic to all neurotypical commands. "The task of schizoanalysis is to tirelessly undo egos and their presuppositions; to liberate the prepersonal singularities they enclose and repress; to mobilize the flows they would be capable of transmitting, receiving or intercepting; to establish always further and more sharply the schizzes and the breaks well below conditions of identity; to mount the desiring machines that cut across each and group it with others. For each is a groupuscule and must live as such. . . . Schizoanalysis is so named because throughout its entire process of treatment it schizophrenizes, instead of neuroticizing, like psychoanalysis" (Deleuze and Guattari 1983: 434, translation modified).

To push experience to its schizoid pole is to take seriously the way in which modes of existence are multiple, uncountable in their potential expressivity. Where the shape of enthusiasm is most palpable, this multiplicity is often decried as "too much," "too noisy," "too uncontained," as though a return to the solitary individual will provide solace. Certainly, it helps to have access to motor skills that can dependably find the right letter on the keyboard, but surely this is not enough to convince us that multiplicity is a travesty. And yet this is what we say every time we bemoan the fate of autistics, or when we speak disparagingly about the complexity of neurologies that evade the comfortable center where existence tends to be most valued.

Anti-Oedipus remains a revolutionary book, and a current one. Taking the force of desire as its mantra, it speaks not of pathologies that are disabling, but to the very potential of moving away from what Guattari calls "normopathy." It's amazing what a group of depressives can do! Just watch the news: demonstrations are happening everywhere, and with each of them we see a reorienting of modes of existence that challenge the neoliberal politics which frames our existence. Mobilizations in Turkey (Gezi Park, 2013) may begin to save a park, but very soon they are about political reform, about neoliberal dominance, about new forms of life-living. And this is not an isolated case. In the 2012 Montreal student strike we saw a similar emphasis not on discrete demands but on a wider rethinking of what it means to learn, to live, and to live well. This, it seems to me, discredits Bifo's suggestion that "the global movement against capitalist globalization reached an impressive range and pervasiveness, but it was never able to change the daily life of society. It remained an ethical movement, not a social transformer. It could not create a process of social recomposition, it could not produce an effect of social subjectivation" (Berardi 2011: 12). For Bifo, if demonstrations do not produce something recognized as a different social system, they have made no difference. What about the *what else* of the in-act? What about the unwieldy effects of their continuing activity? Doesn't this separation between the ethical and what Bifo calls "a social transformer" miss the point of the desiring machine that cuts to recompose? Sure, the effects have not been felt in every corner of daily life. *But they are felt*: a change can be felt in the poststrike classroom in Montreal, in the students' commitment to study and to the undercommons.[17] A change can be felt since the wave of Occupy movements.[18] A change can be felt across America in the wake of Ferguson.[19] Are things rough? Yes, absolutely. Neoliberalism strangles potential every day. But new techniques for life-living are also being invented every day, activated by minor gestures that continuously transform what it means to act.

ACTIVISM

In a bid to do away with activism, Bifo writes:

> The term "activism" became largely influential as a result of the antiglobalization movement, which used it to describe its political communication and the connection between art and communicative action. However, this definition is a mark of its attachment to the past and its inability to free itself from the conceptual frame of reference it inherited from the 20th century. Should we not free ourselves from the thirst for activism that left the 20th century to the point of catastrophe and war? Shouldn't we set ourselves free from the repeated and failed attempt to act for the liberation of human energies from the rule of capital? Isn't the path toward the autonomy of the social from economic and military mobilization only possible through a withdrawal into inactivity, silence, and passive sabotage? (2011: 36–37)

I would like to address Bifo's remarks through a return to *Wretches and Jabberers*, turning to a few scenes where conversations about activism take place. Shortly after having arrived in India, in dialogue with Chammi, Larry types: "I think we are big time movers making a difference in peoples' lives who can't talk." The words don't come easily, and Larry has to fight a meltdown to get them out, but still he finds a way to turn the conversation to what is most important: the activist movement for neurodiversity. A similar encounter happens in Japan. Naoki, a prolific autistic writer and artist who lives in Tokyo, runs up and down the stairs and seems to jump off the walls before he can sit down to write. But then the words come, without pleasantries, immediately addressing the urgent questions at hand. From Larry to Naoki: "Mobilize letters like patterns of thought like proud autistics we are." No time for small talk: every word an effort. Writing, thinking, is in the act. And necessarily so, for the stakes are clear. Tracy, who travels around the world with Larry for the making of the film, does not at the time of the filming have a home: living conditions for autistic adults are extremely precarious. Even though he serves on two state-level advocacy committees, he depends on people who are paid to take care of him, and wonders every day whether he will be able to continue to afford to pay them. And yet his commitment to neurodiversity is unwavering. Depression, anxiety, the agony of difference—these all remain. But they are not decisive in the way Bifo suggests they are. Rather, they are productive, expressive of the multiplicity of experience out of which the movement for neurodiversity composes. "Let's begin the world's intelligence magnified organization," Tracy types in conversation with Naoki and Larry. In Finland, a similar encounter occurs. In their first conversation, again without preamble, Antti, who spends his days in a care center folding towels and doing other kinds of busywork, types: "I'm interested in talking about our current experience, how we have changed as people. . . . I think now is a good time to bind the strings of friendship between us strong people who will pass the message." Later Tracy adds: "We are a perfect example of intelligence working itself out in a much different way."

In the act—the force of activism, of activist philosophy—is not about the individual. At its best, it is about how the collective operates as a group-subject. This is what resonates in *Wretches and Jabberers*, not *despite* their anxiety, their unwieldy oversensing movements, their depression, but *with* this difference, in the shape of its enthusiasm, *because* of it, in the urgency of expression that is spoken in images that pull us into the movement of thought. Larry, Chammi, Tracy, Naoki, Antti, and also DJ, Tito, Emma, Ido, and so many others feel they have work to do, and they are doing it. This, again, not *despite* the exuberant, frustrating, excessive, deactivating, joyful interruptions to the flow of words, but *with*, in the act. Desire is revolutionary not when it is individualized (or turned against itself, as in Bifo's account of depression), but when it creates differential effects. "And if we put forward desire as a revolutionary agency, it is because we believe that capitalist society can endure many manifestations of interest, but no manifestation of desire, which would be enough to make its fundamental structures explode" (Deleuze and Guattari 1983: 455, translation modified). What is revolutionary is not the act in itself, but the opening of the act to its ineffability, to its more-than.

When the more-than is explored in its effects, a schizoanalytic process has begun. This process, as Deleuze and Guattari demonstrate, is not a method, nor is it a therapy in any conventional sense. It is an emergent attunement to the precarious range of petrification and spark, a tuning toward both the frenzied vocalizations of the autistic and the rock-like silence of the depressive (who may inhabit one and the same bodying). There is no hierarchy here—just a set of productive effects from the disarray of a field in motion. The purpose is not to organize or select, but to make the way for something else to emerge—a collective oinking, an engaged discussion, a mobile patterning. From here, new modes of existence begin to take form.

Neurodiverse modes of existence must be created, and they must compose across difference in ways that remain mobile, in the act. Pathology is not the answer. Co-composition across the spectrum is necessary, as much between the precarity of the shape of enthusiasm at its two poles as on the spectrum of our collective difference, autistic or not. For we all have access to autistic perception, and we are all susceptible to falling into depression. For those of us for whom autistic perception comes less quickly, less easily, perhaps, as I've suggested before, it's time to learn to chunk less, to refrain from quick categorization. This will likely not end neoliberalism, but it will continue the engaging process of inventing what life can do when it composes across collective resonances that listen to dissonance.

Bifo writes: "We have today a new cultural task: to live the inevitable with a relaxed soul. To call forth a big wave of withdrawal, of massive dissociation, of desertion from the scene of the economy, of nonparticipation in the fake show of politics" (Berardi 2011: 148). Wouldn't such a task be the very recipe for the kind of depression Bifo forecasts? To act must not be overlaid with capitalism's call to do, to make. In the act is something different altogether: precarious, but creative. Not creative of capitalism's "newest new," but creative of new forms of value, new ways of valuing modes of existence in their emergence and dissolution, new alignments to the time of the event. The challenge: to maintain the schism between the in-act and the act. Systems are quickly formed, as are our habits of existence. And if these systems, these habits, reorient toward the individual in the mode of the preconstituted subject, we can be sure that there will be a deadening of the operations of the movement for neurodiversity. But this isn't where I think we're headed. I prefer to listen to the autistics named above, most of them young adults. For they reassure me: the in-act is where the joy is, where the minor gestures tune experience to its more-than, where activity is not yet dedicated to a cause, or to an effect, but open for the desiring.

WHAT A BODY CAN DO

A Conversation with Arno Boehler

ARNO BOEHLER (AB): Do we know what a body can do?

ERIN MANNING (EM): For me, what a body can do has been a key question for the past decade. My own approach to the question has been to move toward the prelinguistic and ask how movement activates a body in the midst of a process of becoming. I call this bodying. Working through a lexicon of movement in its preacceleration—before displacement as such—I have wanted to explore how movement activates a modality of thought that is of the becoming-body. Such a thinking cannot be directly articulated in language, and yet it is a thinking (or a thinking-feeling) in its own right. A thinking in the moving. What's interesting about this is that it moves thought from a category of organization toward an expression of difference. Thought in the moving is the activation of a differential. It is the making-felt of a changing relationscape. So, I suppose the first answer I could give is that what a body can do is think, in the moving.

I spend a lot of time watching bodies move—in the subway, on the street, in the classroom, in the studio. And I ask myself two questions: what makes us so certain that thinking is not in-the-moving, or in-the-feeling; and what makes us so certain that we can define a body in time and space as a separate and individual entity? These are old Cartesian categories, the first putting thought in the mind, out of the body; the second placing the body outside of its relation to the world. Whatever makes it possible for us to think of a body as defined apart from its participation in the world is the same thing that allows us to believe that thought can be contained by language, apart from the movements that generate it.

In my account of what a body can do, I therefore begin with an attention to the question of the "in-act" of the doing. This emphasizes the microgestures of becoming that are in the bodying. These microgestures are a thinking-in-the-act, I argue, not in the sense that they resolve into this or that conscious thought, but in the sense that they are replete with intensity and directionality. Bodying does resolve into this or that form, eventually, but it does not begin there, nor does it remain there. A body is the metastability of those microgestures more than it is a form as such. If we begin with the microgesture, it becomes clear that a body is more associated milieu (Simondon) than form. What a body does is ecological: it becomes in relation to a changing environment, and what it *does* in that relation is what it is. A body is a tending, an inflection, an incipient directionality. And this incipiency includes a thinking in its own right.

Of course, what a body does always has a place and a time. People often ask how such an account of the body has agency. I prefer the notion of *agencement* to agency—the sense of directionality occasioned by movement rather than a subject-based intentionality—but however you define this moment of "making a difference," there is no question that how it individuates in this time and place, in co-composition—or how it matters, here and now—belongs to what a body can do. A body makes a difference in terms of how this or that vector, this or that inflection, alters the conditions of this or that event. So, that a body is black or white or female or transgender does make a difference. Of course it does! But these are less "states" of an existing body than vectors of a becoming-body that themselves change over time. Identity, like individuation, is emergent. What a body can do is change.

AB: So you suggest that bodies envelop a certain field which we and other bodies already share. This means that one cannot separate the question of what a body can do from the milieu in which it dwells in relation with others. During your workshop with Brian (Massumi) you presented a beautiful picture: What happens when there is light coming through a window and it affects you? Being *in touch* with the sun is more than being a subject contemplating an external object. One is becoming sun-like in this moment?

EM: Yes, that's a beautiful way of putting it. As an artist, I have always been very interested in these kinds of threshold effects. Like that moment when you are sitting at a café and you have been in an intense conversation and suddenly you look up and you notice that it got dark, but you cannot say when the light changed. And yet, upon noticing the shift in light you immediately know that the changing conditions affected how the conversation progressed. Threshold effects make a difference, and yet they are rarely experienced as such.

AB: Would this not mean that bodies are "worldwide entities"? Singularities of a manifold, worldwide field, shared not only with other human bodies, but with innumerous nonhuman bodies as well? Like our liaisons with the sun, for instance? An intimate relationship between our human body and a nonhuman body? Or the special liaison of plants with the sun?

EM: William James said that the relations are as real as the terms of the relation. That is how he defines radical empiricism. So yes, the relation-scape of the bodying is worldwide, even otherworldly, in the sense that it invents worlds. A body is a field of relation out of which and through which worldings occur and evolve. We know neither where a world begins nor where a body ends. What is real, what we know, are relations. This is speculative pragmatism: relations are real, here and now, but what they can do is unknowable in advance, must continuously be invented.

What is at stake in the field of relation is how the relation evolves, how it expresses itself, what it becomes, what it can do. The relation can never be properly called human. It may pass through the human or connect to certain human tendencies, but in and of itself, it is always more-than human.

The question of the nonhuman or the more-than-human is of central importance as regards what a body can do. A bodying begins and returns to the midst, to the relational field that is more-than human. A focus on the middling of experience leads us toward a modality of thinking the becoming-body in a directly ecological sense in terms of an ecology of practices that *includes* the human but is not limited to the human.

One of the ways I have tried to address this directly ecological experience of the world is through what I have called autistic perception. I define autistic perception as a direct experience of emergent field effects. When autistics first perceive, they do not tend to see forms as nonautistics do. Instead, they see perception's very emergence: edges, shadows, colors, shapes. What takes a half second for a neurotypical to perceive as form can take up to five minutes for an autistic. This lag in the taking of form allows autistics to perceptually dwell in the shape-shifting of experience and gives them a lived sense of the malleability of form. This is not completely outside neurotypical experience, it is simply less often directly experienced—artists hone such perceptual tendencies, and they are not unfamiliar to those who drink or take drugs, or those who experience extreme states due to shock or love or fear. However we come to autistic perception, what is important, I think, is the taking account of a phase of experience where it is the associated milieu of relation which is at the forefront not only conceptually, but perceptually. Were we to honor such a perceptual account of process, I think we might come to see the everyday quite differently. This would then have important effects not only on our experience of the world, but on what we do collectively, politically.

To experience the world in its shape-shifting alerts us to the realness of relation and connects to a more-than-human horizon, I think. It allows us to think ecologically, from the middle. And from there, there is an opening to the felt expression of thought-in-the-moving, to language's prelinguistic expressions—what I have elsewhere called prearticulation—to the complex rhythms of what lies between the conscious and the nonconscious at the interstices of the human and the nonhuman, the more-than-human.

AB: So how I understand you is that it is not enough to speak only in the name of the other things, but really to change, or to open up a space in which another form of relationality with other nonhuman things becomes possible. So it is not only a matter of language and a matter of morality to take care of other nonhuman things, and give them a voice, but to work on the level of affection, of affect, of being affected, of what you and Brian also called tendencies which show up in relation to others and to change our behaviors. Or, as you beautifully said before, to care for the event.

EM: Yes, I think that there can be a tendency when we talk about the nonhuman to assume we are talking about the animal or the vegetal, which we are not necessarily doing at all. When you speak about the field, what you are taking into account is the more-than-human of the animal, the more-than-human of the oxygen, the more-than-human of the human. I call this speciation, as opposed to species. Relational fields rather than categories. Emergent constellations. A constellation meets a constellation rather than a particularity meeting a particularity. If you begin to think in terms of that kind of multiplicity, then immediately, I think, there is that sense of *the care for the event,* because the constellation is already eventful. As Whitehead would say, an event always carries with it concern for its eventness. Self-enjoyment of the event, in the event. This is punctual, of course. A constellation or speciation is emergent here and now, this or that way. Pragmatic, yet speculative.

One way I think about the care for the event in the event is in terms of what I call the dance of attention. Not human attention, but *field attention*—the event's attention to its own development, its own concrescence. When it is strong, that's when we leave a dance performance, for instance, and say: "Wow, that really worked!" What is felt in such instances is the lived intensity of the event's capacity to create a field of experience. There is little in our everyday lives that facilitates this kind of dance of attention, but it does take place. It seems to me that it would be important to work harder to develop techniques that allow for that dance of attention to be awakened or energized, to be made possible. It is there, it is latently there, I think, all the time. But it can be overcoded by the habitual tendencies of subject-centered intentionality that work continuously to take us out of the field of relation and into the individual, as though the individual could be cordoned out from the event. The techniques to be invented are ones that open the perceptual register beyond intentionality to the thought-in-the-moving of the complex emergent patterns of our daily lives.

AB: If we take bodies as worldwide entities, the global field, which they share, becomes one of the most important features of any body. Deleuze even speaks of a transcendental field, the all-oneworld which any body shares with all others by populating it.

EM: I think of this as worlding, and it reminds me of the necessity to consider the body always from the perspective of the collective, or the transindividual. I am thinking of an example here. In disability activism it is often said that disability is not what happens to the body—it is not about the state of the body. Disability is about a culture that does not accommodate diversity. So it is not the body (alone) that is disabled; the culture is disabled in its incapacity to create accommodations that allow for difference—different kinds of bodying—to exist. I am thinking about a disability activist, Harriet McBryde-Johnson, a lawyer. She once was invited by the *New York Times* to do a spread on her work for Not Dead Yet, an organization very much against euthanasia and assisted suicide. At first, when I was reading Harriet McBryde-Johnson as part of my ongoing research into disability politics, it was to better understand why it was that so many disability activists were so adamantly against assisted suicide. Because, from my perspective, it seemed that what a body can do is also choose to die. What I learned through my research was that not every body is given the same right to live. A disabled body is often a body seen by the medical establishment as not worthy of life. So a disabled person who has cancer doesn't necessarily get the same kind of care as a nondisabled person. This happens in subtle ways—for instance, a doctor might be quicker to speak to the disabled person about palliative care, assuming that their quality of life is already jeopardized by their disability and that the further strain of treatment may not be worthwhile. This example, which comes up very often in disability activist blogs (see, for instance, Bad Cripple), emphasizes the way disability is taken as an individual rather than as a collective, cultural problem—an ecology of practices. To turn this around, it is necessary to keep asking not how this or that body performs, but how this singular field of relation opens itself to the complexity of bodying. In the case of disability, too often an individual normative standard is imposed that presumes able-bodiedness as the very definition of a body, ignoring the complexity of evolution within all bodyings.

Lately I've been trying to understand accommodation within this context of transindividual bodying. Within disability politics, as I mentioned, there tends to be an understanding that it is the lack of accommodation that creates the category of disability. This is no doubt true and needs to change: there needs to be a general understanding that making our worlds accessible to difference is to enrich them. But I want to push the term even further beyond the able-bodied/disabled divide, always keeping in mind that the disability cannot be reduced to the person; that it is rather the lack of accommodation in the everyday environment that creates the rift between the so-called able and the disabled. Everywhere I turn within the complex work that unfolds within disability activism, I find accounts of the frustrations of accommodation as it plays out in everyday life. The concerns are often pragmatic, though always engaged with philosophical questions about why accommodation is so difficult to fold into our cultural landscapes as both concept and act: why is it that the tables that "accommodate" wheelchairs in a restaurant tend to be in the worst possible places (beside the bathroom, out of sight), why is it that "accommodating" entrances are in the back of hotels or in the bowels of buildings rather than out there in the open? Why isn't every entrance designed to accommodate difference, and why is it that there is a sense, still very strong within architecture (and within so many of our practices) that accommodation is a nasty afterthought? The issue also goes deeper, touching on what is imaginable (thinkable, perceivable) within the field of experience—I wonder here, for instance, about the way in which thresholds between rooms become apparent if you're in a wheelchair, or if you're blind, but otherwise may not "appear" in experience. Without underestimating these important pragmatic issues, I wonder whether there might be a way to take back the term "accommodation" to speak about *all* bodyings, thereby opening up the question beyond the categories of the able and the disabled. Is there any event that does not require accommodation? Are we willing to think of what a body can do in a way that takes seriously how the event accommodates its shifting ecologies?

What would it mean to become aware, for instance, of how a lack of accommodation impedes the dance of attention of an event from being felt? What might it mean to make accommodation, seen as a collective engagement that tends fields of relation, a central concern of the everyday, in all instances, at all times, including accommodation in the strictest physical, architectural sense, but also accommodation to neurodiverse forms of perception and attention? The absence of a robust engagement with accommodation has to do with a practiced ignorance of the complexity of differentials at the heart of speciations. Elsewhere I have argued that this practiced ignorance is at the heart of neurotypical identity politics and its unwavering belief in the volition-intentionality-agency triad.

Accommodation understood this way is not an individual concern. It is a care for the event in its modulation. How the event accommodates is not separate from what a body can do.

Some people might say that this sounds utopian. I don't actually think that we are talking about something utopian. The seeds for this are everywhere present. This already happens in pockets of existence; it happens in the corners, sometimes quite obviously, sometimes much less so. The trick is, I think, to make those corners matter.

AB: You founded a SenseLab to make *the care of the event* matter? What kind of territory, what kind of accommodation, what kind of hospitality, of care, *cura, curie,* and courting takes place there?

EM: You touched on the core concept of the SenseLab, which is hospitality. But it isn't an intersubjective hospitality, as you pointed out. It is
an *event-based hospitality*. To create a thought-experiment, an action-
experiment like the SenseLab, the event has to be hospitable to learning,
to thinking, and to the collaborative gesture that feeds both.

Eleven years into it, what I can say is that the event-based hospitality at the heart of our collective practice has made it possible for us to
engender a culture of affirmation. I hadn't really seen it this way until
I heard a SenseLabber explain to someone else that what we do at the
SenseLab is say *yes*! I loved this description and wondered how this
practice of saying yes has fed our modes of collaboration, allowing us
to develop ways of collective decision-making that are not based in a
kind of Habermasian consensual politics. Thinking it through, it became
clear to me that creating an affirmative practice doesn't mean simply
saying "Yes, I follow you through every aspect of this idea." It means
"Yes, we'll try this and collectively hone the effects." The question thus
moves beyond how this or that is a "good" idea to what the idea can do
in relation to the event with which it co-composes. The selection of one
idea from the many becomes not a decision-making practice that takes
place outside the event, but an emergent tuning from within the event.
We follow the idea that best takes us wherever the event needs to go.
This means that there is very little sense of who "owns" the idea. The
idea becomes a proposition in the Whiteheadian sense: it does something, and that something has effects. If what it does is invigorate, intensify, make itself hospitable to the other event-based inflexions and
tendencies, the idea takes hold. If not, that particular idea simply tends
not to be developed then and there. But ideas do get re-taken-up later,
suddenly reemerging in new contexts, often brought forward by different people than those who might originally have offered them up.
What I like about this approach—an approach that emerged organically
over time—is that it makes apparent that for an event to do its work, the
event-potential of the idea must get taken up over the individual's stake
in it. This allows for forms of collaboration to emerge at the level of the
incipiency of thought—in retrospect we often can't remember whose
idea it was in the first place.

This affirmative stance allows us, I think, to be sensitive to the demands of the event in its unfolding while also collectively orienting
it. This is complex because we are so accustomed to working with the
competing tendency, wherein we separate the individual subject from

the event, assuming an individual intentionality. At the SenseLab we've been able to sidestep this tendency for the most part by using the event as a training ground for the invention of techniques coming out of a collective experimentation with the idea as affirmative proposition. Our process is to work together to mold an idea into a technique that can affect the conditions of the event, altering how the event comes to expression, affecting its dance of attention. Techniques we develop usually center on the event's thresholds—the moving across registers of the event: in a given event this could include the shift from small groups to large groups, shifts in location, shifts in speed or intensity. For instance, for each event we plan we set up modes of introduction and contact that seek to intensify existing shifts in register, and then we participate in these shifts to see whether the conditions we are co-creating, with the event, make a difference in how the event unfolds and what it facilitates.[1] Our approach involves a kind of structured improvisation that builds on an acute form of listening to the unfolding of a process in real-time. Having established what we call enabling constraints, having prepared the threshold, having created the conditions for a coming-together in the mode of affirmation, we then explore how the event facilitates the creation of what Guattari calls "a group-subject," an ecological subjectivity in-formed by the event. There are many failures, of course, some of which we take to be enabling constraints toward the future creation of techniques. Usually a failure is experienced by a resubjectifying on the figure of the individual. The problem with that is that it reestablishes the status quo, foregrounding the individual as the center of performativity rather than making the event the site of care and hospitality.

Over the years, as we have honed our practice, we have moved beyond asking how events are created (what makes an event an event) to asking what an event needs to be able to do. An event-based practice needs to reinvent itself continuously, and it needs to resist becoming institutionalized. It needs to have necessity, in the Nietzschean sense. It needs to create its own value, its own modes of evaluation. Regularly we ask ourselves whether the SenseLab still creates modes of inquiry that are productive of effects that surprise us and move us toward modes of existence that are qualitatively different from ones we have become accustomed to. Do our events still produce thought? Are they still capable of making felt the thinking-in-the-moving I discussed earlier? So far, I think they are, and I believe this is largely due to the fact that we've never had a concept of membership. To be part of the SenseLab is simply to want to participate. The more you're involved, the more you affect our practices, but there is no ideal amount of involvement and no ideal time to get involved. Everything makes a difference.

AB: Very beautiful, very beautiful! What you said is also important for Susanne [Valerie] and me. Susanne comes from the arts and is highly interested in philosophy, and I come from philosophy and am highly interested in the arts. For us it was always important to do both, philosophy *and* art, or, what we call "philosophy on stage," a mode of arts-based philosophy. Something we are hungry for and think is necessary. Today traditional academic philosophers have a lot of problems with bringing the arts together with philosophy. They think that "mixing" the arts with philosophy makes philosophy unserious. So would you—this is my last question—say something about your experience bringing art and philosophy together?

EM: Through the SenseLab, I've found an ever-evolving community of people who think at the interstices of thought-in-the-making (like you and Susanne, like Brian and so many others) and I've found that it is possible, through a transdisciplinary perspective, to reinvent what it means to create in the interval of making and thinking. This has made it easier not only to overcome the closed-mindedness of disciplinary boundaries but also to develop techniques that assist me in both becoming more rigorous as a philosopher and to have a more sustained practice as an artist. It's taken time because the practices are not necessarily complementary, at least not in the way they make or take time in my own experience of them. What I mean by that is that I can't easily move from writing to artmaking, or vice versa, because their ways of making and taking time are so different. I need to create holes of time that can be populated by each practice—holes that can capture the failures in the thinking and the making that are at the heart of creating new ways of approaching each medium. So a busy back-and-forth produces only frustration. Over the years the best approach I have found is to work in chunks, spending a period of two to three months reading and writing, and then changing gears completely and spending time in the studio. I rarely understand the link between the two practices while I am in the making, and I don't try to impose one.

One technique I am using at the moment to try to make a bridge between practices is to allow projects to develop without necessarily deciding what form they will eventually take. This involves allowing the project to investigate its own ways of generating itself before deciding how it comes to expression. In the past months, this led me to work mostly in the studio, developing the conditions for a participatory textile work I am calling *The Smell of Red*, but lately it has moved me back to my desk to explore the concept of the minor gesture, a concept I am working to define in relation to what I think of as the "artful" within the participatory. This is rare for me—to find a passage between writing and art where the writing actually feeds the artmaking and vice versa.

In the end, though, each practice has to be able to do its own work: the philosophy and the art have to stand on their own. And so the rigor of each practice has to be honed, and this is of course difficult with the time constraints we all have. But the SenseLab functions as a good conduit, as does the teaching I do, which both involve close philosophical readings paired with work in the artist studio.

Perhaps one of the most concrete ways art and philosophy come together in my practice is around the question of value. Brian and I did a TEDx talk some time ago called "For a Pragmatics of the Useless," where we were trying to create a vocabulary for a valuing of experience that is not allied to either capitalist market-value or prestige-value.[2] Philosophy and art both sit on the side of prestige-value more than on the side of market-value. But the prestige-value obviously has market effects. Some philosophers and artists have chosen a kind of nondoing as a way of responding to the prestige-value of art and philosophy. The problem with this approach is that it simplifies the act, reducing it to a dichotomy (to act or not to act). I would rather operate within a Spinozist frame, where there is an emphasis on rest in movement and movement in rest. I think that there is a lot of doing in the nondoing and a lot of nondoing in the doing. We need to keep that complexity there, focusing perhaps more on the subtleties of the in-act of autistic perception, an in-act that cannot be reduced so easily to form and category, to intentionality and volition. In our TEDx talk, we proposed the reinvigoration of the concept of *uselessness*, emphasizing a kind of doing, an in-act, where value is not preinscribed but created in the event.

I hope that both the philosophy and the art I do are useless in this sense. As more and more of us actively—activistly—reframe the useless in a speculatively pragmatic sense, perhaps we can redefine value outside of a capitalist mandate. In so doing, perhaps we'll even be able to come back to the original idea of philosophy, which, as you know, had nothing to do with a discipline. Philosophy was what you did in relation to other practices, it was what emerged from practices that remained other, such as art, mathematics, physics. It was never meant to be a field that needed to separate itself out. What if we took philosophy and art not as disciplines but as forms of thinking in the making, and making in the thinking? What if the thinking-doing were conceived as a value in itself, independent of what form it takes?

AB: Thank you!

EM: Thank you! It was a real pleasure.

Into all abysses I still carry the blessings of my saying Yes.
—Friedrich Nietzsche, *Thus Spoke Zarathustra*

WHAT IF (BEYOND GOOD AND EVIL)

The minor gesture is an operative cut that opens experience to its potential. This operation is affirmative to its core—it affirms the field in its transformation, and it affirms the way this transformation emboldens the in-act of experience in the making. Affirmation is the creative force of a reorientation in the event. What affirmation *does, how* it effects the cut, is what gives it affective valence in the event. The affirmative cut of the minor gesture catalyzes a reordering. Cuts are not good or bad. It is what they *do* that makes a difference. The affirmative cut is not the bestowing of a value judgment onto experience. Affirmation is not good or evil, optimistic or cruel.[1]

Nietzschean affirmation counters the Hegelian dialectic. Where the dialectic builds on contradiction and opposition, affirmation refuses to stand against. Critique is not its motor, but neither is acceptance. Affirmation does not do its work according to the either-or of a field predetermined. Nor does it seek to counter (or accept) the *it is* of the given. Cutting into the event is not a process of negation or dialectical synthesis. Affirmation moves at the pace of the differential, aligning to the event's points of inflection, to its operative tangents, where the form of experience has not yet quite emerged.

Affirmation does not yet know what the field can do, and so it neither predicts nor (de)values it in advance of its coming to be. Affirmation does not position: it experiments. It is pragmatic in its speculation. Speculative pragmatism is experimental to its core, asking at every stage how the cut makes a difference. Speculative pragmatism does not comply with the existing parameters of experience. It does not stand outside them to judge. Speculative pragmatism, in the name of affirmation, invents, doing its work at the limit where *what if?* becomes *what else?*

For Nietzsche, affirmation is never reactive. Reactivity is a secondary gesture. It is an interpretation of the cut. Though it seems to coincide with the cutting, in effect reactivity stands just outside its momentum, peering in from the edges. In the interpreting or judging stance, reactivity mutes the minor gesture. It cements the field, holds it to what it is. Interpretation-as-judgment only asks *what if* from the solid stance of the *it is*. It does not risk the *what else*. The categories are clear even when they are being challenged. This is not to suggest that there is no work to do in interpretation. Nor does it suggest that in interpretation all potential is cast aside: interpretation can certainly be affirmative, curious, and creative. It is to say that when interpretation becomes judgment and thus takes the place of affirmation, the event is held in place and its potential tunes toward reactivity. With judgment, the work of thinking, of encountering, is laid out in terms of a field already oriented. Once judgment takes over, it takes a lot to reenergize the field, to move it toward its minor quality.

THE AS IS OF THE WHAT WAS (*RESSENTIMENT*)

Affirmation's movement toward the world is one of mutual inclusion. In a logic of both-and it facilitates modes of coexistence for difference. Its work is not to resolve contradiction. This does not mean that affirmation is comfortable or comforting. Its work is to invent conditions for new ways of activating the threshold of experience, new ways of experimenting in the complexity of what does not easily fold into a smooth surface. Affirmation is striating more than smoothing, its operative potential more at the level of the crease than the stable ground. Affirmation is the push, the pull that keeps things unsettled, a push that ungrounds, unmoors, even as it propels.

Because of how it makes the threshold operative, affirmation is negation's most powerful enemy. Negation's work involves deactivating the threshold. Where negation stops, turning the field inward, affirmation moves, propelling it elsewhere. There is affinity between affirmation and negation, but as Deleuze writes, there is no confusion (2002: 54). Where negation remains so certain of the stakes of the encounter, affirmation delights in the creativity of *what else* that encounter could do. Where negation is content to dwell in the judgment of the *it is*, affirmation is too curious to stay within the already-defined now. This is what makes negation reactive, and affirmation active. "Only active force asserts itself, it affirms its difference and makes its difference an object of enjoyment and affirmation. Reactive force, even when it obeys, limits active force, imposes limitations and partial restrictions on it and is already controlled by the spirit of the negative" (Nietzsche 1968 in Deleuze 2002: 55–56). Two versions of the in-act: one heavy with the weight of its delimitations, the other exuberantly reaching-toward.

> As long as we remain in the element of the negative it is no use changing values or even suppressing them, it is no use killing God: the place and the predicate remain, the holy and the divine are preserved, even if the place is left empty and the predicate unattributed. But when the element is changed, then, and only then, can it be said that all values known or knowable up to the present have been reversed. Nihilism has been defeated: activity recovers its rights but only in relation and in affinity with the deeper instance from which these derive. Becoming-active appears in the universe, but as identical with affirmation as will to power. (Deleuze 2002: 171)

This is not to say that there isn't activity in negation. Negative critique's work is to actively trace what the event cannot do. This is an acting, but one that knows, in advance, what the orientation will be. For negative critique can only be for or against. For-against is the gesture of the either-or. The stakes are clear. This makes negative critique deeply complicit with the way things are. It is in this sense that negation remains, always, in the *it is*, even when its stance may be heard as the *it is not*.

Affirmation does not do its work in the register of contradiction. It does not dwell in the either-or. It does not set up the stage in advance and work backward from its position-taking. This is why for affirmation, it is never a question of making-active from the perspective of reactivity. In affirmation there is no reactivity. Affirmation activates in the activity of the event. It activates in the folds of the event's creases, connecting with their own becoming-active. There is always more for affirmation, more-than.

Affirmation does not see negation as its other. It operates in a completely different logic. Affirmation creates the trajectory, and from there the potential of the *what else* emerges. Negation, on the other hand, travels a closed circle predictable in its choreography. Though there is movement, it goes only where it has gone before. Negation's act is ultimately empty: it tends only to what it knows it knows. Setting what is against what is, there is no desire for difference. There is no desire. This sterility keeps it safe. From its vantage point of the safety of the well-trodden path, negation observes: it does not engage except to deny, to close down, to set apart, to name the stakes, deintensifying the threshold of encounter, of difference. At its limit, it does not even give in to this gesture. It simply closes the door.

Because of its reactivity, negation is stifled in its capacity for creativity. This makes it susceptible to what Nietzsche calls *ressentiment*—the deep resentment of the world as it is and the tireless wish for the *what was*. Of course negation would deny any commitment to the *what was*. Negation is anything but nostalgic. And yet its logic is deeply aligned with that of Nietzsche's last men, who decry the future, wishing that the *what is* were not. In a negative alignment to the futurity in the present, the last men work to keep the *what was* alive, turning their back on change, on difference. While negative critique's skepticism of the *what is* and by extension the *what was* is rooted in a different set of values, what makes negative critique an ally of the last men is the disavowal of the cut of affirmation and its potential to shift the course of time. For both the last men and the critic, time's differential is the enemy. This makes the last men the best allies of negative critique. Listen as the last men sit around the table and you will hear the voice of the critic among them, decrying the world as it is. The critic is most comfortable where *ressentiment* dwells.

Ressentiment creeps up on you. What seemed active soon leads you to the same old, tired values. The worn paths become the only ones in sight, and what seemed like a taking-of-position now looks more like a dead end. Negation is, in the end, predictable, and this predictability tends to close in on itself. Resentment builds, and with it a loss of intensity, a kind of apathetic anxiety that keeps us in our place. "It is as it is," we sigh. It would be a waste of energy to want it to be otherwise.

Is it? Is this path, this architecture, this choreography, truly "as it is"? Hasn't even this worn path changed since yesterday? Can't you see the brush of new growth? The problem with *ressentiment* is that it drags its feet in the same ruts day after day. It doesn't want to feel the new growth.

GIVE ME CREDIT (STAY IN DEBT)

Ressentiment is particularly invested in framing memory: memory is what holds the *what was* in place. The ills, the mistreatments, the judgments and abuses, these become an echo chamber that resonates in the taut alignment between past and present, the worldview always over the shoulder. In the context of the debt owed to African Americans, Fred Moten writes: "There's a very important, and let's call it righteous strain, of Afro-American and Afro-Diasporic studies that we could place under the rubric of debt collection. And it's basically like, 'we did this and we did that, and you continue not to acknowledge it. You continue to mis-name it. You continue to violently misunderstand it. And I'm going to correct the record and collect this debt.' And there's a political component to it, too. Maybe that's partly what the logic of reparations is about" (Moten and Harney 2013: 151). To remember becomes a daily practice. The horror of oppression soon occupies the whole of remembrance. The weight of debt choreographs this circuit. The debt is real, as is the memory. The resentment is justified. A repayment would make a difference. But would it take us out of the cycle? And is this cycle not, despite its urgency, reactive? In operating so firmly against, does this cycle not also deintensify the not-yet of experience in the making? Moten continues: "They want an acknowledgement of the debt because it constitutes something like a form of recognition, and that becomes very problematic because the form of recognition that they want is within an already existing system. They want to be recognized by sovereignty as sovereign, in a certain sense" (2013: 152). The debt, as framed by *ressentiment* becomes the credit that keeps a certain version of life going. A debt remains to be paid, a debt the future cannot rectify. Debt creates a cycle we resent. This cycle is what is familiar, safe in its predictability, and so we continue to dwell in its closed loop, even though it makes us miserable. We'd like to move on, to be elsewhere, but the threshold of past to present always seems to open to the same conditions of indebtedness. If only we could get rid of that debt, we know we would feel better. If only we could get enough credit.

Nietzschean affirmation energizes that threshold. It creates the conditions for another way of entering, another way of walking. A different path reveals itself. The affirmative path is rocky and unsteady. No well-trodden ruts here. This path doesn't know where it's headed. It promises nothing. It gives no credit, and repays no debt. This is what affirmation knows: credit is what keeps us indebted. "They say we have too much debt. We need better credit, more credit, less spending. They offer us credit repair, credit counseling, microcredit, personal financial planning. They promise to match credit and debt again, debt and credit. But our debts stay bad" (Moten and Harney 2013: 61).

Our debts stay bad because we are owed as much as we owe. We are owed a better world. We are owed reparations for the racism, for the sexism, for the horrors of the genocides we have survived, for the sexual abuse we have lived through. We are owed for the judgments we face each day in a world that refuses to accommodate us, a world that excludes us from proper education. And we owe. We owe the environment better conditions for surviving, for thriving. We owe our children more opportunities for movement, for independent exploration. We owe the woman who sleeps on the street. We owe the drug addict who suffers from mental illness. We owe the black man who can't walk safely at night. We owe the Indigenous women who keep disappearing.[2] None of this is in question. We are owed. And we owe.

A culture of affirmation does not deny that there is an infinite debt to be repaid. The difference is that the response to the debt, to the indebtedness, isn't reactive. What keeps it from falling into *ressentiment* is that it refuses to dwell in the unfulfillable wish. Instead, it moves elsewhere, asking, as Moten and Harney do, *what else?* What else can we do in the face of this unpayable debt? What else can we do in this culture of credit which breeds *ressentiment*? How else can the suffering be mitigated? Because let's be clear: repayment can never undo deep and life-changing suffering. It can only recognize it. And while this recognition is definitely something, is it enough? I don't believe it is. It keeps us within the same tight circle. It holds us to the crafting of experience as oriented by the perpetrator: the repayment of the debt is, after all, always done in the name of the sovereign who now holds the power to repay or bestow apology. To believe that payment is possible, to believe that payment will do the job, that payment will still the anguish and change the stakes, that recognition of our pain by the dominant class will fundamentally alter our conditions, is still, no matter how important, to return us to the dialectic.

BAD DEBT (WILL TO POWER)

Fred Moten writes:

> I feel like I want to be part of another project. Which is to say I'm not acceding to the fact; it's not like I'm just trying to turn my eye from it. I don't want to accept in silence without protest all the different forms of inequality and exploitation that emerge as a function of the theft and of the failure to acknowledge the debt. . . . But I also know that what it is that is supposed to be repaired is irreparable. It can't be repaired. The only thing we can do is tear this shit down completely and build something new. (Moten and Harney 2013: 151–152)

How to will something new? Nietzsche's will to power is often misunderstood as the force of an individual will. This misunderstanding turns the will into the volitional act of a preexisting subject. The will to power is not that. It is what brings out the difference in the event. It is the force through which experience tunes and orients. Gilles Deleuze writes: "The question which Nietzsche constantly repeats, 'what does a will want, what does this one or that one want?,' must not be understood as the search for a goal, a motive or an object for this will. What a will wants is to affirm its difference. In its essential relation with the 'other' a will makes its difference an object of affirmation" (2002: 9). The will to power activates the field of relation by shifting its relations of power. This power is directed by the force of affirmation itself.

What moves affirmation is not the subject. Affirmation is in the event, activated and motivated by a will to power that orients the event to its incipient tendency. The will to power is the push-pull within affirmation that forces the event to act. From this act, subjects and objects emerge, but they *are* never in advance of it. A philosophy of the event is never an ontology, never a story of being before becoming. A philosophy of the event is ontogenetic: *it moves* before *it is.*

Nietzsche talked of the will to power as the *feeling of power*. "Will" may just be the wrong word: too quickly aligned to volition, too quickly connected to the subject. Certainly here, in a book skeptical about the place of volition within subject formation (and agency), "will" would seem an odd word to use. Deleuze writes: "For Nietzsche, the capacity for being affected is not necessarily a passivity but an affectivity, a sensibility, a sensation. It is in this sense that Nietzsche, even before elaborating the concept of the will to power and giving it its full significance, was already speaking of a feeling of power. Before treating power as a matter of will he treated it as a matter of feeling and sensibility" (2002: 62).

The event is alive with affective tonality. Its power is its capacity to feel. Its moods, its colors, its tones—all of these contribute to its leanings, to what it can do. Feeling is not after the fact—it is what moves the act. The will to power, the feeling of power, is similarly what directs the event, what propels the event to land in just this or just that way. Whitehead speaks of how an event has a concern for its unfolding. The feeling of power: the activation of a differential sensibility in the event.

This differential sensibility is more-than-human. Nietzsche writes: "The fact is that the will to power rules even in the inorganic world, or rather that there is no inorganic world. Action at a distance cannot be eliminated, for one thing attracts another and a thing feels itself attracted. This is the fundamental fact. . . . In order for the will to power to be able to manifest itself it needs to perceive the things it sees and feel the approach of what is assimilable to it" (Nietzsche 1968 in Deleuze 2002: 63). Action at a distance means that the event does not begin or end with the human. The human can be and often is an aspect of the more-than that pulses through the event, but the event is not delimited by the human. In this worlding, in the ecology of events pulsing from force to form, before there is a fully defined human, there is what Whitehead calls the self-enjoyment of the occasion. The event is replete with feeling, feeling not a subjective, conscious trait, but a mobile directionality, a potentializing tendency, in the event. How the event enjoys its coming-to-be will give it the color that will subsequently define it. This color will affect how the subject—or the superject, as Whitehead would say—comes to expression. The feeling of power is one way of articulating the qualitative complexity of what comes to be. Without the feeling of power, without the notion of the event's self-enjoyment, the only qualitative potential lies in the human's subjective judgment of the event. We are back at the dialectic.

Reactivity, *ressentiment*—these are human traits. Similarly, the cycle of debt and credit is profoundly human. Despite increased speculation on more-than-human elements such as weather, air, and water, the benefit is meant to be ours. Sure, we speak in the name of the environment, of "its" needs, but nevertheless, our habit is not to affirm, but to react: Look what the world is coming to! Look at what it's doing to me, to my life, to my future! Sure, we take responsibility. We feel compelled. But too often we work only within the confines of the given.

Affirmation is always endangered by the reappropriation of the event by the forces that would make it reactive, that would undo it of its generative activity. It is very tempting to see ourselves at the center, directing experience. In fact, this reorienting gesture toward our own needs has become second nature in many if not most of our cultures: our education, our training has led us to believe that this is about us, about our feelings, about our identity, and that it is our judgment that matters most. We associate reason with objectivity, and objectivity with knowledge.

Second nature is reactive. Why not dwell instead in first nature? In affirmation? Why give in to second nature? Why succumb to reactivity?

Reactivity does not happen in the event: it happens in the event's aftermath. It happens in the ways in which the event is taken up, reappropriated. It happens when the event is asked to pay a debt to the world "as we know it." The becoming-reactive cuts into the in-act. Since the in-act cannot properly be stopped, what occurs is the formation of a double perspective, a second nature, one foot in the world and the other at its edges, as though one could be both outside looking in and in the midst. Since this is not really possible, since the event still agitates (us) no matter what we do, we must deaden it, deny it its potential, undo it of its agility. When this happens the in-act gets backgrounded in the name of the *it is*. This creates what Spinoza would call sad affects: affects that close the event to its potential. Reactivity is a mechanism of capture.

Sad affects are not the result of a sad situation any more than joy in Spinoza is about happiness. Sad affects are created when an accounting takes place after the fact that negates bare activity, the agitation of all that comes to be.[3] Soon nostalgia will follow (even if it is negated). For the settling of accounts will never really order experience as it is becoming: only experience as it was can be encapsulated (and then only fleetingly, for it too, is replete with bare activity). The backgrounding of the in-act in the name of an ordering of experience produces sad affects because this cannot but create a deadening, in the event, of what might come to be.

SUPERABUNDANCE (BEYOND GOOD AND EVIL)

Affirmation is the *yes* of the child's *"again!"* ("Was that life? Well then, once more!"). This *yes* is not a simple acquiescence—Nietzsche warns us of becoming the donkey who is willing to carry any and every load. Affirmation's *yes* is a pull to engage with the operative tendencies of a fissure in the field of existence. It is an affirmation of the *what if* at the heart of the *what else. Yes!* does not mean "anything goes." The affirmative *yes* enjoys the stakes of the event's process, enjoys the unknowability of the operative cut that moves experience to that which cannot be known in advance. *Yes!* is an enabling constraint that promises nothing except a pragmatic stance of experimentation, a speculative pragmatism. From this *yes!*, many *nos* will follow, but *no* will never lead the way, for *no* has too much of a habit of knowing in advance.

Nietzsche writes of two kinds of suffering. There are those "who suffer from the superabundance of life" (Nietzsche 1968 in Deleuze 2002: 16). This suffering says *yes!* in a way that does not exclude the pain of the everyday. This *yes!* is not a masochism. It is an affirmation of the force of superabundance. It is a *yes!* to the more-than. The superabundance is a weight, but it is not the any-weight the donkey carries. It is a weight claimed and made operational in the context not of what life *is*, but what life *can do*. It is the weight of a debt unpayable, a debt without credit. The second kind of suffering is consumed with "an impoverishment of life." Those who suffer this way "make intoxication a convulsion, a numbness; they make suffering a means of accusing life, of contradicting it and also a means of justifying life, of resolving the contradiction" (Nietzsche 1968 in Deleuze 2002: 16). The first is affirmative, the second steeped in *ressentiment*. The first lives in the in-act of existence unfolding, the second feels the weight of existence's debt and carries it even while reacting against it.

Existence's debt recognizes itself in the shape preformed of the human. When we imagine what is owed to us, we imagine it taking the shape of an individual or a collection of individuals. This kind of debt grows around the individual and is contained by the individual. Harney writes: "There has to be a way in which there can be elaborations of unpayable debt that don't always return to an individualization through the family or an individualization through the wage laborer, but instead the debt becomes a principle of elaboration" (2013: 151). What would it look like to think of debt without a subject?

Debt without a subject would spin centrifugally. Debt would become a figure uncontainable, an ungraspable force. As a principle of elaboration, debt would become the motor of another kind of process, one that doesn't always lead back to us, to the human as central pivot of experience. Debt would instead become the unfathomable superabundance we carry not because we have no choice, but because, as more-than, we can share the weight, and we welcome that sharing.

"Credit keeps track. Debt forgets" (Moten and Harney 2013: 62). A shared debt would be a debt forgotten, a debt that forgets itself. It would be what Moten and Harney call bad debt. Debt forgotten is bad because its point of inception can no longer be traced. It exists in the world in a way that does not lead back to the individual.

Active forgetting is the ultimate affirmation in Nietzsche. "A specific active force must be given the job of supporting consciousness and renewing its freshness, fluidity and mobile, agile chemistry at every moment. This active super-conscious faculty is the faculty of forgetting" (Deleuze 2002: 113). Forgetting, for Nietzsche is "a plastic, regenerative and curative force" (Nietzsche 2002 in Deleuze 2002: 106). To forget debt does not mean to forgive it. The forgiveness of debt is still in the logic of credit. Credit "is a means of privatization and debt a means of socialization. . . . Debt is mutual. Credit runs only one way" (Moten and Harney 2013: 61). Credit keeps us cagey. Debt must be forgotten in order to leave behind the very idea of credit, the very idea that what we owe can be privatized.

> To forget debt is to invent a new kind of justice, a justice that is only possible where debt never obliges, never demands, never equals credit, payment, payback. Justice is possible only where it is never asked, in the refuge of bad debt, in the fugitive public of strangers not communities, of undercommons not neighborhoods, among those who have been there all along from somewhere. To seek justice through restoration is to return debt to the balance sheet and the balance sheet never balances. It plunges toward risk, volatility, uncertainty, more credit chasing more debt, more debt shackled to credit. To restore is not to conserve, again. There is no refuge in restoration. Conservation is always new. It comes from the place we stopped while we were on the run. It's made from the people who took us in. (Moten and Harney 2013: 63)

This new justice counters *ressentiment*. Here, where the time of the event is not measured in advance, we are alive in a sociality as yet unscripted, a black sociality, as Moten might say. Yes, we are owed, yes, we owe, but we have somewhere else to go, somewhere else to be. The feeling of power, the force of will, moves the event, and with it, we are moved. Being moved does not mean being happy. In affirmation, we are not in the midst of a simple acquiescence. Affirmation is not about following along. A culture of affirmation socially, collectively, makes its own path, and it does not bray: its noises are not so easily parsed as positive or negative, not so easily positioned or understood. In a culture of affirmation there are screams, there are squeaks and moans. There is the unmitigated noise of ecologies under destruction, the silence of the missing bees, the pounding heat of too many untreed sidewalks. There is also love, and laughter.

A culture of affirmation does not seek to contain these sounds. It recognizes that they orient more than they position, and it allows them to do so. How the orientation happens depends on the minor gestures. Minor gestures inflect the event toward a different sounding. Not happier or sadder, but more actively joyful in the ethological Spinozist sense: more-than.

RETURNING IS EVERYTHING (JOY)

Writing about Nietzsche's alignment of joy to tragedy, Deleuze asks:

> Can everything become an object of affirmation, that is to say of joy? We must find, for each thing in turn, the special means by which it is affirmed, by which it ceases to be negative. The tragic is not to be found in this anguish or disgust, nor in a nostalgia for lost unity. The tragic is

only to be found in multiplicity, in the diversity of affirmation as such. What defines the tragic is the joy of multiplicity, plural joy. This joy is not the result of a sublimation, a purging, a compensation, a resignation or a reconciliation. (2002: 16)

For Nietzsche, joy is tragic. It is tragic in that it cannot be contained, cannot be categorized in advance. Joy is tragic in the sense that it does not find its limit in the *it is*. "It is joy that is tragic. But this means that tragedy is imme- diately joyful, that it only calls forth the fear and pity of the obtuse specta- tor, the pathological and moralizing listener who counts on it to ensure the proper functioning of his moral sublimations and medical purgings" (2002: 16). Joy: the active dramatization, in the event, of the more-than.

Joy is tragic in Nietzsche because it touches on the most sensitive nerve, sparking the event toward a transformation that is often painful, and always jarring. Joy is tragic because it touches at the limit where life is most un- bearable, exposing life's inexhaustible vitality. Joy is tragic because it does not hide from death and destruction, because it still says *yes!* in the face of that which most terrifies. It says *yes!* (and is thus tragic) not because it wants to carry the burden but because it refuses to be passively trans- formed by a silence that would render it complicit with the nostalgia for the *what was*.

> Saying Yes to life even in its strangest and most painful episodes, the will to life rejoicing in its own inexhaustible vitality even as it witnesses the destruction of its greatest heroes—that is what I called Dionysian, that is what I guessed to be the bridge to the psychology of the tragic poet. Not in order to be liberated from terror and pity, not in order to purge oneself of a dangerous affect by its vehement discharge—which is how Aristotle understood tragedy—but in order to celebrate oneself the eternal joy of becoming, beyond all terror and pity—that tragic joy included even joy in destruction. (Nietzsche 2008: 5)

Another word for the tragic Deleuze uses is "dramatization." The way the event activates the field of relation can be thought of as a dramatization of that field. How the will to power *acts* dramatizes the stakes, in the event, of the occasion's coming-to-be. Each activation, each act, is dramatic in that it lays claim to having become in *just this way*. "Nietzsche creates his own method: dramatic, typological and differential" (Deleuze 2002: 197).

The will to power, the feeling of power, dramatizes the stakes of the event.

"What do you will?" Ariadne asks Dionysus. What a will wants—this is the latent content of the corresponding thing. We must not be deceived by the expression: what the will wants. What a will wants is not an object, an objective or an end. Ends and objects, even motives, are still symptoms. What a will wants, depending on its quality, is to affirm its difference or to deny what differs. Only qualities are ever willed: the heavy, the light. . . . What a will wants is always its own quality and the quality of the corresponding forces. (Deleuze 2002: 78)

Dramatization is the operation through which a will affirms itself. What dramatization does is reveal the dynamic nature of the field of relation. Dramatization is the motor of differentiation. It is what moves the event toward its pragmatic singularization, asking not "what is" but "in which case, who, how, how much?" (Deleuze 2002: 101). "What are the forces which take hold of a given thing, what is the will that possesses it? Which one is expressed, manifested and even hidden in it?" (Deleuze 2002: 77).

This "tragic method" is tragic because it does not know in advance how difference will be affirmed. It is joyful because it activates an eternal mobility, a mobility alive with difference: the eternal return, a spiraling that never eats its tail.

A culture of affirmation is always spiraling, always reconnecting to a return that does not seek resemblance. When Nietzsche calls it the eternal return of the same, he does not mean the self-same. What returns is not the *it is*, but the *what else*. For the *what else* to return, a motor must make the event operational. This motor is necessity, as affirmed of chance. "Necessity is affirmed of chance in exactly the sense that being is affirmed of becoming and unity is affirmed of multiplicity" (Deleuze 2002: 26). Necessity funnels experience toward the points of inflection (the minor gestures) that tune the event, giving it its color, its tone, its shape. Affirmation creates the conditions for necessity and the will to power mobilizes necessity through the *yes!* of joy, activating the quality in the event. The eternal return then makes time for the event's unfolding, *just this way*.

The spiral, the eternal return, is how the event activates the being in becoming. This is why Nietzsche speaks of the eternal return in terms of selection. The eternal return is the parsing mechanism that gives time, that creates the time of the event. The eternal return gives rhythm to the in-act, tuning it not to a measure so much as to a cadence. For what returns is always more quality than quantity. What returns is not metric time, but the feeling of time, the feeling of power. When a selection happens that creates this or that occasion of experience, and when this selection is affirmed by the will to power, time spirals. Affirmation is a becoming-active precisely in its affirmation of time in its spiraling return. It is this tuning to time in its difference that preserves affirmation's untimeliness. All of this "at once moment and cycle of time" (Deleuze 2002: 25). This is the eternal return: the double affirmation that at one and the same moment—in the cycle of time of its immanent invention—activates *and* contemplates the action. "Eternal return is the distinct return of the outward movement, the distinct contemplation of the action, but also the return of the outward movement itself and the return of the action" (Deleuze 2002: 25).

The eternal return is a synthesis, but nothing like a dialectical one. It is, as Deleuze writes, "a synthesis of time and its dimensions, a synthesis of diversity and its reproduction, a synthesis of becoming and the being which is affirmed in becoming, a synthesis of double affirmation" (2002: 48). The eternal return is active in each moment. "Returning is everything but everything is affirmed in a single moment" (Deleuze 2002: 72).

PLANNING (IN THE ACT)

The figure of the student is a good starting point for thinking debt. Moten and Harney write: "Credit pursues the student, offering to match credit for debt, until enough debts and enough credits have piled up. But the student has a habit, a bad habit. She studies. She studies but she does not learn. If she learned they could measure her progress, establish her attributes, give her credit. But the student keeps studying, keeps planning to study, keeps running to study, keeps studying a plan, keeps elaborating a debt. The student does not intend to pay" (2013: 62). She studies. She learns for learning's sake. She learns beyond credit. She learns to forget. She learns by heart, beyond the page. She takes the risk of knowing differently. She cannot pay because she will never have stopped studying, will never have stopped inventing what it means to study.

She is a fugitive public. Fugitive because she keeps bad debts, fugitive because she does not begin her encounter by identifying herself. Fugitive because she is unrecognizable. Only the credited are known to us, for they are the private individuals, the counted ones. She is beyond count, beyond position. She's too busy moving to where the studying takes her. She is of the undercommons, the fragile net that sometimes grows around her, the place where debts are gathered and shared, but never paid off. The undercommons is not a community, and nor is the fugitive public. Temporary, uneasy, surprising, these are emergent collectivities that become active in the untimeliness of an eternal return. For they are always there, and always new.

> Fugitive publics do not need to be restored. They need to be conserved, which is to say moved, hidden, restarted with the same joke, the same story, always elsewhere than where the long arm of the creditor seeks them, conserved from restoration, beyond justice, beyond law, in bad country, in bad debt. They are planned when they are least expected, planned when they don't follow the process, planned when they escape policy, evade governance, forget themselves, remember themselves, have no need of being forgiven. They are not wrong though they are not, finally, communities; they are debtors at distance, bad debtors, forgotten but never forgiven. (Moten and Harney 2013: 64)

Fugitive publics do not wait for a space to present itself for their gathering. They invent the spacetimes of study's composition. They invent the university.

> They study without an end, play without a pause, rebel without a policy, conserve without a patrimony. They study in the university and the university forces them under, relegates them to the state of those without interests, without credit, without debt that bears interest, that earns credits. They never graduate. They just ain't ready. They're building something in there, something down there. Mutual debt, debt unpayable, debt unbounded, debt unconsolidated, debt to each other in a study group, to others in a nurses' room, to others in a barber shop, to others in a squat, a dump, a woods, a bed, an embrace. . . . And in the undercommons of the university they meet to elaborate their debt without credit, their debt without count, without interest, without repayment. Here they meet those others who dwell in a different compulsion, in the same debt, a distance, forgetting, remembered again but only after. (2013: 67–68)

Study does not evaluate from outside its process. It values in the doing. Its plan involves creating conditions for an encounter that has not prechoreographed what it can do. "But if you listen to them they will tell you: we will not handle credit, and we cannot handle debt, debt flows through us, and there's no time to tell you everything, so much bad debt, so much to forget and remember again. But if we listen to them they will say: come let's plan something together. And that's what we're going to do" (2013: 68).

This planning does not work from the perspective of the *ressentiment*-clad *it could be*. *It could be* is too passive. Study affirms, and in the affirmation it asks not *what could we do*, but *how do we do*, how *else* do we do. Planning in the undercommons is the setting into place of techniques that open the event to its more-than, the setting into place of conditions through which the minor gesture expresses itself, tuning the event to its potential. The planning in the undercommons, the planning in the event—this is affirmation. This is not policy-making. This planning is the creating of techniques for worlds to come. It is planning as affirmation, planning that does not set apart the field of action from the welling event, planning that does not rely on either/or but moves instead at the speed of the eternal return.

BEYOND INTERPRETATION, TOWARD VALUING (ACTIVIST PHILOSOPHY)

Affirmation is activist philosophy. It doesn't believe in one speed. It doesn't see the in-act only as purposeful activity. Nor does it prioritize a smooth process. It sees activity as rhythm. Affirmation operates at the differential where rhythms co-compose. Cutting across refrains in the making, affirmation intensifies. This intensification is a "becoming-active personified," a becoming-active that acts from the perspective of the in-act itself. From the perspective of the in-act is another way to say from the perspective of individuation. Individuation is the operational flow of a process. Affirmation cuts into individuation. The cutting affects the process, activating what Simondon calls a dephasing. The dephasing is how the individuation personifies. It is how the individuation makes its conditions of existence known. The dephasing creates the conditions for quality to become felt as such. In the transduction that ensues—the shift in level that creates a new process—the process's differential comes to the fore. Key to affirmation is this dephasing of the in-act, the differential rhythm that activates a new process. Each dephasing opens the way for a new qualitative field, and it is this qualitative difference that affirmation affirms.

The question of the in-act, of activist philosophy, of the becoming-active, is tied to quality-as-difference. Quality as difference is opposed to quality that succumbs too quickly to measure. Such quality is in the service of quantity: it serves only to qualify the *it is*. When quality is perceived only from the perspective of what can be measured, quality is limited to the pregiven realm of what can be accounted for in advance. This is apparent in stereotyping. When we speak, for instance, of the litheness of a dancer, the assumption is that all dancers are lithe. Quality is here more a framing device than an open orientation. The quality of litheness is held together by the preestablished notion not only of what a dancer is, but also of what litheness means in the context of a body predisposed to dancing. Litheness becomes a way of reifying the allure of a dancing body, thereby reducing both litheness and the dancing body to a set of predictable figures (thinness, able-bodiedness, youth). This puts quality at the service of quantity, limiting the force both of what the dancing body can do and how litheness might correspond to this doing. There are of course an infinity of ways this relation could play out, beyond measure, beyond stereotype. But for this to happen, quality would have to be affirmed beyond its relation to form. Form would have to become the afterthought of how quality lands, *this* time, *this* way. Quality as activated in the affirmation is not yet contained by a preexisting relation. The quality of affirmation is beyond measure. It operates, it tunes and attunes, it orients, but it does not set up the frame in advance. Litheness without a subject takes on a completely different sense, opening itself to an emergent shaping that does not yet know how to take hold, how to become-form. The dancing body is invented in affirmation, not reified.

Stereotype tunes quality to a becoming-reactive. We know in advance what the black body, the female body, the animal body can do. We attribute quality to form, and even as we tell ourselves that we are open to variation, the pull of the established relation between the quality and the measure directs our perception. *What was* is a powerful lure.

Becoming-active does not ignore inheritance. It sees it elsewhere—not in the *it was*, but in the planning of the not-yet. It creates value in the moving. It proceduralizes. It evaluates from the perspective of the event's necessity, activated by the pulse of affirmation that opens the event to its qualitative difference. Affirmation is a qualitative valuation that alters the field. Because its will to power is active and not reactive, it never works *against*. *Against* would reorder the event into parts, staging one set of conditions for experience against the other. Affirmation does not stage—it fields. This fielding, as mentioned above, is before all else a tuning of affective tonality. *This* willing feeling, felt in the event, colors experience. There is no sense here of an external purview.

Quality-as-difference is allied, in Nietzsche, with transmutation. Transmutation is the process through which the field values difference. Like transduction, it involves a singularization of the field that reorients it. Transmutation, also called transvaluation, involves "a change of quality in the will to power" (Deleuze 2002: 175). This technique, in the event, is what allows the stakes of the event to express themselves. This creates new values, values that exceed use-value, values that have not yet invented their use. They don't yet know what they owe. "Values and their value no longer derive from the negative, but from affirmation as such. In place of a depreciated life we have life which is affirmed—and the expression 'in place of' is still incorrect. It is the place itself which changes, there is no longer any place for another world. The element of values changes place and nature, the value of values changes its principle and the whole of evaluation changes character" (Deleuze 2002: 175).

Affirmation can no more be "in place of" than it can be quantified. Always without credit, it never knows where it will land, or what its debt will be. Once affirmation takes over, what is left is not reactivity, but risk— the risk of the not-yet, of not knowing, of not even knowing how to know. Study is all we have—the curious exploration of what the in-act can do. This is activist philosophy.

THE POWER OF THE FALSE (BEYOND GOOD AND EVIL)

Beyond interpretation means beyond an analysis that would seek to measure only according to the given. Evaluative judgment is too content with the *it is*, too sure in advance of what the stakes are. Between an incipient valuation and judgment-oriented evaluation, two kinds of truth are at work. One is a truth that puts its faith in the past and feels accountable to that past. A process of excavation is often necessary to reveal it. This process of excavation, directed as it is toward a unifying event, is perilously close to what creates *ressentiment* in Nietzsche's last men, for it is concerned first and foremost with *what was*. In a gesture similar to that of the nostalgic harking back that breeds a lackluster relationship to the affirmation of life in the making, this excavation of the past relies on the belief that the truth will forever stay the same. The work of the excavator is to build resistant tunnels into the past so that this unwavering truth can easily be reached. Life is attended to in reverse, with the past as the barometer for the present. The second kind of truth, allied to Deleuze's concept of the power of the false, is serial. Here narration is mutational and the posture is less the crawl down the tunnel than the Nietzschean leap from peak to peak. "Narration is constantly being completely modified . . . not according to subjective variations, but as a consequence of disconnected places and de-chronologized moments" (Deleuze 1989: 133). Time serially folding onto itself in an eternal return of difference.

These two truths are often at battle in therapeutic settings. Take the example of childhood abuse returned to later in life. One ubiquitous technique is to dig into the past to find the truth of the event. This technique aims to site the originary event as the cut after which everything changed. The therapy builds its narrative around this cut, returning to it as the symptom of all that follows. The tunnel becomes a regular passageway as memory becomes more and more stabilized. Cause-effect scenarios are inevitable here where the light is dim and the paths are straight. The problem is that knowing the truth of the event is rarely much help in alleviating the pain. This is why schizoanalysis takes a different approach, allying itself not to the excavation of truth and with it the thickening of the solitary tunnel walls, but to a collective architecting of mobility that is capable of creating new encounters with life-living. Schizoanalysis does not deny the past but nor does it seek to perseveratively return to it. Instead, it seeks modes of encounter that allow the narration to mutate, to fabulate.

Fabulations are lively with the power of the false. They distance themselves from the truth of first principles (including first cuts). They do so not to discount the pain and the horror of the abuse but to invest in the collective exploration of what life can be, here, now. For they recognize that what is most likely causing the unbearable pain is not only the truth of this "first" cut, but the myriad imperceptible cuts that followed and are still following, cuts that complicate the narration of the event precisely because the event is continuing and the life that is growing around it is changing. The excavation of a truth that would live in a past that could be located cannot account for these thousands of subsequent variations on the pain, variations that pass by almost imperceptibly but nonetheless deeply alter the color of experience. Nor can they account for the ways the variations may have included glimpses of other affective tonalities. The pain that is felt might also be more-than what it seems, including contrasts open to potentials too ineffable to articulate. Attuned to these incipient variations, to these minor gestures, techniques of schizoanalysis refrain from settling back into the *what was* not because they seek to ignore what happened but because the ecologies of experience that co-compose with life-living have already radically changed the stakes of *what was*. To affirm life-living is to affirm the difference that settles itself into life through these minor variations. What emerges from this affirmative stance is not a denial of the abuse, but a technique for composing with the complex patterns of a life capable of including more than one truth: valuation of life-living necessarily means growing truths for life. These truths, alive in the interstices of the imperceptible, are now recognized for the difference they make as incipient tendencies toward a different kind of accounting.

Truths-in-the-making are fabulations: they are affirmative intercessors into the everyday that come alive at the interstices where narration composes with the ineffable. These truths, these fabulations, are too often silenced by the "first" cut which holds the power to create a tight circle that only leads us back to one narrative, to one way of accounting for experience. Fabulation tells life differently. Beyond interpretation.

What the force of fabulation draws out, what it makes felt, is that there was not really a "first" cut. This "first" cut was just the most intensive of the myriad cuts that propel experience. It may be the cut that mattered most, in retrospect, but has its mattering too forcefully backgrounded the ecological nature of experience? Has it silenced the minor gestures that choreograph life-living? When the first is transduced into the myriad, when the ecology of practices is foregrounded and the event opens itself to the not-yet of experience in the making, there may be the potential of a shift that, while not denying the horrors, perceives the more-than that was always also alive in the cut. This more-than may be the motor for another kind of refrain. A refrain that honors the horror, but this time in the tragic joy of a dramatization that affirms difference. Schizoanalysis.

Cuts orient process. They dramatize it. When the dramatization is allied to the power of the false, a new contour emerges that undoes the cut of its hold on the *what was*. "A new status of narration follows from this: narration ceases to be truthful, that is, to claim to be true, and becomes fundamentally falsifying. This is not at all a case of 'each has its own truth,' a variability of content. It is a power of the false which replaces and supersedes the form of the true, because it poses the simultaneity of incompossible presents, or the coexistence of not-necessarily true pasts" (Deleuze 1989: 131). This qualitative shift in the way narrative understands itself tunes truth toward a rhythm of serial complexity that brings to the fore the "undecidable alternatives and differences between the true and the false, and thereby imposes a power of the false as adequate to time, in contrast to any form of the true which would control time" (1989: 132). The mutational rhythm this incites makes felt how the field moves, moved not only by what is known, but also, and even especially, by what cannot yet be known. The power of the false is an intercessor into the field of expression that makes it uneasy, that pushes it to its limit. It is not a lie—that would be too simple. It is the ineffable, the unknowable at the core of the *what if* as experimented in *what else*'s fabulations. "Beyond the true or the false, becoming as power of the false" (Deleuze 1989: 275).

Deleuze connects the will to power with the power of the false. "The other quality of the will to power is a power through which willing is adequate to the whole of life, a higher power of the false, a quality through which the whole of life and its particularity is affirmed and has become active" (2002: 185). It is through the power of the false that another kind of valuing is set into motion. "To affirm is still to evaluate, but to evaluate from the perspective of a will which enjoys its own difference in life instead of suffering the pains of the opposition to this life that it has itself inspired" (2002: 185). The power of the false does not offset responsibility—it reorients it toward the ability, in the not-yet, to respond from the perspective of the event's own unfolding. "To affirm is not to take responsibility for, to take on the burden of what is, but to release, to set free what lives. To affirm is to unburden: not to load life with the weight of higher values, but to create new values which are those of life, which make life light and active. There is creation, properly speaking, only insofar as we make use of excess in order to invent new forms of life rather than separating life from what it can do" (2002: 185).

With the power of the false, *no* reorients itself and develops a new relationship to the *yes!* of affirmation. No longer its adversary, *no* now becomes another kind of limit, an affirmative limit that refuses to choreograph experience according to preexisting narratives of truth, of debt, of credit. No becomes a new kind of truth in the making. *No!* Not the *what was!*

THE UNDERCOMMONS (BECOMING-ACTIVE)

Every time affirmation creates new forms of value, an undercommons is potentialized. This undercommons is less form than force. The undercommons: a field of relation fabulated at the interstices of the now and the not-yet.

The undercommons is alive with minor gestures. But like the minor gestures, the undercommons also often remains on the edges of imperceptibility. Grand gestures overshadow it.

Grand gestures operate within the bounds of the possible. They mobilize around the solidity of narratives already composed. These grand gestures, as mentioned in the introduction, are often seen as the site where true political change occurs, but in fact the grand gesture only upholds the status quo. Unlike the minor gesture, which unsettles the field through its affirmation of difference, the grand gesture choreographs the field around a truth that seeks to justify the *it is*.

Our world is replete with grand gestures. These gestures have as their goal to rally the masses into a common truth. Take the example of Prime Minister Stephen Harper's grand gesture of reconciliation to the First Nations about the residential school system. In the name of the Canadian government, his speech reads:

> To the approximately 80,000 living former students, and all family members and communities, the Government of Canada now recognizes that it was wrong to forcibly remove children from their homes and we apologize for having done this. We now recognize that it was wrong to separate children from rich and vibrant cultures and traditions, that it created a void in many lives and communities, and we apologize for having done this. We now recognize that, in separating children from their families, we undermined the ability of many to adequately parent their own children and sowed the seeds for generations to follow, and we apologize for having done this. We now recognize that, far too often, these institutions gave rise to abuse or neglect and were inadequately controlled, and we apologize for failing to protect you. Not only did you suffer these abuses as children, but as you became parents, you were powerless to protect your own children from suffering the same experience, and for this we are sorry.
>
> The burden of this experience has been on your shoulders for far too long. The burden is properly ours as a Government, and as a country. There is no place in Canada for the attitudes that inspired the Indian Residential Schools system to ever prevail again. You have been working on recovering from this experience for a long time and in a very real sense, we are now joining you on this journey. The Government of Canada sincerely apologizes and asks the forgiveness of the Aboriginal peoples of this country for failing them so profoundly.[4]

This statement of reconciliation, in its acknowledgment of the unspeakable suffering of the First Nations, outlines the responsibility of all Canadians in the forced sequestering of children into Indian Residential Schools and acknowledges the irreparable pain that caused.[5] It also acknowledges the failure of the nation-state to give reparations to the First Nations. In all of these ways, it speaks the truth. But what does this truth do other than restratify the uneven relations between the First Nations and those who have the power to apologize? And whose truth is it?

The gesture of reconciliation claims to give voice to the Indigenous people. Through the reconciliatory rhetoric, Harper asks forgiveness in the name of Canadians. He claims to recognize that there are ongoing effects of what amounts to cultural genocide. But what does the act actually give voice to? What does it mobilize? What work does this grand gesture do other than get us, we the ones who stand firmly on the side of nonvictims in the indigenous context, off the hook? For doesn't it simply once again set the stage into two camps—those who have the power to speak, and those who must listen (and forgive)? Doesn't this grand narrative that puts the abuses in the past risk silencing the indigenous, for whom the either/or option of forgiveness may just not be an option, especially given the context of ongoing practices of colonization?

There is the grand gesture of reconciliation, and then of course there are the minor gestures that push through the process and move it in ways unchoreographed. The Truth and Reconciliation hearings, by all accounts, were replete with such minor gestures. Many First Nations people who testified speak of the healing that ensued from the act of sharing. Vincent Yellow Old Woman puts it this way: "Now that we've acknowledged it, we're beginning to deal with it. And then we can work together on how to move forward."[6] But what changes in the process does not change thanks to the grand gesture. What changes does so because another movement begins to affect the field, a movement harder to pinpoint, a movement less allied to the either/or, good/evil narrative of Harper's speech. It does so because it acknowledges that reconciliation means an infinity of things in the context of colonization, many of these impossible to account for, impossible to count. No grand gesture can settle the score. There is no simple "first" cut that can be magically healed. The conditions can only be shifted through minor gestures that make the field more pliable, more fertile for the sort of planning Moten and Harney see as key to the undercommons.

Planning and fabulation are inextricably linked. In a pull to a futurity active in a time too cyclic to narrate vertically across linear time, fabulation energizes the past, retelling pastness at those junctures that connect it to the ineffable not-yet. It speaks in the between of what is usually considered important and retells stories from perspectives that make felt the complexity of the ecologies operative in the inheritances that carry us forward. It recognizes that something else is at stake here, another kind of power. Planning takes this power, this power of the false, and moves it in a direction as yet unqualified. What is planned in the undercommons of fabulation are the conditions for an action as yet unmappable. For inheritance as lived from the perspective of the undercommons brings past and future into a mobile coexistence. No history only knows itself from one perspective, and no history writes itself without fabulation. Fabulation activates, in the historical record yet to be mobilized, *again*, the force of deviation within the strands of how experience accounts for itself.

Despite its splash, the grand gesture of reconciliation in the end cannot open up experience to the force of its ineffability because it does not make way for a fabulation that could expose it to these activating deviations. Instead, it reduces the field to the either/or scenario of acceptance or denial, firmly positioning power stakes that continue unaltered. Experience is contained: "If I tell you I am sorry, then surely you must accept my apology, and now we can get on with things. If not, that's your choice—I've done what I can." But what of the thousands of fissures, complex and untimely, that make up our collective experience? What of the truths that have grown and mutated over the years of our collective experience? What if we began there, in the complexity, in the proliferation? How else could we proceed without reducing experience to its common denominator? How else could we consider healing without asking you, the victim, to reconcile yourself to our uneasy continued complicity? How else could we collectively invent modes of existence without reducing experience to that first wound that has already been worried enough? First Nations have been clear: self-determination is the recognition they require, on their terms, in their way. It is not for us to excavate their past. It is for them to create their future.[7]

I am not saying the apology is worthless. It was high time for it. I am just saying that the politics of reconciliation are mired in reactivity. This has become starkly apparent in the Canadian context. How else to understand the Harper government's studied disinterest in the continued disappearance and murder of Indigenous women? Over the past thirty years more than twelve hundred Indigenous women have gone missing in Canada. Indigenous women are three times more likely to experience violence than non-Indigenous women. The Harper government's response: it's not a systemic racial issue, but simply a criminal one. The grand gesture has been done, he seems to be saying—isn't that enough?[8]

I am wary of the grand gesture, wary of how it seeks to choreograph the field, wary of how it cements the narrative of the *it is* in its alignment with

the *what was*. What the grand gesture does, it seems to me, is further solid-
ify the becoming-reactive on both ends. The victim, who has been haunted
by the *what was*, must now be content, forever more, with the *it is*. "Get on
with it!" reconciliation announces. "We've paid our debt! You are again in
our debt, the cycle of credit healthy once more."

I am not alone in my wariness. The First Nations listened to the apology, recognized the debt, acknowledged it, but refused the credit.[9] Instead
they continued the mobilizations that have become part of the activism
of indigenous necessity, and they made themselves heard, again (we have
never been good at listening). The power of the false, it turns out, was alive
and well within Indigenous communities, vivid in the fabulations passed
from generation to generation in the oral histories that are there not only
to weave the traces of the past into the present, but to turn time on itself.
With the force of fabulation as the motor, new stories were generated and
shared, and with them a process of emergent planning was born. Idle No
More was born.[10]

FABULATION (TRUTH'S FUTURITY)

Idle No More did not come out of nowhere. And yet it did. This is the
strange thing about affirmation—that it is always wholly new, and always
already present, for all time.[11] This untimeliness reveals another kind of
history than that penned for reconciliation, a history fabulated in the retelling, invented in the interstices of what cannot yet be spoken, played at
the junctures where rules are invented in the event of the game. This we
learn from our children whose games morph in the playing, and for whom
the art of fabulating is still very much alive. In the midst of the play, in the
game whose rules would keep changing on the fly, Idle No More at once
revealed itself and was born, inventing its history with the words of the
future, receptive, from the moment of its inception, to the cycle of eternal
return already so much a part of First Nations culture.[12]

Idle No More began as teach-ins throughout Saskatchewan in the fall
of 2012, sparked by three First Nations women and one non-Native ally.
The original aim of Jessica Gordon, Sylvia McAdam, Sheelah McLean, and
Nina Wilson was to provide Canadians with information about the im-
pending Bill C-45 and its impacts on Aboriginal Rights and Protections.
Soon thereafter, Chief Theresa Spence of the Attawapiskat Cree Nation
announced that she would add her support to the movement with a hunger
strike on Parliament Hill, hoping to also bring attention to the deplorable

housing conditions on her reserve. An undercommons was born—a field without firm limits, an opening for thought, an environment for action of all speeds and slownesses. Its net soon widened. Others began to see their place in it, their nonplace.

From the start Idle No More refused categorical breakdowns based on identity. Its focus was education, forward-thinking, not bloodlines. It was concentrated around Indigenous issues, but it knew the field needed to be everything but either/or. The teach-ins that at first focused on parliamentary bills that would continue to erode First Nations sovereignty, that would continue to undo existing environmental protections, soon became teach-ins that included broader issues of Indigenous rights. These teach-ins and the ones they bred truly became study: I felt their effects in my classes, on the street. More people joined, in Canada and beyond. Some walked sixteen hundred kilometers across Canada to protest with Chief Spence and to support the hunger strike she was undertaking based on "a historical survival diet for indigenous communities facing food shortages and land loss in colonial policies" (Simpson 2013).[13] Chief Spence hoped to convince Prime Minister Harper and Governor General David Johnston to meet with her to discuss First Nations leadership. She implored the government to have a "nation-to-nation" meeting about the James Bay Treaty (Treaty 9), signed by communities in 1905 and 1906, that promised that the communities would receive benefits that served to balance anything that they were giving."[14] She felt strongly, as did other supporters of Idle No More, that Bill C-45, the Conservative government's omnibus budget bill, which contained changes to the Navigable Waters Act, including waterways in First Nations territory, would affect ecological conditions and make it easier to sell reserve land to non-Natives.[15] Each one of us who considers themselves an activist became involved, even those among us who didn't participate in the walk or the teach-ins, recognizing in perhaps a new way that there can be no cause that does not in some way connect to the injustices First Nations have suffered, and continue to suffer. As the website says: "Everyone is invited to join the movement."[16]

Idle No More is about the in-act. It is about rhythms of difference that open up experience to its minor gestures. Idle No More began in a movement, in a walk, and this walk has refused to stop, despite the fact that the government didn't listen to the 270 Nishiyuu Walkers who arrived at Parliament Hill after trekking across Canada in the cold of winter.[17] In the end Theresa Spence had to stop her hunger strike because her health was failing. The government still wasn't listening.

The walk of Idle No More is still creating pockets of undercommons. The point is not to be "faithful" to one particular iteration of Idle No More, but to create with it, to invent how else we can walk, how else we can idle no more. Speculating on the future of Idle No More in March 2013, Leanne Simpson writes:

> It's difficult to say where the movement will go because it is so beautifully diverse. I see perhaps a second phase that is going to be on the land. It's going to be local and it's going to be people standing up and opposing these large-scale industrial development projects that threaten our existence as Indigenous peoples—in the Ring of Fire [a region in northern Ontario], tar sands, fracking, mining, deforestation. . . . But where they might have done that through policy or through the Environmental Assessment Act or through legal means in the past, now it may be through direct action. Time will tell.[18]

Idle No More makes debt social by recognizing that there is no repayment that will do justice to the pain. There is no repayment that can absolutely undo the effects of environmental degradation, no repayment that can still the history of human suffering in the disenfranchised communities of the Canadian North. There is no way to bring back the families destroyed by the residential schools. But there are ways of being rhythmically, differentially in-act, of idling no more and asking, collectively, *what else?* What else can be imagined? What else can we walk toward, or around, or behind? There is a way to claim the stories, and to continue to write them. There is a way to compose the speech, a speech that would sound very different from Harper's because it knows the way the fissures of experience crowd the surface, it knows about the tricksters and their ability to jump onto the *what if* and fly with it, it knows about the power of fabulation.

Fabulation, it bears repeating, is not the denial of the truth. It is another species altogether, a dramatization born of joy that composes at the limits of experience in the making. Fabulation is true! Absolutely true, in the only register of truth affirmation knows: the pragmatically speculative. Pragmatic because it does what it does, it mobilizes *just this way*, under just these conditions. And speculative because how it will unfold, what it can do, what else it will be, remains unknowable in advance of the doing.

Fabulation is replete with bad debt, or affirmation without credit. Fabulation makes no absolute promises. It does not hold to the *what was*. Fabulation is the language spoken by the fugitive public, the public that does not know its place.

The place of refuge is the place to which you can only owe more and more because there is no creditor, no payment possible. This refuge, this place of bad debt, is what we call the fugitive public. Running through the public and the private, the state and the economy, the fugitive public cannot be known by its bad debt but only by bad debtors. To creditors it is just a place where something is wrong, though that something wrong—the invaluable thing, the thing that has no value—is desired. Creditors seek to demolish that place, that project, in order to save the ones who live there from themselves and their lives. . . . But all of a sudden, the thing credit cannot know, the fugitive thing for which it gets no credit, is inescapable. (Moten and Harney 2013: 61–62)

There is no repayment. Only *more*: more fabulation, more walking, more debt. "We saw it in a step yesterday, some hips, a smile, the way a hand moved. We heard it in a break, a cut, a lilt, the way the words leapt. We felt it in the way someone saves the best stuff just to give it to you and then it's gone, given, a debt. They don't want nothing. You have got to accept it, you have got to accept that. You're in debt but you can't give credit because they won't hold it" (Moten and Harney 2013: 61–62).

Idle No More affirms its debt. It knows the debt it's owed. But it doesn't seek credit. It knows credit would only silence it. In its affirmation, it activates the minor, and minor gestures abound. Some of them are immediately captured. There is often exhaustion, dismay. But there is also laughter, and play. "The transition is going to be hard, but from my perspective, from our perspective, having a rich community life and deriving happiness out of authentic relationships with the land and people around you is wonderful. I think where Idle No More did pick up on it is with the round dances and with the expression of the joy. 'Let's make this fun.' It was women that brought that joy."[19]

The place of refuge feels more livable when we remember that no movement, no fugitive public, is held by individuals. It is held by a multiplicity larger than anyone alone, larger than identity. It is held by that round dance in the shopping center that became the image of Idle No More, by a collective gesture infinitely more complex than any individual gesture could be.[20] This is what returns: the multiplicity, the ineffability of an exhaustion, of a tragic joy that teaches us new ways of moving, new rhythms for bare activity. For the in-act, like affirmation, is not just about forward movement. In the undercommons, the place we cannot know, movement is before all else quality—it is the affective tonality of a shift in cadence, a barely perceptible sounding that propels a thought, a lulling that makes us dream and gives us the courage to dance. This is affirmation, a gift without limit.

THE MANY BECOME ONE (AND ARE INCREASED BY ONE)

Affirmation is always more-than-human, always across registers vegetable and mineral, plant and animal. This is why, for Nietzsche, affirmation is not manifested in "man." Affirmation does not belong to the human, it does not belong to a species. Affirmation cuts across the very idea of species. It conditions openings to the more-than, crafting experimental speciations.

For Nietzsche, the figure of the more-than is the Overman. I would rather keep man out of it. What is important about what affirmation can do is that it does not idle in preexisting categories. The figure I seek does not have a predefined form. It is affirmation itself, affirmation as the force of a becoming.

Being is born of becoming. Affirmation cuts into becoming to create being. This being is always more-than. It is an emergent constellation before it is a form. The field does not begin and end in form: it erupts into form, and then dephases into new processes that create an opening for new deviations. Speciations abound, and with them fugitive publics take form and then move along. Places of refuge grow and are fabulated into new constellations. Undercommons emerge and disappear. When being is born of becoming, the way the event settles has not been choreographed in advance. When being is born of becoming, the deviations of experience have not yet expressed themselves in a form preconstituted. Experience is a univocal force, not a simple unity. It is all that it is, in its full becoming, and always more than one in its full being. Both-and.

Both-and is transvaluing. It is not either/or. It is qualitatively abstract, undefinable in advance, and absolutely what it is when it lands. "Becoming and being are a single affirmation" (Deleuze 2002: 189). This is an affirmative book. It accepts affirmation's mantra: "The whole, yes, universal being, yes, but universal being ought to belong to a single becoming, the whole ought to belong to a single moment" (Deleuze 2002: 72). It builds with the single moment's capacity to shift the register of the *what else*. It choreographs with the single moment of the untimeliness of the eternal return. And it recognizes in that single moment the multiplicity of the open whole. The *it is what it is* is nowhere present.

There is violence here, and to negate the violence would be reactive. Affirmation is tragic. There is no question that the will to power, that the power of the differential, involves an act that could be called violent. The minor gesture is not immune to that violence. Even the most imperceptible forces of change can have great effects, and those effects can be destructive. Think of the way a tsunami erupts from the most indiscernible activity. Affirmation does not deny the violence. On the contrary, the work of affirmation involves affirming the violence in order to activate its more-than, in order to make felt what, in violence, can cause the decisive turn, in the event, that opens it to a qualitative difference that really makes a difference. "Thinking is the n-th power of thought. It is still necessary for it to become 'light,' 'affirmative,' 'dancing.' But it will never attain this power if forces do not do violence to it. Violence must be done to it as thought, a power, the force of thinking, must throw it into a becoming-active" (Deleuze 2002: 108). Transmutation, transvaluation, these are potentially violent acts. Change is violent. Thought too cuts, it skews, it reorients. Reorientation is uneasy-making, and it has effects. But this violence heeds a different call than do grand gestures. This is not a violence that replays itself in the same register. It is a violence that opens the way for techniques that create new conditions, conditions propitious for new ways of crossing the threshold that open the event to the *what else*. The line is fine, of course. Violence turns quickly, and reactivity is always right there, ready to pounce. The potential for the event to sway toward destruction is always present, especially when the stakes are so high and the pain is so raw.

There is a call, an appeal, even a demand that is part of a politics of affirmation, and it is this demand that best counters violence's capture of the *what else* in the name of a nihilism that revictimizes. Fred Moten gives a beautiful account of it through the example of Joe McPhee's playing on *Nation Time*.[21] Using the figure of the soloist in the jazz ensemble to challenge the authoritative voice of the univocal speaker, Moten asks,

> What if authoritative speech is detached from the notion of a univocal speaker? What if authoritative speech is actually given in the multiplicity and the multivocality of the demand? This was something that was also happening at that same moment in the music, so that the figure of the soloist was being displaced. Even if the soloist was, in a certain sense, only temporarily occupying a certain kind of sovereign position, the return to collective improvisational practices was sort of saying, "we are making a music which is complex enough and rich enough so that when you listen to it you are hearing multiple voices, multiply formed

voices. We are sort of displacing the centrality of the soloist." (Moten and Harney 2013: 135–136)

In the multiplicity of the ensemble, the demand becomes an appeal, as Moten says, that opens the field to redefinition. "An appeal, in this delivery—you're making all this sound, you're making all this noise. You're an ensemble, and that's bound up with that notion of study and sociality that we've been talking about" (Moten and Harney 2013: 136). The strength of the demand is its capacity to create a transduction, a transmutation in the field. McPhee "was playing harmonics on the horn, so that the horn itself becomes something other than a single-line instrument; it becomes chordal, social. And that chordal playing shows up for us aurally as screams, as honks, as something that had been coded or denigrated as extramusical—as noise rather than signal. So, what I'm trying to do is to consider this notion of the demand as an appeal, as a claim, where you're not appealing to the state but appealing to one another" (Moten and Harney 2013: 136). What matters is not just how the sound is being played and how it can be responded to by another player. What matters is the more-than, the way the horn "becomes something other than a single-line instrument," the way "it becomes chordal, social." The appeal in the event creates a speciation that shifts not only what the music can do, what the sound can do, but creates an emergent collectivity that cannot be reduced to the sum of its parts.

The appeal is not without its violence, not without its consequences, but it does have the power to counter violence's reactivity precisely because of its capacity to cut into the event to expose its multiplicity, to activate its emergent collectivity. As Moten writes, placing the question of the appeal in the context of blackness and black politics: "But, what we understand as the social zone of blackness and the undercommons is the zone precisely in which you make that claim—so that the demand is a doublevoiced thing, an enunciation in the interest of more than what it calls for. You are saying what you want, though what you want is more than what you say, at the same time that you are saying what you are while in the guise of what you are not" (Moten and Harney 2013: 138).

This is the work of a politics of affirmation: to create the conditions for another way of saying *yes!*, for another kind of appeal. This *yes!* is not the donkey's bray, it is not the victim's burden. This *yes!* is a form of listening that also hears the untimely noises of what cannot be contained in the words that describe the event. It is the *yes!* of the fugitive public, that which runs "through the public and the private, the state and the economy," a public "of strangers not communities, of undercommons not neighborhoods, among those who have been there all along from somewhere" (Moten and Harney 2013: 63).

With Nietzsche, with Moten and Harney, with Idle No More, a politics of affirmation makes an appeal that cannot but be heeded. The response to this appeal may be cynical. With cynicism may come critique. And negation. Followed by reconciliation. And identity politics. An affirmative politics will opt against each of these gestures and propose instead a stance that moves with the painful joy that comes with the being born of becoming. It will propose a thinking that moves to the nth power of thought, a thinking ecological to its core, that spreads from the middle, where speciations have not yet resolved into species. This affirmative politics will walk to the improvised tune of an emergent collectivity, a multiplicity replete with gestures that trouble categories, a multiplicity exuberant with fabulations that dance to the power of the false. "We should consider every day lost on which we have not danced at least once. And we should call every truth false which was not accompanied by at least one laugh" (Nietzsche 1977: 332).

INTRODUCTION

1 The Occupy movement is a good example of this. There is no question, it seems to me, that Occupy has had long-lasting effects. It has affected our belief in mobilization and has resulted in sustained political work at the local scale. Montreal is a good example of this: not only did we see the largest student strike in Quebec history in 2012 (the Maple Spring), but the classroom has palpably changed since the end of the strike: students are much more vocal about their belief in free education and in their critique of neoliberalism. Almost three years later, demonstrations took over the streets once again in March and April 2015 in the hope of reenlivening debate around austerity measures and free education. While this student strike only lasted a few months, there is a sense that the unrest remains active under the surface. Forums for debate and political organizing abound, not only in the student sector, but among primary school teachers and other public sector unions.

 The critique of Occupy is one based on the alignment between politics and the grand gesture. Because the protest was open, because it was lively with minor gestures, because it was capable of morphing, its shape has radically changed in the many iterations it has spawned. When we look at political unrest today, when we look at emergent collectivity around the world, we see not "Occupy" but what Occupy allowed to proliferate. Occupy set into motion something already in act and gave it the momentum it needed to reinvent itself. This is how a politics of the minor gesture does its work.

2 Throughout the manuscript, as I did with my book *Always More Than One* (Manning 2013), I toggle between more-than-human and more-than human. For me, the more-than-human is a way of making operative ways of thinking the nonhuman without excising the force of human complicity from these

worldings. When I speak of the more-than human, I am focusing on the realm of the human, emphasizing that the category of the human is always modulated and affected by the more-than. In *Always More Than One* I develop the concept of speciation to account for the intercession of the more-than in what it means to be human. See "Another Regard" in Manning 2013.

3 For more on the ecology of practices, see Stengers 2010, 2011. My own reading of an ecology of practices in some ways departs from that of Stengers, for whom the ecology has less to do with an exploration of how environments are relational at their core than with how self-defined practices (such as science and philosophy, in her example) come together while retaining their difference. I find these two approaches compatible in the sense that in both cases the ecology of practices is not straining toward homogeneity, but toward a bringing-into-relation of difference. An ecology of practices activates the relational field at its point of inflection, creating a new composition that is capable of keeping difference alive.

4 This of course also stages an unimpeachable separation between the human and the animal, between the human-oriented environment and the wider non-human ecologies. For works that have influenced my thinking on the subject, see Wolfe 2012 and Massumi 2014.

5 For more information from the National Association for Down Syndrome, see http://www.nads.org. See also Buckley and Bird 1993.

6 The issue of accommodation is always present for people with disabilities, but was particularly apparent during a recent (2014) conference, held at Syracuse University (known internationally for its disability studies program). This conference was on disability politics, and yet had not considered several levels of accommodations. For details, see William Peace, "Chronicle of Higher Education Story Features Me on the Lack of Access at Academic Conferences," *Bad Cripple* (blog), June 16, 2014, http://badcripple.blogspot.ca/2014/06/chronicle-of-higher-education-feature.html, as well as an article penned by William Peace, of *Bad Cripple*, entitled "Indifference toward Disabled Scholars Alarms a Disabilities Scholar," at http://chronicle.com/ (accessed May 11, 2015). See also Mark Boatman, "William Peace: Scholar, Advocate," *New Mobility, the Magazine for Active Wheelchair Users*, September 1, 2014, http://www.newmobility.com/2014/09/william-peace/, and Stephen Kuusisto's blog *Planet of the Blind*. On lack of accommodation during a conference, see "Dear Disabled Person, We're Sorry but You're a Real Inconvenience, Signed, (Insert Conference Name Here)," *Planet of the Blind*, February 2, 2014, http://www.stephenkuusisto.com/uncategorized/dear-disabled-person-were-sorry-but-youre-a-real-inconvenience-signed-insert-conference-name-here#comment-103575. On able-bodied blues: "The Able-bodied Blues," *Planet of the Blind*, March 7, 2014, http://www.stephenkuusisto.com/uncategorized/the-able-bodied-blues#comment-103572. Another important arena of accommodation includes sensory accommodations, which are rarely taken into account

despite the way sensory overstimulation affects many people on the spectrum of neurodiversity.

7 For an extreme case, see writing around the death of Tim Bowers, a thirty-two-year-old man who fell out of a tree. The day after his accident, he was taken out of a medical coma and asked to decide whether he wanted his life to be saved or not. He decided not to live. His wife was quoted as saying: "The last thing he wanted was to be in a wheelchair. . . . To have all that stuff taken away would probably be devastating. He would never be able to give hugs, to hold his baby. We made sure he knew that, so he could make a decision. Even if he decided the other thing, the quality of life would've been very poor. His life expectancy would be very low." "Injured Indiana Deer Hunter Chose Death over Paralysis," *Indy Star*, November 6, 2013, http://www.indystar.com/article/20131106/NEWS/311060059/Injured-hunter-chooses-death-over-paralysis?nclick_check=1. Several disability activists used this example to discuss the way disability is viewed. One of their key arguments was that it was unethical not to have someone present at this meeting who lives with disabilities of the kind Bowers would have had. See, for instance, William Peace, "Loneliness, Autonomy, Fear and Tim Bowers," *Bad Cripple*, May 9, 2014, http://badcripple.blogspot.ca/2014/05/loneliness-autonomy-fear-and-tim-bowers.html.

8 See, for instance, Richard Dawkins's tweet on Down syndrome (as well as the fallout that followed as disability activists responded). From Dawkins: "Abortion & Down Syndrome: An Apology for Letting Slip the Dogs of Twitterwar," Richard Dawkins Foundation, August 21, 2014, https://richarddawkins.net/2014/08/abortion-down-syndrome-an-apology-for-letting-slip-the-dogs-of-twitterwar/. In response: Chris Kaposy, "A Response to Richard Dawkins on Down Syndrome," Impact Ethics, September 2, 2014, http://impactethics.ca/2014/09/02/response-to-dawkins/; William Peace, "A Brave New World," *Bad Cripple*, August 24, 2014, http://badcripple.blogspot.ca/2014/08/a-brave-new-world.html; Sean McGuire, "Richard Dawkins: It's Immoral to Bring a Down's Syndrome Child into the World," *My Secret Atheist Blog*, August 23, 2014, http://www.mysecretatheistblog.com/2014/08/richard-dawkins-its-immoral-to-bring.html.

9 Moten and Harney write: "Whom do we mean when we say 'there's nothing wrong with us'? The fat ones. The ones who are out of all compass however precisely they are located. The ones who are not conscious when they listen to Les McCann. The Screamers who don't say much, insolently. The churchgoers who value impropriety. The ones who manage to evade self-management in the enclosure. The ones without interest who bring the muted noise and mutant grammar of the new general interest by refusing. The new general intellect extending the long, extra-genetic line of extra-moral obligation to disturb and evade intelligence. Our cousins. All our friends" (2013: 52). This issue comes up often in thought-provoking ways on Dave Hingsburger's blog, http://davehingsburger.blogspot.ca/ (accessed October 1, 2015).

10　This comment was made by Fred Moten in his review of this manuscript.

11　"Do Black Lives Matter? Robin D.G. Kelley and Fred Moten in Conversation," https://vimeo.com/116111740 (accessed March 15, 2015). Michael Brown was shot and killed by a police officer, Darren Wilson, on August 9, 2014, in Ferguson, Missouri. A federal investigation later cleared Wilson. Eric Garner was killed on July 17, 2014, when a police officer put him in a chokehold for fifteen seconds. Caught on tape, the incident clearly demonstrates that Garner is not fighting. Restrained by four police officers, Garner repeats "I can't breathe" eleven times before he dies, lying face down on the sidewalk. The grand jury ruled it a homicide, and the officer, Daniel Pantaleo, was not indicted. These two events (two of uncountable such events) sparked the Black Lives Matter movement, which has resulted in hundreds of protests and rallies across the United States.

12　"Do Black Lives Matter? Robin D.G. Kelley and Fred Moten in Conversation," https://vimeo.com/116111740 (accessed March 15, 2015).

13　See, for instance, the chapter entitled "Waltzing the Limit" in Manning 2013.

14　Neurodiversity is not about cure. In the words of autistic John Elder Robinson:

> To many neurodiversity proponents, talk of "cure" feels like an attack on their very being. They detest those words for the same reason other groups detest talk of "curing gayness" or "passing for white," and they perceive the accommodation of neurological differences as a similarly charged civil rights issue. If their diversity is part of their makeup they believe it's their right to be accepted and supported "as-is." They should not be made into something else — especially against their will — to fit some imagined societal ideal. . . . After many years of struggle it's against the law to discriminate against someone because of race or faith anywhere in America. Unfortunately we have not come that far in other areas. It's still legal to fire someone for being gay in many states. People who act different by virtue of their neurology have no protections other than those general ones afforded under the Americans With Disabilities Act. . . . The task of changing societal attitudes is complicated by the fact that neurological difference is invisible. . . . We can accept that neurological difference is a natural part of us while still working hard to minimize or eliminate its negative effects. At the same time we should recognize and celebrate the very real benefits difference confers on many of us, and embrace people as they are because that is reality. . . . I believe acceptance of neurodiversity backed up by support for solid research into how we can be our best (least disabled, most productive, etc.) is the most positive position those of us who are different can take. I celebrate all the people who fight for the rights of people who are different, and I look forward to the further fruits of those efforts. Meanwhile, I will use my own differences as I always have — to make a living doing those odd things I do better by virtue of my neurology.

John Elder Robinson, "What Is Neurodiversity," *My Life With Asperger's* (blog), October 7, 2013, Psychology Today, http://www.psychologytoday.com /blog/my-life-aspergers/201310/what-is-neurodiversity.

15 Gary Genosko discusses Guattari's use of this term, initially used by Jean Oury, in Genosko 2002. Guattari thought of normopathy as the most incurable of all diseases.

16 See Deleuze 2005. I also discuss Deleuze's concept of *a life* in detail in "Waltzing the Limit" in Manning 2013.

17 I discuss procedural architecture in chapter 4. See Arakawa and Gins 2002.

18 An encouraging recent trend that would work against the normalization discussed above is the decision, by many US colleges, to get rid of the SAT scores usually necessary in the application to university programs. "Meredith Twombly, Hampshire's dean of admissions and financial aid, says that a college-wide study showed little, if any, correlation between high test scores academic achievement. The tests were eliminated, she says, because they were a 'very poor predictor of success.' 'If we have a success story in a year or two, I fully expect at least a handful of schools to follow us,' Twombly says, noting that getting rid of test scores will help the admissions office place a higher premium on more meaningful areas of college applications, such as extracurricular activities, writing samples and high school GPAs." Justin Peligri, "No, the SAT Is Not Required. More Colleges Join Test-Optional Train," College, USA Today, July 7, 2014, http://college.usatoday.com/2014/07/07/no-the-sat -is-not-required-more-colleges-join-test-optional-train/.

19 For a thorough exploration of research-creation in its alignment to SenseLab practices, see "Propositions for Thought in the Act" in Manning and Massumi 2014.

20 The SenseLab defines itself as a laboratory for thinking and making that works at the intersection of art, philosophy, and activism. I started it in 2004. It is defined in more detail on its website at http://senselab.ca/wp2/ (accessed June 10, 2015).

21 Autistic Perception is a key concept in Manning 2013. See chapters "Toward a Leaky Sense of Self" and "An Ethics of Language in the Making."

22 Throughout, when I discuss consciousness, it is usually with an emphasis on the reflective side of consciousness. Bergson makes a distinction between immediate consciousness and reflective consciousness. Immediate consciousness is closer to the nonconscious as I am using it throughout. It refers to the edge of the nonconscious (where something is felt without a cognitive process taking over). "Awareness" or "field awareness" might be another term for this. In immediate consciousness, representation in language is not yet available. In reflective consciousness, which is closer to consciousness as I am using it, there is a tuning toward cognition and language to represent what is felt. In the citations from Bergson throughout, this distinction is not made, however. I therefore prefer to work with the terms "conscious" and "nonconscious." This

also facilitates the task of linking Bergson's work on the feeling of effort to James's in chapter 6.

23 See "Propositions for the Verge" and the interlude entitled "What Else" in Manning 2013.

24 For current work in the mainstream that makes a similar argument, see Malcolm Gladwell's *Blink* (Gladwell 2006). On the book's back cover it describes itself as "a book about how we think without thinking, about choices that seem to be made in an instant—in the blink of an eye—that actually aren't as simple as they seem. . . . *Blink* reveals that great decision makers aren't those who process the most information or spend the most time deliberating, but those who have perfected the art of 'thin-slicing'—filtering the very few factors that matter from an overwhelming number of variables."

25 Many autistics have argued that person-first language denies the complexity of autism as a way of living, of being in and with the world. For this reason, I never use person-first language (i.e., "person with autism"). Lydia Brown writes:

> At the Adult Services Subcommittee's final meeting last Wednesday, much to do was made about semantic disagreements—"ASD individual" versus "individual with ASD," and of course, the dreaded "person with autism" or "person who has autism" versus "autistic person." These issues of semantics are hot button issues, and rightfully so. . . . When we say "person with autism," we say that it is unfortunate and an accident that a person is Autistic. We affirm that the person has value and worth, and that autism is entirely separate from what gives him or her value and worth. In fact, we are saying that autism is detrimental to value and worth as a person, which is why we separate the condition with the word "with" or "has." Ultimately, what we are saying when we say "person with autism" is that the person would be better off if not Autistic, and that it would have been better if he or she had been born typical. We suppress the individual's identity as an Autistic person because we are saying that autism is something inherently bad like a disease.
>
> Yet, when we say "Autistic person," we recognize, affirm, and validate an individual's identity as an Autistic person. We recognize the value and worth of that individual as an Autistic person—that being Autistic is not a condition absolutely irreconcilable with regarding people as inherently valuable and worth something. We affirm the individual's potential to grow and mature, to overcome challenges and disability, and to live a meaningful life *as an Autistic*. Ultimately, we are accepting that the individual is different from non-Autistic people—and that that's not a tragedy, and we are showing that we are not afraid or ashamed to recognize that difference.

Lydia Brown, "Identity-First Language," ASAN: Autistic Self Advocacy Network, http://autisticadvocacy.org/home/about-asan/identity-first-language/ (accessed October 4, 2015).

This is also an issue in the wider context of disability studies activism. Cara Liebowitz explains:

> Though person-first language is designed to promote respect, the concept is based on the idea that disability is something negative, something that you shouldn't want to see. After all, no one tells me that I should call myself a *person with femaleness* or a *person with Jewishness*. I'm a Jewish woman. No one questions that. Yet when I dare to call myself a disabled person, it seems the whole world turns upside down. That's because gender and religion are seen as neutral, if not positive, characteristics. The idea of separating the disability from the person stems from the idea that disability is something you should *want* to have separated from you, like a rotten tooth that needs to be pulled out.
>
> Disability is only negative because society makes it so. For sure, there are negative aspects of my disability. (For the sake of simplicity, I'm focusing solely on my physical disability, which is both the most visible and the most integrated into my being.) Chronic pain and fatigue are no picnic. But for the most part, my disability is just another thread in the tapestry of my life. Pull it and the whole thing might unravel. Pull it and you might get an ugly hole where something beautiful once was.
>
> Identity-first language is founded upon the idea of the social model of disability. In a nutshell, the social model says that though our *impairments* (our diagnostic, medical conditions) may limit us in some ways, it is the inaccessibility of *society* that actually *disables* us and renders us unable to function. The most basic example is wheelchair accessibility. If I am using my wheelchair and I can't go to a restaurant because it doesn't have a ramp, am I disabled by my cerebral palsy or am I disabled by the inaccessibility of the restaurant?

Cara Liebowitz, "I am Disabled: On Identity-First versus People-First Language," *The Body Is Not an Apology*, March 20, 2015, http://thebodyisnot anapology.com/magazine/i-am-disabled-on-identity-first-versus-people-first -language/ (accessed October 4, 2015).

1. AGAINST METHOD

1 The Social Science and Humanities Research Council, a Canadian government agency, implemented research-creation as a funding category in 2003. Since then, it has continued to honor its commitment to artists, now making it possible to apply for any large grant with a research-creation project. This has certainly been useful for artists within the academy who had formerly been excluded from applying to large grants (if they didn't have PhDs), but it has also had the consequence of segregating research from creation, foregrounding social-science-inflected methodological inquiry over the exploration of how art itself produces knowledge. On the "creation" side, research-creation

as granting category has tended to emphasize industry-oriented knowledge-transfer. What it hasn't been as capable of assessing (and willing to fund) is the kind of speculative knowledge art is best at producing.

2   I am thinking here of two scenarios, both of which I see in the university setting. The first is the general distrust, within studio departments, of practices that have a strong philosophical component. Here, the fear seems to be that the art will be stifled, which does tend to happen when a theoretical model is simply imposed (from outside) onto the art object. Another example of the theory-practice split happens in the wider arena of the humanities, particularly where there are interdisciplinary research-creation programs. Here, I observe professors lamenting the lack of clear articulation of a project, wishing it had a stronger theoretical backbone, which too often means putting the practice aside in lieu of a more art-historical approach. Neither of these tendencies truly engages with the singularity of research-creation, it seems to me. What I am proposing here is quite different: an approach that takes the art process as generative of thought, and that transversally connects that thought-in-the-act to a writing practice, should the need arise for writing to accompany it.

3   The SenseLab (www.senselab.ca) has been a creative incubator for this kind of thinking for the past decade. At the SenseLab, we engage primarily with the question of how events can be created that open themselves to new forms of collaboration not only between different people, but between different kinds of practices.

4   See also Brian Massumi's use of the concept in his introduction to *Semblance and Event* (Massumi 2011).

5   For more on the question of subjectivity understood as generative (active in an ecology of practices), see Guattari 2012.

6   Whitehead writes:

> The range of species of living things is very large. It stretches from mankind throughout all the vertebrates, and the insects, and the barely organized animals which seem like societies of cells, and throughout the varieties of vegetable life, and down to the minutest microscopic forms of life. At the lower end of the scale, it is hazardous to draw any sharp distinction between living things and inorganic matter. There are two ways of surveying this range of species. One way abstracts from time, and considers the variety of species as illustrating various levels of life. The other way emphasizes time, by considering the genetic relations of the species one to another. The latter way embraces the doctrine of evolution, and interprets the vanishing of species and of sporadically variant individuals, as being due to maladjustment to the environment. This explanation has its measure of truth: it is one of the great generalizations of science. But enthusiasts have so strained its interpretation as to make it explain nothing, by reason of the fact that it explains everything. We hardly ever know the definite character of the struggle which occasioned the disappearance. . . . The importance

of the doctrine of the struggle for existence depends on the assumption that living beings reproduce themselves in sufficient numbers of healthy offspring, and that adaptation to the environment is therefore the only decisive factor. This double assumption of prolificness and of healthiness is obviously not always true in particular instances. (1929: 5–7)

7　The use of methodology here raises the issue of the difference between method and methodology. I concur with Whitehead that the line between them is very fine. One need only consider the normative use of the term "methodology" in dissertations and grant applications to become aware that the term is generally conceived not as the reflection on the value of method but as the placeholding of certain disciplinary criteria. I am not saying, of course, that it is not possible to open method to its potential, but my preferred term for this would be "technique," as technique better emphasizes the necessity for a process to itself define the limits of its actualization.

8　Whitehead also refers to Descartes here. He writes: "But the word 'feeling,' as used in these lectures, is even more reminiscent of Descartes. For example: 'Let it be so; still it is at least quite certain that it seems to me that I see light, that I hear noise and that I feel heat. That cannot be false; properly speaking it is what is in me called feeling (sentire); and used in this precise sense that is no other thing than thinking'" (1978: 65).

9　See "Dancing the Virtual" in Manning 2013.

10　This is apparent in both the art market context and in the academic institution. Artistic trajectories that do not map well on existing "disciplinary" trends are often overlooked, as are scholars whose practices are truly transversal. In my experience, it is quite common in a job interview, for instance, to look upon a scholar's work with admiration, even while casting aside his or her application because they are seen not to have the means to adequately fulfill the needs of a given discipline. This always strikes me as odd, given the fact that transdisciplinary thinkers are generally very creative and intelligent, and extremely capable of reorienting themselves where the need surfaces. To turn away transdisciplinary thinkers is to also cast aside the potential for the crafting of unexpected links that open the discipline to new areas of investigation.

2. ARTFULNESS

1　S.v. "art," *Oxford English Dictionary*, http://www.oed.com (accessed April 10, 2014).

2　I have developed relational movement as a concept in both *Politics of Touch* (2007) and *Relationscapes* (2009).

3　I discuss this concept more fully in "Propositions for the Verge" in Manning 2013.

4　For a more in-depth exploration of the concept of likeness, see "The Thinking-Feeling of What Happens" in Massumi 2011. I also explore the relationship between likeness and counterpoint in "Another Regard" in Manning 2013.

5 See "Dancing the Virtual" in Manning 2013 for a more comprehensive reading of technique and technicity.

6 In *Always More Than One* (Manning 2013), I have an interlude entitled *Fiery, Luminous, Scary* that explores these questions in relation to a work of mine entitled *Slow Clothes || Folds to Infinity*. It seems to me that the demands of relational or participatory art are such that the creation of conditions for participation must be crafted with as much attention as the objects themselves receive (if there are objects). The art here is precisely the art of relation.

7 For an account of animality and creativity, see Massumi 2014.

3. WEATHER PATTERNS

1 I discuss this work in some detail in Manning 2013 — see the second section of the chapter entitled "Choreography as Mobile Architecture." The work has been exhibited several times, both as *Slow Clothes* and as *Stitching Time*. The last two iterations of the work were exhibited at the Sydney Biennale (2012) and at the Moscow Biennale (2013). Images of the work can be found at www .erinmovement.com under "Artwork."

2 Objectness would here be allied to the objectile as defined by Deleuze in *The Fold* (Deleuze 1992). I also discuss it in relation to the choreographic object in the chapter entitled "What Else" in Manning 2013.

3 For more on Song Dong's work, see http://ybca.org/song-dong (accessed November 12, 2013).

4 Song Dong's work is very attentive to modes of production (and the excess that results from capitalist production) in China.

5 Leo Kamen, art dealer and ex-owner of the Leo Kamen Gallery in Toronto, speaking of artistic practice, suggests that much art that sells within the contemporary art market is based on conclusions rather than processes. We like conclusions, it seems, but whether conclusions are artful is an open question.

6 For more on the concept of mobile architecture, see "Choreography as Mobile Architecture" in Manning 2013.

7 For Forsythe's definition of the choreographic object, see Forsythe 2008.

8 For a thorough account of presentational immediacy and causal efficacy, two key concepts in Whitehead's account of perception, see Whitehead 1927.

9 I foreground the gallery as a setting for contemporary art throughout not because I think the artful necessarily lives in the gallery setting. In fact, the artful and the gallery have a history of contention. Nonetheless, for most artists the gallery remains a site of experimentation and exhibition, and therefore the question of what the contemporary art gallery can mobilize in the name of the artful is important.

10 Curator Catherine de Zegher is an exception in this regard. Her exhibitions are alive with minor gestures, activated both through the works themselves and in their emergent relations. De Zegher's curatorial technique of choosing artists not based on flashy magazines or fame but by traveling to their places

of work and engaging with them one on one to bring out the relational force of their work is what enables the rare expression of the minor gesture within the setting of the contemporary art gallery. De Zegher's careful attendance to the choreography of exhibition is also key to this process as it allows artists to compose in relation to each other's work, sensitive to the openings created in their physical and conceptual proximity.

4. DRESS BECOMES BODY

1 From "Biotopological Diagramming, A New Procedure/Method for Staying Alive Indefinitely," in Arakawa and Gins 2011.

2 In *Always More Than One*, I speak about the force of relation that constitutes a bodying. I refer to speciations as the form the movement takes, in the bodying. A speciation might be thought of as the active ecology, more-than human, that accompanies a given activity. A writing speciation might involve a finger-chair-sitting constellation, or a pecking-rocking-sounding constellation. Affirmation activates speciations by generating a push in the event that catalyzes a singular constellation that includes us, but is not delimited by any idea of a pregiven form. See the chapter entitled "Another Regard" in Manning 2013.

3 Rei Kawakubo, "Rei Kawakubo's Creative Manifesto," *BusinessofFashion.com*, October 30, 2013, http://www.businessoffashion.com/2013/10/rei-kawakubo -comme-des-garcons.html.

4 Kawakubo, "Rei Kawakubo's Creative Manifesto."

5 There also exist indigenous traditions in garment design that challenge the idea of the predefined shape of a body, inviting the body to define itself through an encounter with the fabric. These include the Indian sari, the Malay or Indo-nesian sarong, and the African *kanga* or *kitenge*, each of which is emergent as garment in the folding.

6 Kawakubo, "Rei Kawakubo's Creative Manifesto."

7 Rei Kawakubo, "Rei Kawakubo in Her Own Words," *AnotherMag.com*, Oc-tober 3, 2013, http://www.anothermag.com/current/view/3075/AnOther _Magazine_18__Rei_Kawakubo_in_Her_Own_Words.

8 Kawakubo, "Rei Kawakubo in Her Own Words."

9 For more on Whitehead's concept of creativity, see Whitehead 1967: 179–180.

10 Adrian Joffe, "The Idea of Comme des Garçons," *Hypebeast.com*, January 10, 2011, http://hypebeast.com/2011/1/adrian-joffe-the-idea-of-comme-des -garcons.

11 Rei Kawakubo and Hilary George-Parkin, "Rei Kawakubo Doesn't Sketch, Use a Desk, or Like Being 'Understood,'" *Styleite.com*, June 3, 2002, http://www .styleite.com/news/rei-kawakubo-nyt/.

12 See Keane and Glazebrook 2013.

13 For a more detailed exploration of how attention dances, see "The Dance of Attention" in Manning 2013.

14 It is important to emphasize that not all collections are primarily designed by Rei Kawakubo, though she does supervise the process. Junya Watanabe has been an important designer for Comme des Garçons, first as a pattern-maker starting in 1984, and then as a designer in 1987. He started designing under his own name in 1992. Other designers include Tao Kurihara and Kei Ninomiya.

15 See, for instance, Derrida 1998, 1983.

16 Rei Kawakubo and Hilary George-Parkin, "Rei Kawakubo Doesn't Sketch, Use a Desk, or Like Being 'Understood,'" *Styleite.com*, June 3, 2002, http://www.styleite.com/news/rei-kawakubo-nyt/ (accessed February 24, 2014).

17 This concept is developed at more length in "Just Like That: William Forsythe, Between Movement and Language" in Manning and Massumi 2014.

18 There is a conceptual connection between the absolute fold or infinite line described above and Deleuze and Guattari's "abstract line." They define an abstract line as "a line that delimits nothing, that describes no contour, that no longer goes from one point to another but instead passes between points, that is always declining from the horizontal and the vertical and deviating from the diagonal, that is constantly changing direction, a mutant line of this kind that is without outside or inside, form or background, beginning or end and that is as alive as a continuous variation—such a line is truly an abstract line, and describes a smooth space. It is not inexpressive" (1987: 498).

5. CHOREOGRAPHING THE POLITICAL

1 Motor apraxia, linked as it is to specific brain function, tends to condense movement difference to a simplified reading of brain damage. It is more interesting, therefore, to consider the movement divergence autistics speak of in terms of "autistic movement disturbance." While some aspects of the pathology are allied to apraxia, current research suggests that what occurs within autistic experience is more global and therefore cannot be reduced to a single pathology. For the purposes of this chapter, while I will hold on to Kedar's use of apraxia, my focus will be on how movement opens up the very question of pathology. For an interesting paper on the topic of autistic motor disturbance, see Torres et al. 2013. Torres et al. write: "Our results suggest that there is a lack of spontaneous autonomy in the autistic system that impedes adaptive and co-adaptive volitional control and that this is largely contributed by corrupted afferent peripheral information, including input from the autonomic and somatic nervous systems of which we specifically tackled hand movement proprioception here. Our work highlights that autism is a systemic neurodevelopmental disorder with concrete, measurable physical bases. Autism should not be exclusively portrayed as a psychological, abstract cognitive/social problem of a 'disembodied' brain. This would be a static snapshot of a person whose sensory-motor systems are clearly evolving and changing in compensatory ways." For more, see Torres et al. 2013.

2 Ido Kedar recounts his experience from ages twelve to fifteen; he wrote *Ido in Autismland* (Kedar 2012) over this period. I mention this both to underline the extraordinary maturity in his writing and to draw attention to the fact that he has perhaps not yet fully come into himself as a thinker of disability or neurodiversity.

3 Deleuze and Guattari's account of the "Body without Organs"—a concept that comes from Antonin Artaud—might be considered a limit condition where neurotypicality meets neurodiversity. See Deleuze and Guattari 1987.

4 About stimming, which is usually described as uncontrollable, involuntary movements that calm down the nervous system, Ido Kedar writes: "Stims have a force that is powerful and compelling. They feel like forces that make resistance futile. It's like resisting hunger or sleep in some ways. They come into my mind so suddenly. Then I feel overwhelmed by the urge to do something like hand flapping, or noises, or spitting out water" (2012: 42).

5 See Manning 2013; "Coming Alive in a World of Neurodiversity" in Manning and Massumi 2014.

6 ABA refers to Applied Behavior Analysis, which is still a dominant therapeutic means for dealing with autistics. Autism Speaks, a highly questionable organization that privileges the model of cure and doesn't allow autistics to speak for themselves, describes it this way: "Behavior analysis focuses on the principles that explain how learning takes place. Positive reinforcement is one such principle. When a behavior is followed by some sort of reward, the behavior is more likely to be repeated. Through decades of research, the field of behavior analysis has developed many techniques for increasing useful behaviors and reducing those that may cause harm or interfere with learning. Applied behavior analysis (ABA) is the use of these techniques and principles to bring about meaningful and positive change in behavior." For more on ABA, see "Applied Behavior Analysis (ABA)," Autism Speaks, http://www.autismspeaks.org/what-autism /treatment/applied-behavior-analysis-aba (accessed March 5, 2015).

7 S.v. "inflection," *Oxford English Dictionary* (accessed April 14, 2014).

8 From "Mouvement total," an unpublished manuscript by Jose Gil (2000).

9 This comes close to the definition of "bare activity," which Massumi develops in several of his essays, most notably in *Semblance and Event: Activist Philosophy and the Occurrent Arts* (Massumi 2011: 1–3, 10–11) and "Perception Attack: Brief on War Time" (Massumi 2010).

10 The concept of the interval is explored in more detail in Manning 2009, particularly the first chapter, "Incipient Action: The Dance of the Not-Yet."

11 For more on cueing and aligning in the context of Bill Forsythe's work, see "Choreography as Mobile Architecture" in Manning 2013.

12 Recent studies have shown that doodling enhances attention. John Cloud writes: "We doodlers, fidgeters and whisperers always get the same jokey, passive-aggressive line from the authority figure at the front of the room: 'I'm sorry, are we bothering you?' How droll. But the underlying message is clear:

Pay attention. . . . In a delightful new study, which will be published in the journal *Applied Cognitive Psychology*, psychologist Jackie Andrade of the University of Plymouth in southern England showed that doodlers actually remember more than nondoodlers when asked to retain tediously delivered information, like, say, during a boring meeting or a lecture." Cloud does go on to suggest that doodling enhances memory because there is no time to daydream. Neurotypicality rears its head even in accounts of how we are now invited to doodle! For more on the question of time and neurodiversity, see John Cloud, "Study: Doodling Helps You Pay Attention," *Time*, February 26, 2009, http://content .time.com/time/health/article/0,8599,1882127,00.html.

13 On the impossibility of standing still, see "A Mover's Guide to Standing Still" in Manning 2009.

14 For a more detailed exploration of the concepts of "preacceleration" and the "elasticity of the almost," see "Elasticity of the Almost" in Manning 2009.

15 See Souriau 2009. For a more detailed exploration of modes of existence in relation to process philosophy, see also Erin Manning, "Body Becomes Dress: Fashioning the Force of Form," *The Funanbulist* (March 2014), http://thefunambulist .net/2014/03/13/the-funambulist-papers-51-dress-becomes-body-fashioning -the-force-of-form-by-erin-manning/.

16 Unable to find a better term, Brian Massumi opted for the already-existent translation. While many people have expressed doubt about the translation, nothing better has yet been found.

17 For a detailed account of techniques invented at the SenseLab, see "Propositions for Thought in the Act" in Massumi and Manning 2014.

18 Although I don't write about the interval per se in *Politics of Touch: Sense, Movement, Sovereignty* (Manning 2007), it was a thinking of the interval in regards to a reaching-toward that was at the heart of the rethinking of the body politic in that book.

19 Much excellent work has been done in this area in the past decade. This includes (but is not limited to) Massumi 2015 and forthcoming; Connolly 2013, 2010; Bennett 2009; and Panagia 2009.

20 For more on machinic animism, see Angela Melitopoulos and Maurizio Lazzarato, "Assemblages: Félix Guattari and Machinic Animism," *e-flux*, 2012, http:// www.e-flux.com/journal/assemblages-felix-guattari-and-machinic-animism/ (accessed January 20, 2015).

21 For a more thorough account of autistic emphasis on the more-than-human and the ways in which autistics are seen as non-human, see my critique of "mindblindness" in "An Ethics of Language in the Making" in Manning 2013. See also Savarese 2015.

22 See more by Amelia Baggs at http://withasmoothroundstone.tumblr.com (accessed March 24, 2015).

23 Massumi develops a similar account of the link between activist philosophy and the theory of value. Central to his argument is a critique of capitalist forms of value, including capitalist surplus-value. See Massumi forthcoming.

1 An incomplete list of the many important accounts of autistic perception and the challenges of crossing the neurodiversity/neurotypical divide include Blackman 2001; Brauns 2002; Gerland 1997; McKean 1994; Miller 2003; DJ Savarese, http://tash.org/breaking-the-barriers/personal-stories/d-j-savarese/ (accessed September 30, 2015); Mukhopadhyay 2000, 2007; Prince-Hughes 2004; Williams 1992; Yergeau 2013.

2 Because the point I am making here concerns the role of the "subject" as an event-based category in Whitehead, I am simplifying the concept of subjective aim, which in Whitehead has a role to play at both the physical and the mental poles. On the one hand, the subjective aim can be understood as the act of "aiming," in the event, that orients how it comes to express itself as such (as subjective form). The subjective aim is "the lure for feeling," the concern, in the event, for how it comes to be (1978: 130). In Bergsonian terms, it might be allied to the concept of sympathy. This gets more complicated when Whitehead delves into what he calls "the category of subjective intensity." Now, aim operates not only as an orientation, but also as a force for the (conceptual) future. He writes: "The subjective aim, whereby there is origination of conceptual feeling, is at intensity of feeling (a) in the immediate subject, and (b) in the relevant future. This double aim at the immediate present and the relevant future is less divided than appears on the surface. For the determination of the relevant future, and the anticipatory feeling respecting provision for its grade of intensity, are elements affecting the immediate complex of feeling. The greater part of morality hinges on the determination of relevance in the future. The relevant future consists of those elements in the anticipated future which are felt with effective intensity by the present subject by reason of the real potentiality for them to be derived from itself" (Whitehead 1978: 41). A new kind of novelty is potentialized here: "Thus a single occasion is alive when the subjective aim which determines its process of concrescence has introduced a novelty of definiteness not to be found in the inherited data of its primary phase. The novelty is introduced conceptually and disturbs the inherited 'responsive' adjustment of subjective forms. It alters the 'values,' in the artist's sense of that term" (1978: 159). Subjective aim brings difference to the fore in the event. The minor gesture works in a similar way, both motivating the event and activating the event's differential.

3 Whitehead writes: "Prehensions are not atomic; they can be divided into other prehensions and combined into other prehensions. Also prehensions are not independent of each other. The relation between their subjective forms is constituted by the one subjective aim which guides their formation. This correlation of subjective forms is termed 'the mutual sensitivity' of prehensions" (1978: 358). There tends to be some misunderstanding about the role of atomicity in Whitehead. The atomic aspect of the event, that the event is, here, now, exactly what it is, does not mean that there was not potential for it to be

something else, nor does it mean that the occasion that follows from it is fixed. It simply means that once the event has found its subjective form, it cannot be unformed. Its orientation is now in the world, of the world. The concept of mutual sensitivity is key. With mutual sensitivity comes mutual inclusion: the time of experience is relational, the occasion alive with incipient futurity.

4 Screening tests are the norm for many in the category considered "at danger" for Down syndrome. Current statistics demonstrate that more than 90 percent of pregnancies in the United Kingdom and Europe with a diagnosis of Down syndrome are terminated, with similar though slightly lower percentages in the United States and Canada. Renate Lindeman writes: "Singling out a condition by offering routine screening and enabling selective abortion sends a strong value judgment about potential quality of life. Trying to predict the future based solely on their genes opens the door to discrimination, anxiety, fears and underestimating social and environmental factors in maintaining health. Progress that was made over many generations, in terms of inclusion and equal rights, could be lost in less than one" (2008).

5 On his blog *Bad Cripple*, William Peace writes as an advocate for disability rights, focusing especially on people with spinal injury. He writes:

> In the last 25 years the statistics associated with unemployment and disability have not changed significantly. Between 66 and 70% of people with a disability are unemployed. These are grim numbers. The reasons for the shockingly high unemployment rates have been keenly debated. Businesses are loath to hire people with a disability. Years ago I had a student who was stunned by these numbers and wanted to do a fieldwork project. She proposed to go to the mall and ask the big national clothing stores, Gap, Banana Republic, American Eagle, Ann Taylor, etc. for a job application. She wore the same clothing and told the same background story each time. On one visit she would simply walk in the store and ask for an application. She got an application 99% of the time. She would return one week later wearing the same clothes but using a properly fitting wheelchair. She was not given one application. Every store told her they were not hiring. The point here is the social bias against hiring people with a disability is overwhelming.

William Peace, "The Return on Disability: A Capitalistic Profit Model I Approve of," *Bad Cripple*, March 1, 2014, http://badcripple.blogspot.ca.

6 Within the community of autistics who argue in favor of neurodiversity, there is a strong movement against the dominant cure-based autism organization Autism Speaks. The Autism Self-Advocacy Network is a strong proponent of this view. "Nothing About Us Without Us" is their mandate (http://autisticadvocacy.org). In a joint letter written on January 6, 2014, they write: "'Autism Speaks' advertising depends on offensive and outdated rhetoric of fear and pity, presenting the lives of autistic people as tragic burdens on our

families and society. In its advertising, Autism Speaks has compared being autistic to being kidnapped, dying of a natural disaster, having a fatal disease, and countless other inappropriate analogies. In one of its most prominent fundraising videos, an Autism Speaks executive stated that she had considered placing her child in the car and driving off the George Washington Bridge, going on to say that she did not do so only because she had a normal child as well. Autism Speaks advertisements have cited inaccurate statistics on elevated divorce rates for parents of autistic children and many other falsehoods designed to present the lives of autistic children and adults as little more than tragedies." For the full letter, see http://autisticadvocacy.org/2014/01/2013-joint-letter -to-the-sponsors-of-autism-speaks/ (accessed June 10, 2014).

7 There remains a gender income gap in the United Kingdom, Canada, the United States, and most countries in Europe and Japan that exceeds 20 percent and can be as high as 29 percent (in Japan).

8 For current movements that combat this infantilization, arguing not only for their rights as nations but also for the recognition of their essential difference, see, for instance, the work of the indigenous movement Idle No More (http:// www.idlenomore.ca). See also the section on affirmation in the postscript.

9 Many authors have written about the so-called "case" of facilitated communication (FC). In "Moral Spectatorship: Technologies of Voice and Affect in Postwar Representations of the Child," Lisa Cartwright writes: "The case against FC was so volatile . . . because the method made absolutely blatant the uncomfortable fact of intersubjectivity and dependency as requisites of sociality in a culture that holds onto a notion of the autonomous subject as the proud cornerstone of democratic freedom even as technological means proliferate" (2008: 161).

10 For a more thorough account of techniques, see "Touch as Technique" in Manning 2009.

11 For an account of chunking, see "Coming Alive in a World of Texture" in Manning and Massumi 2014.

12 For a more in-depth exploration of the prearticulation in relation to the ways in which autistics come to language, and for a closer reading of several autistic writers, see "An Ethics of Language in the Making" in Manning 2013.

13 DJ Savarese spent hours on a trampoline in the periods when his sensory system felt most deregulated. Emily and Ralph Savarese have both given accounts of how confident his movements on the trampoline are as compared to walking on hard ground. I wonder about the necessity for sensory feedback—the trampoline, the swing, water. Even softer ground like grass probably makes movement easier. As discussed in the preceding chapter, the issue is not that autistics can't move or stand still, but that there is such a tendency to think of movement as beginning in stillness.

14 It isn't solely the human that acts as facilitator. Blackman, for instance, also speaks of how water brings relaxation: "Water is a support that makes my body really know where it is" (2013: 36). Water is one site where the latencies in

auditory perception, the "perceptual holes," as she calls them, are more back-grounded, allowing for the felt perception of a certain specificity of edgings into form.

15 See Amelia (formerly Amanda) Baggs's video *In My Language* (2007). For a more detailed engagement with this video, see both "Thought in Motion" in Manning 2009 and "Toward a Leaky Sense of Self" in Manning 2013.

16 Ralph Savarese discusses poetry in relation to Larry Bissonnette's writings in Savarese 2012. See also Larry Bissonnette's paintings: http://www.taaproject .com/portfolio/larry-bissonnette/. For a discussion of Tito Mukhopadhyay's writings, see also Savarese 2014.

17 For Whitehead's discussion of recipient and provoker, see "Subjects and Objects" in Whitehead 1967.

18 For a sustained account of relational movement and preacceleration, see "Incipient Action: The Dance of the Not-Yet" in Manning 2009.

19 See "The Dance of Attention" in Manning 2013.

20 A quick perusal of the Internet will bring up endless sites to "increase your autistic child's attention span." The following type of description abounds: "Sam is a visually distracted 5 year old boy with autism. He interacts and communicates very well but the moment that something catches his eye he is compelled to go and check it out. This can be very frustrating when we are trying to work on his ability to maintain attention and develop a great connection with him. Sound familiar?" Monique, "Nutty Therapy Idea That Worked! Help Improve the Attention Span of Your Child with Autism," Connect Therapy, http://www .autism-essentials.com/blog/improve-attention-span-of-child-with-autism/ (accessed March 15, 2015). What these sites emphasize is a form of attention completely aligned to neurotypical accounts of volitional intentionality. This is not how autistics attend. Autistics engage in a field attention that opens toward the environment. Their way of attending is extremely engaged, though less focused on parsing. It allows them to have extraordinary powers of memory. It is key to learn from autistics themselves how best to create the kind of facilitation that works for their kind of distributed, field attention.

21 *Wretches and Jabberers* (dir. Geraldine Wurzburg, 2011) is a documentary that follows two classical autistics, Larry Bissonnette and Tracy Thresher, on a global journey to address prevailing attitudes about disability and intelligence. They visit autistics in India, Japan, and Finland, and in all of the autie-typing that happens, we hear the familiar lilting, metaphorical (metamorphical), poetic language Savarese calls autie-type.

22 For writing by Emma Zurcher-Long and Ariane Zurcher, see http://emmashop ebook.com/page/2/ (accessed April 12, 2015).

23 For writing by Larry Bissonnette, see http://www.wretchesandjabberers.org /larry/index.php (accessed August 23, 2015).

24 For writing by DJ Savarese, see http://www.ralphsavarese.com/category/djs -writings/ (accessed July 10, 2015).

25 For a discussion of this statement of Mukhopadhyay's, see Savarese 2013.

26 Among several articles written on the subject, see, for instance, Bebko, Perry, and Bryson 1996. The general critique of FC in the literature, particularly from the 1990s, is that it is "not a valid method." Unfortunately (but not surprisingly), when FC proponents have defended FC, they have similarly done it around method, despite both strong evidence that autie-type is singular across cultures and populations (could all facilitators possibly be so poetic?!) and the fact that within the testing models of methods there is no way to account for relation. In fact, to come to a strong account of method, as I argue in chapter 1, relation must be cut out of the equation.

About Rapid Prompting, the kind of facilitated communication Soma Mukhopadhyay uses, the same kinds of issues around methodology arise. Wombles writes: "Though Rapid Prompting Method has been in use for approximately a decade, there are no studies on this method's effectiveness at helping individuals with autism communicate or master academic material; there are only testimonials. Therefore, it is not possible to assess whether individuals with autism legitimately benefit or gain skills from RPM." Kim Wombles, "Questionable Autism Approaches: Facilitated Communication and Rapid Prompting Method," *Thinking Person's Guide to Autism*, June 22, 2010, http://www .thinkingautismguide.com/2010/06/questionable-autism-approaches.html. For the full work, see Wombles 2011.

A bibliography of work that dismisses FC on the basis on method would include, among many others, Finn, Bothe, and Bramlett 2005; Gernsmacher 2004; Green 2007; Kerrin et al. 1998; Mostert 2001; and Myles and Simpson 1996. For his groundbreaking work on FC and a completely different perspective, see Biklen 1993; Biklen and Cardinal 1997.

27 *Drawing Autism*, http://50watts.com/Drawing-Autism (accessed April 22, 2015).

7. IN THE ACT

1 Andrew Solomon, "Notes on Depression," recorded October 29, 2008, posted August 5, 2014, The Moth: True Stories Told Live, http://themoth.org/posts /stories/notes-on-an-exorcism. See also Andrew Solomon, "Naked, Covered in Ram's Blood, Drinking a Coke, and Feeling Pretty Good," *Esquire*, February 28, 2014, http://www.esquire.com/blogs/news/notes-on-an-exorcism.

2 The question of *ressentiment* and its relationship to affirmation (and critique) will be discussed more thoroughly in the postscript, in the "Affirmation without Credit" section.

3 "Neurodiversity Statement," No Stereotypes Here, http://nostereotypeshere .blogspot.ca/p/neurodiversity-statement.html (accessed February 20, 2015).

4 Adrienne Warber, "Time Perception in Autism Spectrum Disorder," Love to Know, http://autism.lovetoknow.com/Time_Perception_in_Autism _Spectrum_Disorder (accessed October 30, 2014).

5 Amanda Leigh Mascarelli, "Time Perception Problems May Explain Autism Symptoms," Spectrum, September 20, 2010, http://sfari.org/news-and-opinion /news/2010/time-perception-problems-may-explain-autism-symptoms.

6 Emily Willingham, "For People with Autism, Time Is a Slippery Concept," Spectrum, August 29, 2014, http://sfari.org/news-and-opinion/blog/2014/for -people-with-autism-time-is-slippery-concept.

7 Steve Connor, "New Forensic Technique for Estimating Time of Death by Checking Internal Clock of the Human Brain," Independent, May 14, 2013, http:// www.independent.co.uk/news/science/new-forensic-technique-for-estima ting-time-of-death-by-checking-internal-clock-of-the-human-brain-8614624 .html.

8 Matthew Radcliffe, "Varieties of Temporal Experience in Depression," Aca- demia, http://www.academia.edu/895934/Varieties_of_Temporal_Experi ence_in_Depression (accessed November 6, 2014).

9 Radcliffe, "Varieties of Temporal Experience in Depression."

10 See "The Shape of Enthusiasm" in Manning 2013.

11 See Amelia Baggs, "A Bunch of Stuff That Needed Saying," Ballastexistenz (blog), April 18, 2013, http://ballastexistenz.wordpress.com/2013/04/18/a -bunch-of-stuff-that-needed-saying/. This website has gone offline, though its archive remains. Amelia Baggs's new blog can be found at http://witha smoothroundstone.tumblr.com (accessed October 6, 2015).

12 Baggs, "A Bunch of Stuff That Needed Saying."

13 Baggs, "A Bunch of Stuff That Needed Saying."

14 See Julia Bascom, "The Obsessive Joy of Autism," Just Stimming . . . (blog), April 5, 2011, http://juststimming.wordpress.com/2011/04/05/the-obsessive -joy-of-autism/.

15 Franco Berardi Bifo, "Reassessing Recomposition: 40 Years after the Publi- cation of Anti-Oedipus," Through Europe, March 12, 2012, http://th-rough.eu /writers/bifo-eng/reassessing-recomposition-40-years-after-publication-anti -oedipus.

16 Bifo, "Reassessing Recomposition."

17 Two years after the student strikes in Montreal (the Maple Spring), demon- strations are starting up again, this time clearly focused on the effects of neolib- eralism: Rachel Lau, "Tens of Thousands Gather in Montreal, Quebec City for Anti-austerity Protest," Global News, November 29, 2014, http://globalnews .ca/news/1699395/anti-austerity-demonstrators-gather-at-place-du-canada/. For more on the Maple Spring, see Theory and Event's supplement on the Que- bec strikes: Theory and Event 15, no. 3 (2012 Supplement), http://muse.jhu.edu /journals/theory_and_event/toc/tae.15.3S.html.

18 See, for instance, Occupy London's recent organizing around austerity mea- sures, http://occupylondon.org.uk (accessed November 23, 2014).

19 The death of Michael Brown, an unarmed black man, on August 9, 2014, in Ferguson, Missouri, created deep political unrest. The issues sparked by the shooting have only become more pressing in the wake of the grand jury's de-

cision not to indict the police officer who shot him (November 24, 2014). This has mobilized social justice groups across the United States and brought a renewed visibility to the use of unwarranted violence against black and brown people across America. While waiting for the verdict in Ferguson, in a strong post called "Why We Won't Wait," Robin D. G. Kelley writes about how Ferguson represents the continuation of a long history of ignoring violence in black and brown communities:

> As we waited, Cleveland cops took the life of Tanisha Anderson, a 37year-old Black woman suffering from bipolar disorder. Police arrived at her home after family members called 911 to help her through a difficult crisis, but rather than treat her empathetically they did what they were trained to do when confronted with Black bodies in Black neighborhoods they treated her like an enemy combatant. When she became agitated, one officer wrestled her to the ground and cuffed her while a second officer pinned her "face down on the ground with his knee pressed down heavily into the back for 6 to 7 minutes, until her body went completely limp." She stopped breathing. They made no effort to administer CPR, telling the family and witnesses that she was sleeping. When the ambulance finally arrived twenty minutes later, she was dead.
>
> As we waited, police in Ann Arbor, Michigan, killed a fortyyearold Black woman named Aura Rain Rosser. She was reportedly brandishing a kitchen knife when the cops showed up on a domestic violence call, although her boyfriend who made the initial report insisted that she was no threat to the officers. No matter; they opened fire anyway.
>
> As we waited, a Chicago police officer fatally shot 19yearold Roshad McIntosh. Despite the officer's claims, several eyewitnesses reported that McIntosh was unarmed, on his knees with his hands up, begging the officer to hold his fire.
>
> As we waited, police in Saratoga Springs, Utah, pumped six bullets into Darrien Hunt, a 22 year old Black man dressed kind of like a ninja and carrying a replica Samurai sword. And police in Victorville, California, killed Dante Parker, a 36yearold Black man and father of five. He had been stopped while riding his bike on suspicion of burglary. When he became "uncooperative," the officers repeatedly used Tasers to try to subdue him. He died from his injuries.
>
> As we waited, a twenty eight year old Black man named Akai Gurley met a similar fate as he descended a stairwell in the Louis H. Pink Houses in East New York, Brooklyn. The police were on a typical reconnaissance mission through the housing project. Officer Peter Liang negotiated the darkened stairwell, gun drawn in one hand, flashlight in the other, prepared to take down any threat he encountered. According to liberal mayor Bill DeBlasio and police chief Bill Bratton, Mr. Gurley was collateral damage. Apologies abound. He left a two yearold daughter.

As we waited, LAPD officers stopped 25yearold Ezell Ford, a mentally challenged Black man, in his own South Los Angeles neighborhood and shot him to death. The LAPD stopped Omar Abrego, a 37yearold father from Los Angeles, and beat him to death.

And as we waited and waited and waited, Darren Wilson got married, continued to earn a paycheck while on leave, and received over $400,000 worth of donations for his "defense."

You see, we've been waiting for dozens, hundreds, thousands of indictments and convictions. Every death hurts. Every exonerated cop, security guard, or vigilante enrages. The grand jury's decision doesn't surprise most Black people because we are not waiting for an indictment. We are waiting for justice or more precisely, struggling for justice. We all know the names and how they died. Eric Garner, Kajieme Powell, Vonderitt D. Meyers, Jr., John Crawford III, Cary Ball Jr., Mike Brown, ad infinitum. They were unarmed and shot down by police under circumstances for which lethal force was unnecessary. We hold their names like recurring nightmares, accumulating the dead like ghoulish baseball cards. Except that there is no trading. No forgetting. Just a stack of dead bodies that rises every time we blink. For the last three trayvonsgenerations, Eleanor Bumpurs, Michael Stewart, Eula Love, Amadu Diallo, Oscar Grant, Patrick Dorismond, Malice Green, Tyisha Miller, Sean Bell, Aiyana StanleyJones, Margaret LaVerne Mitchell, to name a few, have become symbols of racist police violence. And I'm only speaking of the dead not the harassed, the beaten, the humiliated, the stoppedandfrisked, the raped.

Robin D. G. Kelley, "Why We Won't Wait," Portside, November 25, 2014, http://portside.org/2014-11-27/why-we-wont-wait. For more on Ferguson, see https://twitter.com/ds4si; Kenneth Bailey and Lori Lobenstine, "We Are in a Social Emergency. Now What?," Design Studio for Social Intervention, http://us2.campaign-archive1.com/?u=0ede54f6027b2abf3b7f48607&id=16a3e30b6e&e=7700a36aa9 (accessed November 30, 2014); "Protesters Shut Down Three New York City Bridges in Reaction to Ferguson Decision," *Huffington Post*, November 25, 2014, http://www.huffingtonpost.com/2014/11/25/nyc-ferguson-protests_n_6216528.html; Syreeta McFadden, "Ferguson, Goddamn: No Indictment for Darren Wilson Is No Surprise. This Is Why We Protest," *Guardian*, November 24, 2014, http://www.theguardian.com/commentisfree/2014/nov/24/ferguson-no-indictment-darren-wilson-protest.

8. WHAT A BODY CAN DO

1 Brian Massumi and I discuss this in more detail in our chapter "Propositions for Thought in the Act" in Manning and Massumi 2014.

2 For Brian Massumi's and my TEDx talk, see https://www.youtube.com/watch?v=D2yHtYdI4bE (accessed October 4, 2015).

Epigraph: "Rei Kawakubo: Exclusive Q&A," *WWD*, November 19, 2012, http://
www.wwd.com/fashion-news/fashion-features/rei-kawakubo-qa-6486260.

1   For Laurent Berlant cruel optimism is a desire that is an obstacle to flourishing.
Her project is one of accounting for what I would call a reactive tendency in
the register of the affective. She does write about the gesture, however, in ways
very much in tune with the project here laid out: "The gesture is a medial act,
neither ends- nor means-oriented, a sign of being in the world, in the middle
of the world, a sign of sociability. To elaborate, this version of the gesture is not
a message; it is more formal than that—the performance of a shift that could
turn into a disturbance, or what Deleuze would call a 'problem-event.' The gesture does not mark time, if time is a movement forward, but makes time, holding the present open to attention and unpredicted exchange. The grimace is
such a gesture. So is a deadpan response. A situation can grow around it or not,
because it makes the smallest opening, a movement-created space. The gesture
is thus only a potential event, the initiation of something present that could
accrue density, whether dramatic or not" (2011: 198–199). I find real complicity in this account of the gesture, but would emphasize that the minor gesture
makes a difference whether or not this difference is *actually* perceived. It is not,
to my mind, a question of "a situation [growing] around it *or not*" but more a
question of degree. Many minor gestures never cross the threshold into actualization. These gestures remain potentialized, as Berlant says, but that does not
mean their effects aren't felt in other registers than that of the actual. To make
it an either/or situation keeps it within the register of the given. An affirmative
politics emphasizes this point: all cuts make a difference. See Berlant 2011.

2   Amnesty Canada reports:

> In a 2009 government survey of the ten provinces, Aboriginal women
> were nearly three times more likely than non-Aboriginal women to report
> being a victim of a violent crime. . . . RCMP statistics released in 2014 show
> that Indigenous women are four times more likely to be murdered than
> non-Indigenous women. . . . Some patterns of violence facing Indigenous
> women and girls are different from those facing non-Indigenous women.
> For example, according to the RCMP report released in May 2014, Indige-
> nous women are more likely than non-Indigenous women to be murdered
> by what the police call acquaintances—friends, colleagues, neighbors and
> other men who are not intimate partners or spouses. . . . A report released
> by the RCMP in May 2014 states that 1,017 Indigenous women and girls were
> murdered from 1980 to 2012. Because of gaps in police and government re-
> porting, the actual numbers may be much higher.

See http://www.amnesty.ca/our-work/issues/indigenous-peoples/no-more
-stolen-sisters (accessed November 30, 2014).

3   See Spinoza 2009.

4 "Statement of Apology to Former Students of Indian Residential Schools,"
Indigenous and Northern Affairs Canada, https://www.aadnc-aandc.gc.ca
/eng/1100100015644/1100100015649 (accessed December 2, 2014).

5 Glen Sean Coulthard, in *Red Skin, White Masks: Rejecting the Colonial Politics
of Recognition*, frames his whole narrative around the rejection of recognition
as a dominant trope of liberal politics, going into much further detail than is
possible for me here. About Stephen Harper's apology to the First Nations,
he writes: "Although there was a great deal of skepticism toward the apology
in the days leading up to it, in its immediate aftermath it appeared that many,
if not most observers felt that Harper's apology was a genuine and necessary
'first step' on the long road to forgiveness and reconciliation. The benefit of
the doubt that was originally afforded the authenticity of the prime minister's
apology has since dissipated. . . . On September 25, 2009, . . . Harper made the
somewhat astonishing (but typically arrogant and self-congratulatory) claim
that Canadians had 'no history of colonialism'" (2014: 105–106). Coulthard
then goes on to weave his analysis around "the current entanglement of settler
coloniality with the politics of reconciliation" (2014: 206).

In "Restitution Is the Real Pathway to Justice for Indigenous Peoples,"
Taiaiake Alfred also upholds a strong critique of the politics of recognition,
suggesting that "genuine reconciliation is impossible without recognizing
Indigenous peoples' right to freedom and self-determination, instituting restitution by returning enough of our lands so that we can regain economic
self-sufficiency, and honoring our treaty relationships. Without these com-
mitments reconciliation will remain a 'pacifying discourse' that functions to
assuage settler guilt, on the one hand, and absolve the federal government's
responsibility to transform the colonial relationship between Canada and
Indigenous nations, on the other" (in Coulthard 2014: 127).

Another important voice on this issue is that of Leanne Simpson. On reconciliation and the politics of recognition, she writes: "Indigenous people attempted to reconcile our differences in countless treaty negotiations, which
categorically have not produced the kinds of relationships Indigenous people
intended. I wonder how we can reconcile when the majority of Canadians
do not understand the historic or contemporary injustice of dispossession
and occupation, particularly when the state has expressed its unwillingness to
make any adjustments to the unjust relationship. . . . If Canadians do not fully
understand and embody the idea of reconciliation, is this a step forward?"
(2011: 21).

There are many other important voices. Among them I would strongly rec-
ommend Kulchyski 2013.

6 Caley Ramsay, "Residential School Survivors Share Stories during Truth and
Reconciliation Event," *Global News*, March 28, 2014, http://globalnews.ca
/news/1238064/residential-school-survivors-share-stories-during-truth-and
-reconciliation-event/.

7 Leanne Simpson writes: "The process of resurgence must be Indigenous at its core in order to reclaim and re-politicize the context and the nature of Nishnaabeg thought" (2011: 20).

8 Hana Shafi, "For Canada's Indigenous Women, Going Missing Is a Terrifying Possibility," *The Blog, Huffington Post*, November 4, 2014, http://www.huffing tonpost.ca/hana-shafi/missing-and-murdered-indigenous-women_b _6097234.html.

9 For an important and beautiful account of the kinds of issues discussed here, see Simpson 2011. The question that frames Simpson's book is what reconciliation means to Indigenous peoples. Simpson argues that reconciliation can do its work only if it honors the traditions of governance of First Nations peoples, as well as their languages and oral cultures. Her argument, that reconciliation has always been a part of First Nations culture, places reconciliation within the context of affirmation rather than reactivity. She writes: "Reconciliation must move beyond individual abuse to come to mean a collective re-balancing of the playing field," and "this idea is captured in the Anishnaabeg concept aanji maajitaawin: to start over, the art of starting over, to regenerate." Leanne Simpson quoted in Christine McFarlane, "Path to Reconciliation Means Educating Canadians," AMMSA: Aboriginal Multi-Media Society, http://www.ammsa.com /publications/windspeaker/path-reconciliation-means-educating-canadians (accessed November 28, 2014). Speaking as a member of the Anishnaabeg nation, Simpson emphasizes that "our systems are designed to promote more life," which can be achieved through "resisting, renewing, and regeneration." In a politics of affirmation, she continues: "I also think it's about the fertility of ideas and it's the fertility of alternatives. One of the things birds do in our creation stories is they plant seeds and they bring forth new ideas and they grow those ideas. Seeds are the encapsulation of wisdom and potential and the birds carry those seeds around the earth and grew this earth. And I think we all have that responsibility to find those seeds, to plant those seeds, to give birth to these new ideas. Because people think up an idea but then don't articulate it, or don't tell anybody about it, and don't build a community around it, and don't do it." Leanne Simpson in Naomi Klein, "Dancing the World into Being: A Conversation with Idle No More's Leanne Simpson," *Yes! Magazine*, March 5, 2013, http://www.yesmagazine.org/peace-justice/dancing-the-world -into-being-a-conversation-with-idle-no-more-leanne-simpson.

On the question of the politics of affirmation and Indigenous resurgence, see "Five Theses on Indigenous Resurgence and Decolonization" in Coulthard 2014: 165–179.

10 Leanne Simpson writes about the politics of love at the heart of Idle No More. "That was the difference with Idle No More because there were so many women that were standing up. Because of colonialism, we were excluded for a long time from that Indian Act chief and council governing system. Women initially were not allowed to run for office, and it's still a bastion of patriarchy.

But that in some ways is a gift because all of our organizing around governance and politics and this continuous rebirth has been outside of that system and been based on that politics of love." Referring to a lake that is no longer clean enough to swim in, and thereby connecting a politics of love to a politics of affirmation, Simpson writes: "If you can't swim in it, canoe across it." Klein, "Dancing the World into Being."

11 Leanne Simpson writes: "Over the past 400 years, there has never been a time when indigenous peoples were not resisting colonialism. Idle No More is the latest—visible to the mainstream—resistance and it is part of an ongoing historical and contemporary push to protect our lands, our cultures, our nationhoods, and our languages. To me, it feels like there has been an intensification of colonial pillage, or that's what the Harper government is preparing for—the hyper-extraction of natural resources on indigenous lands. But really, every single Canadian government has placed that kind of thinking at its core when it comes to indigenous peoples." Klein, "Dancing the World into Being."

12 In a conversation with Naomi Klein, Simpson describes the cosmology of the Nishnaabeg:

> Because within Anishnaabeg cosmology, this isn't the First World, maybe this is the Fourth World that we're on. And whenever there's an imbalance and the imbalance isn't addressed, then over time there's a crisis. This time, there was a big flood that covered the entire world. Nanabush, one of our sacred beings, ends up trapped on a log with many of the other animals. They are floating in this vast sea of water with no land in sight. To me, that feels like where we are right now. I'm on a very crowded log, the world my ancestors knew and lived in is gone, and me and my community need to come up with a solution even though we are all feeling overwhelmed and irritated. It's an intense situation and no one knows what to do, no one knows how to make a new world.
>
> So the animals end up taking turns diving down and searching for a pawful of dirt or earth to use to start to make a new world. The strong animals go first, and when they come up with nothing, the smaller animals take a turn. Finally, muskrat is successful and brings her pawful of dirt up to the surface. Turtle volunteers to have the earth placed on her back. Nanabush prays and breaths life into that earth. All of the animals sing and dance on the turtle's back in a circle, and as they do this, the turtle's back grows. It grows and grows until it becomes the world we know. This is why Anishnaabeg call North America *Mikinakong*—the place of the turtle.
>
> When Edna tells this story, she says that we're all that muskrat, and that we all have that responsibility to get off the log and dive down no matter how hard it is and search around for that dirt. And that to me was profound and transformative, because we can't wait for somebody else to come up with the idea. The whole point, the way we're going to make this better, is

by everybody engaging in their own being, in their own gifts, and embody this movement, embody this transformation.

Klein, "Dancing the World into Being."

13 This diet was composed of sips of lemon water, medicinal teas, and fish broth. See "Think Chief Spence Is on a 'Liquid Diet'? You're Ignorant," *Huffington Post*, January 20, 2013, http://m.huffpost.com/ca/entry/2517450.

About the way the media portrays the indigenous in Canada, Leanne Simpson writes:

> While many of our communities are economically impoverished in a Western sense, they are far from poor. Our northern communities are rich because they know their languages. They are rich because they have strong connections to their land. They are rich because at least some of their lands exist in a natural state. They are rich because they live in the same community as their grandparents, aunties, uncles, cousins, and extended families. They are rich because they do not rely on material wealth to bring them happiness. They are rich because, despite years of disrespect, they have survived and in many ways flourished.
>
> The mainstream media does not see this richness, nor do they take a step back to examine the broader set of forces that has led to the crisis in Indigenous-state relations. And so, the well-meaning solution to Indigenous poverty becomes economic development, which to me is tremendously misguided.
>
> Our people have repeatedly been shown that industrial development does not solve our economic development problems. The diamond mine hasn't helped Attawapiskat. Yet over and over, settler governments, which are primarily concerned with opening up Indigenous territories to development, paint the choice as either protecting Indigenous territories and living in abject poverty, or sacrificing the territory to hyperdevelopment by multinational corporations in exchange for jobs. Community-controlled, local, sustainable, and small-scale economic development is almost never discussed. Indigenous economies, the ones that kept our nations strong for tens of thousands of years, are erased and deemed a relic of the past.

Leanne Simpson, "Attawapiskat, Revisited," *Briarpatch Magazine*, May 1, 2012, http://briarpatchmagazine.com/articles/view/attawapiskat-revisited. See also Alanis Obomsawin's film *People of Kattawapiskak River* (http://www.nfb.ca/film/people_of_kattawapiskak_river/) and Kulchyski 2013.

14 For a general overview, see "How the Idle No More Movement Started and Where It Might Go from Here," White Wolf Pack, http://www.whitewolfpack.com/2012/12/how-idle-no-more-movement-started-and.html (accessed October 7, 2015). For more on treaty 9, see "Treaty," Matawa: First Nations Management, http://www.matawa.on.ca/66-2/ (accessed October 7, 2015), and Grand Chief Stan Louttit, "'The Real Agreement as Orally Agreed To':

The James Bay Treaty—Treaty No. 9," http://www.mushkegowuk.com /documents/jamesbaytreaty9_realoralagreement.pdf (accessed October 7, 2015).

15 Teresa Smith, "Justin Trudeau Meets with Hunger Striking Chief Theresa Spence," *National Post*, December 26, 2012, www2.nationalpost.com/m/wp /blog.html?b=news.nationalpost.com/2012/12/26/theresa-spence-justin -trudeau.

16 Naomi Klein writes: "Though sparked by a series of legislative attacks on indigenous sovereignty and environmental protections by the Conservative government of Stephen Harper, the movement quickly became about much more: Canada's ongoing colonial policies, a transformative vision of decolonization, and the possibilities for a genuine alliance between natives and non-natives, one capable of re-imagining nationhood." Klein, "Dancing the World into Being."

17 "'Nishiyuu Walkers' Complete 1,600 km Trek to Ottawa," *CTV News*, March 25, 2013, http://www.ctvnews.ca/canada/nishiyuu-walkers-complete-1–600-km-trek-to-ottawa-1.1209929#.

18 Klein, "Dancing the World into Being."

19 Klein, "Dancing the World into Being."

20 For a video of the round dance, see http://www.youtube.com/watch?v= x2Nx4jUEZfc (accessed November 30, 2014).

21 For a version of Joe McPhee's *Nation Time*, see http://www.youtube.com /watch?v=EmPW0AO2gnU (accessed November 10, 2014).

Arakawa and Madeline Gins. 2002. *Architectural Body*. Tuscaloosa: University of Alabama Press.

—. 2011. "Arriving Soon—Biotopological Diagramming, a New Procedure/Method for Staying Alive Indefinitely from Alive Forever, Not If, But When." Unpublished manuscript.

—. 2014. "Alive Forever, Not If, But When." Unpublished manuscript.

Baggs, Amanda [Amelia]. 2010. "Up in the Clouds and Down in the Valley: My Richness and Yours." *Disability Studies Quarterly* 30, no. 1, http://dsq-sds.org /article/view/1052/1238.

Bebko, James M., Adrienne Perry, and Susan Bryson. 1996. "Multiple Method Validation Study of Facilitated Communication: II. Individual Differences and Subgroup Results." *Journal of Autism and Developmental Disorders* 26, no. 1: 19–42.

Benjamin, Walter. 1973. "Some Motifs in Baudelaire." In *Charles Baudelaire: A Lyric Poet in the Era of High Capitalism*. London: New Left Books.

—. 2008. *The Work of Art in the Age of Mechanical Reproduction*. Translated by J. A. Underwood. London: Penguin Classics.

Bennett, Jane. 2009. *Vibrant Matter: A Political Ecology of Things*. Durham, NC: Duke University Press.

Berardi, Franco (Bifo). 2008. *Felix Guattari: Thought, Friendship, and Visionary Cartography*. Translated by Giuseppina Mecchia and Charles J. Stivale. London: Palgrave.

—. 2011. *After the Future*. Edited by Gary Genosko and Nicholas Thoburn. Oakland, CA: AK Press.

Bergson, Henri. 1998. *Creative Evolution*. Translated by Arthur Mitchell. New York: Dover.

————. 2001. *Time and Free Will—an Essay on the Immediate Data of Consciousness*. Translated by F. L. Pogson. New York: Dover.

————. 2004. *Matter and Memory*. New York: Dover.

————. 2007. *The Creative Mind: An Introduction to Metaphysics*. New York: Dover.

Berlant, Lauren. 2011. *Cruel Optimism*. Durham, NC: Duke University Press.

Biklen, Douglas. 1993. *Communication Unbound*. New York: Teachers College Press, Columbia University.

Biklen, Douglas, and Donald Cardinal, eds. 1997. *Contested Words, Contested Science: Unraveling the Facilitated Communication Controversy*. New York: Teachers College Press, Columbia University.

Blackman, Lucy. 2001. *Lucy's Story: Autism and Other Adventures*. London: Jessica Kingsley.

————. 2013. *Carrying Autism, Feeling Language*. Edited by and with contributions by Mary Jane Blackman ("Jay"). Los Gatos, CA: Smashwords.

Bogdashina, Olga. 2005. *Communication Issues in Autism and Asperger Syndrome: Do We Speak the Same Language?* London: Jessica Kingsley. Kindle version.

Bousquet, Marc, Stefano Harney, and Fred Moten. 2009. "On Study: A *Polygraph* Roundtable Discussion with Marc Bousquet, Stefano Harney, and Fred Moten." *Polygraph* 21: 159–75.

Brauns, Axel Buntschatten. 2002. *Fledermäuse—Leben in einer anderen Welte*. Munich: Goldmann Wilhelm.

Buckley, S. J., and G. Bird. 1993. "Teaching Children with Down Syndrome to Read." *Down Syndrome Research and Practice* 1, no. 1: 34–39, http://www.down-syndrome.org/perspectives/9/, doi:10.3104/perspectives.9.

Cartwright, Lisa. 2008. *Practices of Looking: An Introduction to Visual Culture*. Oxford: Oxford University Press.

Caspersen, Dana. 2000. "It Starts from Any Point: Bill and the Frankfurt Ballet." "William Forsythe," edited by Senta Driver, special issue, *Choreography and Dance* 5, no. 3: 25–40.

Connolly, William. 2010. *A World of Becoming*. Durham, NC: Duke University Press.

————. 2013. *The Fragility of Things: Self-Organizing Processes, Neoliberal Fantasies, and Democratic Activism*. Durham, NC: Duke University Press.

Coulthard, Glen Sean. 2014. *Red Skin, White Masks: Rejecting the Colonial Politics of Recognition*. Minneapolis: University of Minnesota Press.

Deleuze, Gilles. 1972. *Proust and Signs*. Translated by Richard Howard. New York: George Braziller.

————. 1978. *Difference and Repetition*. Translated by Paul Patton. New York: Columbia University Press.

————. 1983. *Nietzsche and Philosophy*. Translated by Hugh Tomlinson. New York: Columbia University Press.

————. 1988. *Spinoza: Practical Philosophy*. Translated by Robert Hurley. New York: City Light Books.

————. 1989. *Cinema 2: The Time-Image*. Translated by Hugh Tomlinson and Robert Galeta. Minneapolis: University of Minnesota Press.

————. 1991. *Bergsonism*. Translated by Hugh Tomlinson and Barbara Habberjam. New York: Zone Books.

————. 1992. *The Fold*. Translated by Tom Conley. Minneapolis: University of Minnesota Press.

————. 2002. *Nietzsche and Philosophy*. Translated by Janis Tomlinson. New York: Columbia University Press.

————. 2005. *Pure Immanence: Essays on a Life*. New York: Zone Books.

————. 2007. *Dialogues—with Claire Parnet*. Translated by Hugh Tomlinson and Barbara Habberjam. New York: Columbia University Press.

Deleuze, Gilles, and Félix Guattari. 1983. *Anti-Oedipus*. Translated by Robert Hurley and Mark Seem. Minneapolis: University of Minnesota Press,

————. 1986. *Kafka: Toward a Minor Literature*. Translated by Dana Polan. Minneapolis: University of Minnesota Press.

————. 1987. *A Thousand Plateaus*. Translated by Brian Massumi. Minneapolis: University of Minnesota Press.

Derrida, Jacques. 1983. *Dissemination*. Translated by Barbara Johnson. Chicago: University of Chicago Press.

————. 1998. *Of Grammatology*. Translated by Gayatri Spivak. Baltimore: Johns Hopkins University Press.

Finn, P., A. Bothe, and R. Bramlett. 2005. "Science and Pseudoscience in Communication Disorders: Criteria and Applications." *American Journal of Speech-Language Pathology / American Speech-Language-Hearing Association* 14, no. 3: 172–186.

Forsythe, William. 2008. *Suspense*. Zurich: JRP, Ringier Kunstverlag.

Genosko, Gary, ed. 1996. *The Guattari Reader*. Oxford: Blackwell.

————. 2002. *Felix Guattari: An Aberrant Introduction*. Edinburgh: Continuum.

Gerland, Gunilla. 1997. *A Real Person: Life on the Outside*. London: Souvenir Press.

Gernsmacher, M. A. 2004. "Language Is More Than Speech: A Case Study." *Journal of Developmental and Learning Disorder* 8: 81–98.

Gil, Jose. 2000. "Mouvement Total." Unpublished manuscript.

————. 2001. *Movimento Total*. Lisbon: Antropos.

Gins, Madeline. 1994. *Helen Keller or Arakawa*. New York: Burning Books.

Gladwell, Malcolm. 2006. *Blink: The Power of Thinking without Thinking*. New York: Back Bay Books.

Glowczewski, Barbara. 1988. *La loi du rêve: Approche topologique de l'organisation sociale et des cosmologies des Aborigènes Australiens*. Thèse d'Etat ès lettres et Sciences Humaines, University of Paris I Sorbonne.

Green, V. 2007. "Parental Experience with Treatments for Autism." *Journal of Developmental and Physical Disabilities* 19, no. 2: 91–101.

Guattari, Félix. 1984. *Molecular Revolution: Psychiatry and Politics*. Translated by Rosemary Sheed. Harmondsworth, Middlesex, UK: Penguin.

————. 1996. *The Guattari Reader*. Edited by Gary Genosko. Oxford: Blackwell.

————. 2012. *Chaosmosis: An Ethico-Aesthetic Paradigm*. Seattle: University of Washington Press.

————. 2013. *Schizoanalytic Cartographies*. Translated by Andrew Goffey. New York: Bloomsbury.

Higashida, Naoki. 2013. *The Reason I Jump*. Translated by David Mitchell and K. A. Yoshida. Introduction by David Mitchell. Toronto: Alfred A. Knopf. Kindle version.

James, William. 1969. "The Feeling of Effort." In *Collected Essays and Reviews*. New York: Russell and Russell.

————. 1996. *Essays in Radical Empiricism*. Nebraska: University of Nebraska Press.

Keane, Jondi, and Trish Glazebrook, eds. "Arakawa and Gins." Special issue, *Inflexions: A Journal for Research-Creation* (January 2013), www.inflexions.org.

Kedar, Ido. 2012. *Ido in Autismland: Climbing Out of Autism's Silent Prison*. Sharon Kedar.

Kerrin, R., J. Murdock, W. Sharpton, and N. Jones. 1998. "Who's Doing the Pointing? Investigation Facilitated Communication in a Classroom Setting." *Focus on Autism and Other Developmental Disabilities* 13, no. 2: 73.

Kulchyski, Peter. 2013. *Aboriginal Rights Are Not Human Rights: In Defense of Indigenous Struggles*. Winnipeg: Arbeiter Ring.

Lapoujade, David. 2008. "Intuition et Sympathie chez Bergson." *Eidos*, no. 9 (July–December): 10–31.

————. 2010. *Puissances du temps, versions de Bergson*. Paris: Editions Minuit.

Lindeman, Renate. 2008. "Take Down Syndrome Out of the Abortion Debate." CMAJ 179, no. 10, http://www.cmaj.ca/content/179/10/1088.short, doi:10.1503/cmaj.081583.

Manning, Erin. 2007. *Politics of Touch: Sense, Movement, Sovereignty*. Minneapolis: University of Minnesota Press.

————. 2009. *Relationscapes: Movement, Art, Philosophy*. Cambridge, MA: MIT Press.

————. 2013. *Always More Than One: Individuation's Dance*. Durham, NC: Duke University Press.

Manning, Erin, and Brian Massumi. 2014. *Thought in the Act: Passages in the Ecology of Experience*. Minneapolis: University of Minnesota Press.

Massumi, Brian. 2010. "Perception Attack: Brief on War Time." *Theory and Event* 13, no. 3 (October), http://muse.jhu.edu/journals/theory_and_event/vo13/13.3.massumi.html.

————. 2011. *Semblance and Event: Activist Philosophy and the Occurrent Arts*. Cambridge, MA: MIT Press.

————. 2014. *What Animals Teach Us about Politics*. Durham, NC: Duke University Press.

————. 2015a. *Ontopower: War, Power and the State of Perception*. Durham, NC: Duke University Press.

————. 2015b. *The Power at the End of the Economy*. Durham, NC: Duke University Press.

————. Forthcoming. "Virtual Ecology and the Question of Value." In *On General Ecology: The New Ecological Paradigm in the Neo-Cybernetic Era*, edited by Eric Hörl. London: Bloomsbury.

McKean, Thomas. 1994. *Soon Will Come the Light: A View from Inside the Autism Puzzle*. Arlington: Future Horizons.

Miller, Jean Kearns. 2003. *Women from Another Planet? Our Lives in the Universe of Autism*. Bloomington, IN: Authorhouse.

Moisseeff, Marika. 1989. "Représentations non figuratives et singularité individuelle: Les churinga du désert central australien." In *Anthropologie de l'art: Faits et significations (Arts de l'Afrique, de l'Amérique et du Pacifique)*, edited by L. Perrois. Paris: ORTSOM.

————. 2002. "Australian Aboriginal Ritual Objects, or How to Represent the Unrepresentable." In *People and Things: Social Mediations in Oceania*, edited by M. Jeudy-Balini and B. Juillerat, 239–263. Durham, NC: Duke University Press.

Mostert, M. 2001. "Facilitated Communication since 1995: A Review of Published Studies." *Journal of Autism and Developmental Disorders* 31, no. 3: 287–313.

Moten, Fred, and Stefano Harney. 2013. *The Undercommons: Fugitive Planning and Black Study*. New York: Minor Compositions.

Mukhopadhyay, Tito Rajarshi. 2000. *Beyond the Silence: My Life, the World and Autism*. London: National Autistic Society.

————. 2007. *The Mind Tree*. New York: Riverhead.

Myles, B., and R. Simpson. 1996. "Impact of Facilitated Communication Combined with Direct Instruction on Academic Performance." *Focus on Autism and Other Developmental Disabilities* 11, no. 1: 37.

Nietzsche, Friedrich. 1954. *Thus Spoke Zarathustra*. Translated by Walter Kaufmann. New York: Penguin.

————. 1968. *The Will to Power*. Translated by Walter Kaufmann. New York: Vintage.

————. 1977. *The Portable Nietzsche*. Translated by Walter Kaufmann. New York: Penguin.

————. 1996. *Philosophy in the Tragic Age of the Greeks*. Washington, DC: Gateway Editions.

————. 2002. *Beyond Good and Evil: Prelude to a Philosophy of the Future*. New ed. Edited by Rolf-Peter Horstmann and Judith Norman. London: Cambridge University Press.

————. 2003. *Writings from the Late Notebooks*. Edited by Rüdiger Bittner; translated by Kate Sturge. Cambridge: Cambridge University Press.

————. 2008. *Twilight of the Idols*. Translated by Duncan Large. London: Oxford.

Panagia, Davide. 2009. *The Political Life of Sensation*. Durham, NC: Duke University Press.

Pelbart, Peter Pál. 1994. "Un droit au silence." *Chimères*, no. 23: 1–10.

Portanova, Stamatia, Bianca Scliar, and Natasha Prevost. 2009. "Rhythmic Nexus: The Felt Togetherness of Movement and Thought." *Inflexions: A Journal for Research-Creation*, no. 2, www.inflexions.org.

Prince-Hughes, Dawn. 2004. *Songs of the Gorilla Nation: My Journey through Autism*. New York: Broadway Books.

Rissanen, Timo. 2007. "Types and Fashion Design and Patternmaking Practice." *Design Inquiries. Nordic Design Research*, no. 2: 1–5.

Russell, Bertrand. 1996. *History of Western Philosophy*. London: Routledge.

Ruyer, Raymond. 1958. *La genèse des formes vivantes*. Paris: Flammarion, 1958.

Savarese, Ralph. 2008. "The Lobes of Autobiography: Poetry and Autism." *Stone Canoe*, no. 2.

———. 2010. "More Than a Thing to Ignore: An Interview with Tito Mukhopadhyay." *Disability Studies Quarterly—Autism and the Concept of Neurodiversity* 30, no. 1, http://dsq-sds.org/article/view/1056/1235.

———. 2012. "Gobs and Gobs of Metaphor: Dynamic Relation and a Classical Autist's Typed Massage." "Simondon: Milieu, Techniques, Aesthetics," special issue, *Inflexions: A Journal for Research-Creation* (March): 184–223, www.inflexions.org.

———. 2013. "Moving the Field: The Sensorimotor Perspective on Autism." *Frontiers in Integrative Neuroscience* 7, no. 6, http://www.ncbi.nlm.nih.gov/pmc/articles/PMC3578197/.

———. 2014. "The Critic as Neurocosmopolite; Or, What Cognitive Approaches to Literature Can Learn from Disability Studies: Lisa Zunshine in Conversation with Ralph Savarese." *Narrative* 22, no. 1 (January): 17–44.

———. 2015. "I Object: Autism, Empathy, and the Trope of Personification." In *Rethinking Empathy through Literature*, edited by Sue Kim and Meghan Marie Hammond, 74–92. New York: Routledge.

Simondon, Gilbert. 2005. *L'individuation à la lumière des notions de forme et d'information*. Grenoble: Editions Jérôme Millon.

Simpson, Audra. 2014. *Mohawk Interruptus: Political Life across the Borders of Settler States*. Durham, NC: Duke University Press.

Simpson, Leanne. 2011. *Dancing on Our Turtle's Back: Stories of Nishnaabeg Re-creation, Resurgence and a New Emergence*. Oakland: AK Press.

———. 2013. *Islands of Decolonial Love*. New York: Arbeiter Ring Publishing.

Solomon, Andrew. 2014. *The Noonday Demon: An Atlas of Depression*. New York: Simon and Schuster.

Souriau, Étienne. 2009. *Les Différents modes d'existence suivi de l'oeuvre à faire*. Edited by Isabelle Stengers and Bruno Latour. Paris: Presses Universitaires de France.

Spinoza, Baruch. 2009. *The Ethics*. Floyd, Virginia: Wilder.

Stengers, Isabelle. 2010. *Cosmopolitics 1*. Minneapolis: University of Minnesota Press.

———. 2011. *Cosmopolitics 2*. Minneapolis: University of Minnesota Press.

Taussig, Michael. 1995. "The Sun Gives without Receiving: An Old Story." *Comparative Studies in Society and History* 37, no. 2 (April): 368–398.

Torres, Elizabeth B., Maria Brincker, Robert W. Isenhower, Polina Yanovich, Kimberly A. Stigler, John I. Nurnberger, Dimitris N. Metaxas, and Jorge V. José. 2013. "Autism: The Micro-Movement Perspective." *Frontiers in Integrative Neuroscience* 7, no. 32, http://www.ncbi.nlm.nih.gov/pmc/articles /PMC3721360/.

Whitehead, Alfred North. 1927. *Symbolism*. New York: Fordham University Press.

———. 1929. *The Function of Reason*. Boston: Beacon.

———. 1938. *Modes of Thought*. New York: Free Press.

———. 1967. *Adventures of Ideas*. New York: Free Press.

———. 1978. *Process and Reality*. New York: Free Press.

Williams, Donna. 1992. *Nobody Nowhere: The Extraordinary Autobiography of an Autistic*. New York: Times Books.

———. 1996. *Autism: An Inside-Out Approach*. London: Jessica Kingsley.

———. 1998. *Autism and Sensing—the Unlost Instinct*. London: Jessica Kingsley. Kindle version.

Wolfe, Cary. 2012. *Before the Law: Humans and Other Animals in a Biopolitical Frame*. Chicago: University of Chicago Press.

Wombles, Kim. 2011. "Questionable Autism Approaches: Facilitated Communication and Rapid Prompting Method." In *Thinking Person's Guide to Autism: What You Really Need to Know about Autism, from Autistics, Parents, and Professionals*, edited by Shannon Des Roches Rosa, Jennifer Byde Myers, Liz Ditz, Emily Willingham, and Carol Greenburg, 153–158. Redwood City, CA: Deadwood City Publishing.

Yergeau, Melanie. 2013. "Clinically Significant Disturbance: On Theorists Who Theorize Theory of Mind." *Disabilities Studies Quarterly—Improving Feminist Philosophy and Theory by Taking Account of Disability* 33, no. 4, http://dsq-sds .org/article/view/3876/3405.

dance, 19, 59, 121, 153, 169–170, 216–217, 228–229, 232; of attention, 104–105, 110, 120, 154–155, 158, 193, 195, 197; choreography and, 106, 127; perception and, 60, 62, 116, 170; technique, 40, 126

debt, 205–211, 214–215, 218, 221, 225–228

deconstruction, 104, 106

Deleuze, Gilles, 27, 46, 50, 51, 65–66, 72, 84–85, 165, 180; actual-virtual and, 29–30; affirmation and, 202; *agencement* and, 123; belief and, 93; desire and, 168, 182–183, 193; dramatization and, 211–212; inflection and, 117; "a life" and, 7–8; minor and, 1, 66, 72, 74–75; power and, 207; schizoanalysis and, 173, 187. *See also* Guattari, Félix

depression, 166–168, 173, 182, 184; anxiety and, 178, 186; autism and, 174–175, 180; neoliberalism and, 171–172

Derrida, Jacques, 105

desire, 167–168, 171, 182–183, 188, 204

de Zegher, Catherine, 242n10

diagram, 89

dialectic, 201–204, 206, 208, 214

difference, 1, 8, 22–24, 39, 47, 51, 65, 100, 118–119, 247n2; accommodation and, 3–5, 128, 186–187, 202; activist philosophy and, 129–130; affirmation and, 6, 203–207, 213; *agencement* and, 125; architecture and, 88; cut of, 32, 34, 40, 201; differential, 11, 13–14, 21–23, 33–35, 48, 50–52, 57–58, 60, 63–64, 66, 68, 72, 81, 85, 87, 90, 93, 96, 104, 117, 163, 201, 230; emergent, 15; eternal return and, 218; fashion and, 92–97, 108; intuition and, 57, 60; movement and, 156, 189–190; neurological, 9; pathologization of, 174; quality and, 216–217; repetition and, 89; rhythm and, 226

discipline (academic), 27–29, 31, 38–39, 43; of art, 58; interdisciplinarity, 198; of philosophy, 41, 198, 200

Donnellan, Anne, 179

Down syndrome, 3, 136, 235n8

dramatization, 212–213, 220, 227

duration, 47, 50–51, 65, 67, 117–118, 127

echolalia, 144, 174

ecology of practices, 3, 8, 53, 76, 91–92, 99, 102, 115, 117, 123, 128, 191; research-creation and, 13

ecosophy, 127

elasticity, 246n14

emotion, 20

enabling constraint, 88–91, 197, 209

entertainment, 81, 84

environment, 76–79, 81, 83, 85, 88, 91, 96, 109, 208; body and, 114–115; degradation of, 226–227; modulation of, 162, 164

essence, 50–51

eternal return, 213–214, 216, 218, 225, 229

ethics, 127, 149, 159, 161, 185

ethnicity, 96

event: affirmation of, 232; agency and, 154; of art, 58; of attention, 121, 153; collaboration and, 196; concern/care for, 90, 192–193, 195, 197; of creation, 91, 94; cut and, 219; of destruction, 230; dramatization and, 213; event design, 95; event-time, 22, 24, 50, 65, 81–83, 85, 96, 103, 122–123, 127, 171–172, 174, 211, 214; experience and, 2–3, 15, 29, 34, 36, 38, 50, 61, 64, 150–151, 175; fashion as, 98; feeling and, 133, 145; freedom and, 23; hospitality and, 196, 197; joy and, 211; of life-living, 104; movement of, 118–119, 150, 156; participation and, 55, 79, 197; procedure and, 93–94, 101; schizoanalysis and, 171; subjective form of, 134; sympathy for, 57; technique and, 125; transvaluation

event (*continued*)
and, 218; volition and, 17–21; will to power and, 207–208; of writing, 162

experience, 17, 27–29, 34, 38–41, 50, 64, 112, 134, 208, 229; aesthetics of, 44; affective tonality and, 30; architecture and, 86–89; art and, 47–49, 59–60, 81; carrying, 135, 145; collective, 181; of communication, 137; desire and, 183; ecology of, 84; everyday, 100; fabulation and, 124; in-act, 30, 36, 47, 201; individuation and, 53; limits of, 96; mentality and, 35; minor gesture and, 1–3, 7, 13; neuro-diverse, 14–15, 22, 114–115, 136, 140, 142, 144–145, 147, 157, 160, 172, 174–175, 186, 188, 191–192; neurotypical, 6, 111, 115, 117, 129–131, 140, 146, 150–151, 154, 162, 191–192; practice and, 53; pure, 29, 138–139; reason and, 31; ritual and, 171; study and, 12; technique and, 125; time of, 50–52, 173; volition and, 19–21, 23–25, 149

fabulation, 219–221, 223–225, 227–228, 232

facilitation, 158. *See also* communication, facilitated

fashion, 75, 86, 90–108

feeling, 131–134, 162–163, 177–178; of effort, 152, 155, 157

First Nations, 4, 222–226; cosmology, 258n12

fold, 110

Folds to Infinity (Erin Manning), 67, 76–77

force: affect and, 20, 23, 49, 162; of affirmation, 211, 229–230; of art, 54, 58–59, 61, 71–73, 81, 84, 149, 161, 178–179; a-signifying, 43; of autistic perception, 158; of debt, 210; decisional, 33, 88; of difference, 118, 203; of dramatization, 213; duration and, 47, 50–53, 56; of fabulation, 220, 224–225;

of form, 22, 27, 53, 68–69, 88–96, 99, 104–110, 122–123, 126, 128–129, 134, 150–157, 208, 221, 229; freedom and, 23; of life, 8; mentality and, 35; minor gesture and, 1–2, 6–7, 13, 24, 57, 60, 64, 75, 84, 100, 163, 172, 201, 217; neurotypicality and, 3, 5, 137–138, 142, 168, 207; of philosophy, 41; of radical empiricism, 30–31, 40; of schizoanalysis, 168–170, 173, 181–184; speculative pragmatism and, 15, 42, 52, 209; virtuality and, 153

form, 8, 48, 68; affirmation and, 229; architecture and, 88–89, 103; art form, 13–14, 28, 47, 49, 65, 81, 91, 138; choreography and, 114, 127; and content, 15, 28, 47, 49, 56, 58, 81, 89; event and, 134; of experience, 138, 141; fashion design and, 95–96, 99, 105–106, 108, 110; of knowledge, 8–13, 26–27, 29–35, 42; language and, 158; matter-form, 65, 73, 75, 84; milieu and, 190; minor and, 2, 23; movement and, 18–19, 53; process and, 53, 57; of time, 52; undercommons and, 221; virtual and, 30. *See also* force

Forsythe, William, 106, 126, 157

freedom, 18, 23–25, 95, 163

futurity, 23

Garner, Eric, 4–5, 254n19

gender, 96, 249n7

Gil, Jose, 117

Gill, Simryn, 72–75

Gins, Madeline, 86–90, 93–94, 98, 100–106, 109

Goodman, Andrew, 79–81

Gordon, Jessica, 225. *See also* Idle No More

Guattari, Félix, 1, 6, 42–44, 65–66, 72, 74–75, 84, 89, 123, 127–128, 165–173, 180–184, 187–188, 197. *See also* Deleuze, Gilles; La Borde

mental illness, 128. *See also* depression
mentality, 35
metamodel, 43–44
metamorphosis, 107, 124
method, 26–27, 31–38, 40–43, 45, 105–106, 212; depression and, 167, 187; facilitated communication as, 163; tragedy and, 213
milieu, 107, 158, 190; relational, 94, 192
minor gesture: architecture and, 94, 103; of art, 51–52, 62, 72–76, 81–83, 85, 198; art gallery and, 71–72; desire and, 183; event and, 2–3, 7, 13, 15, 24, 37, 211; experience and, 65, 162, 140, 188, 201; freedom and, 23; grand gesture and, 223–224; imperceptibility of, 81; life-living and, 8; major and, 1, 7, 66; marginal and, 7; memory and, 73; microgesture, 190; modes of existence and, 96; necessity and, 213; neoliberalism and, 172, 185; potential and, 75; reactivity and, 202; ritual and, 170–171; schizoanalysis and, 6, 219; sympathy and, 39, 57, 60; technique and, 125–127; technology and, 84; time and, 2, 51, 65; undercommons and, 221, 228; volition and, 19–20, 22; weather patterns and, 64–65
modes of existence, 90, 92–93, 95–96, 100, 103, 108, 110, 123–124, 171, 173, 184, 187
more-than, 29–31, 33, 35, 53, 55–59, 61, 119, 130, 176, 219, 231; affirmation and, 230; art, 49, 51–52, 81, 83, 191–192, 207–208; of becoming, 173; of choreography, 127, 130; debt, 210; desire and, 183, 187; of event, 170, 212; experience, 131, 158, 171; of fashion, 88, 93; of form, 122, 138; human, 3, 59–60, 76, 85, 94, 119, 126–127, 229; one, 147; procedure and, 89
Moten, Fred, 4–5, 8–12, 27, 71, 205–206, 210–211, 214–215, 223, 228, 230–232
motor apraxia, 111

movement: architecture and, 102; autism and, 132, 142–143, 147, 151, 153, 177–178; collective, 120, 163; depression and, 178; disturbance, 111; effort and, 152, 156–157; emergent, 118; immanent movement, 59; nonvoluntary, 158; of poetry, 161; relational, 47, 106, 121–122, 153–154, 156, 163; stimming, 245n4; technique and, 126; of thought, 116, 120–127, 146, 155, 176–177, 180, 182, 189–190, 193, 232; total movement, 117–119, 122; undercommons and, 228
Mukhopadhyay, Tito, 31, 112, 149, 160–161
multiple, 66–67, 69
Murphie, Andrew, 43
mutual inclusion, 202

narration, 218–221, 223–224
Nation Time (Joe McPhee), 230
natural selection, 136
negation, 202–204, 218, 229, 232
neoliberalism, 166, 172, 184–185, 187
neurocosmopolitanism, 160
neurodiversity, 5, 174; activist philosophy and, 129, 132; blackness and, 4–5; cure and, 136, 236n14; depression and, 168, 172, 174, 186; movement and, 188; pathology and, 171, 187; perception and, 14, 59, 101, 111–112, 121; spectrum of, 142, 161; subjectivity and, 128; voluntarism and, 150. *See also* autism; autistic perception
neuroscience, 111, 148
neurotypicality, 3–6, 21, 28, 99, 111–112, 114, 121, 123, 129–132, 135–138, 140–141, 149, 151–152, 157, 159–160, 162, 180; communication and, 177; depression and, 168; pathologization and, 174; politics of, 163
Nietzsche, Friedrich, 6, 34–37, 152, 172, 197, 201–213, 217–218, 229, 232

truth, 218–224, 227
Truth and Reconciliation Commission (Canada), 223

Ulysses, 32
unconscious, machinic, 166–167
undercommons, 8–10, 27, 39, 43, 53, 71, 130, 185, 214, 216, 221, 223, 229, 231–232; Idle No More and, 226–228; study and, 13
university, 9, 146, 185, 215
untimeliness, 24, 50, 103, 175

value, 203–204, 228; of animal life, 234n4; of art, 75, 247n2; capitalist, 44, 187, 198; and evaluation, 27; of event, 130; fashion and, 95; judgment, 57, 201; of knowledge, 9, 11, 31, 42, 66; of neurodiverse life, 3–4, 15, 21, 123, 138, 150, 184, 194, 248n4; of pathology, 167; prestige value, 71, 198; of rituality, 69–71; of time, 49; transvaluation, 217–218, 221, 230; use-value, 9, 11, 62, 116, 199–200
Vicuña, Cecilia, 31
violence, 230
virtual, 68, 122; actual and, 29–30, 117–118; event, 155; excess and, 53; milieu and, 158
volition, 195; depression and, 166, 168; freedom and, 23, 117; inhibition and, 157; movement and, 15–19, 21, 114, 117–121, 137, 143, 152–153, 244n1; neurotypicality and, 123, 130, 136–

137, 140, 147, 149, 155–157; passivity and, 174; reason and, 20–21; subjectivity and, 3, 6, 112, 130, 207
Volumetrics (Erin Manning), 76–80

Waste Not (Song Dong), 69–71
weather, 64, 76, 78, 83–85
Weather Patterns (Erin Manning), 75–78, 81–83
Whitehead, Alfred North, 57–58, 61–62, 95, 133–135, 150, 182, 207–208; actual occasion and, 2–3, 90; decision and, 20, 88; in-act and, 47–48; instauration and, 100; method and, 26, 28–36, 163; negative prehension, 119; nonsensuous perception and, 96, 135; presentational immediacy and, 81; self-enjoyment and, 193. *See also* superject
will. *See* volition
Williams, Donna, 136, 141, 155, 157, 163–164
Willingham, Emily, 175
will to power, 206–207, 211–213, 221
Wilson, Darren, 5, 254n19
Wilson, Nina, 225. *See also* Idle No More
Wretches and Jabberers (Geraldine Finn), 176, 185–186

Yamamoto, Yohji, 92, 105, 107
Yergeau, Melanie, 31

Zurcher-Long, Emma, 158